NON-HODGKIN'S LYMPHOMAS

Making Sense of Diagnosis, Treatment & Options

NON–HODGKIN'S LYMPHOMAS

Making Sense of Diagnosis, Treatment & Options

Lorraine Johnston

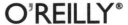

Beijing · Cambridge · Farnham · Köln · Paris · Sebastopol · Taipei · Tokyo

Non-Hodgkin's Lymphomas: Making Sense of Diagnosis, Treatment, and Options
by Lorraine Johnston

Copyright © 1999 O'Reilly & Associates, Inc. All rights reserved.
Printed in the United States of America.

Published by O'Reilly & Associates, Inc., 101 Morris Street, Sebastopol, CA 95472.

Editor: Linda Lamb

Production Editor: Claire Cloutier LeBlanc

Printing History:

> May 1999: First Edition

Library of Congress Cataloging-in-Publication Data:

Johnston, Lorraine.
    Non-Hodgkin's lymphomas: making sense of diagnosis, treatment, and options /
       Lorraine Johnston.
       p.   cm.—(Patient-centered guides)
    Includes bibliographical references and index.
    ISBN 1-56592-444-4 (pbk.)
    1. Lymphomas—Popular works. I. Title. II. Series.
R280.L9J64   1999
616.99'446—dc21

                               98-55468
                                   CIP

To my wonderful husband, Larry

Table of Contents

Foreword ix

Preface xv

1. Symptoms and Diagnosis 1

2. Finding the Right Oncologist 16

3. What Are the Non-Hodgkin's Lymphomas? 27

4. Prognoses 51

5. Tests and Procedures 69

6. How the NHLs Are Treated 113

7. What to Expect During Chemotherapy 142

8. What to Expect During Radiotherapy 157

9. Side Effects of Treatment 165

10. If You're Hospitalized 189

11. Stress and the Immune System 205

12. Interacting with Medical Personnel 234

13. Getting Support 248

14. Insurance, Finances, Employment, Record-Keeping 281

15. After Treatment Ends 297

16. Late Effects, Late Complications 312

17. Sexuality, Fertility, and Pregnancy 331

18. Relapse 348

19. Clinical Trials 358

20. Transplantation 381

21. Traveling for Care 410

22. If All Treatments Have Failed 418

23. The Future of Therapy 432

24. Researching Your Lymphoma 459

A. Resources 481

B. Blood and Marrow Test Values 505

C. Body Surface Area in Square Meters 507

D. Classification Systems 509

E. Common Chemotherapies 520

Notes 527

Glossary 529

Bibliography 535

Index 541

Foreword

The present book is a timely addition to the available literature for patients suffering from serious medical problems. The non-Hodgkin's lymphomas are among the most common malignant tumors throughout the world, and, for reasons that are not clear, are increasing in incidence by a few percent per year. In the United States, their incidence (the number of new cases per 100,000 of the population per year) increases markedly above the age of 65 years. They account for almost 4 percent of all cancers, and the actual number of new cases is approaching 40,000 per year. The median age of patients who die from these illnesses is over 70 years; as a whole, these diseases are more likely to occur in the elderly, although they can occur at any age.

It is important to understand that the term non-Hodgkin's lymphoma encompasses a large number of subtypes with a broad range of behavior patterns, ranging from those that may lie "dormant" for many years, to rapidly growing tumors that can double in size in a matter of days and, if untreated, will rapidly lead to death. The good news, however, is that a significant fraction of these tumors can be cured, while many of those that are incurable can be controlled for long periods of time with appropriate therapy.

Moreover, recent research has identified a number of new treatment approaches that show considerable promise. Thus, not only is there much that can be done for patients with a non-Hodgkin's lymphoma today, but there is every reason to believe that even more effective treatment approaches will be developed in the future. Such treatments depend, of course, upon the conduct of research, including clinical trials, in which the usefulness of a particular treatment approach is explored, or in which different treatment approaches are compared in patients. Without research, we would be doomed to remain frozen with respect to our knowledge or the treatment approaches available to us. If no research had been conducted in the last hundred years, we would have no effective treatments available to us at all.

Fortunately, we live in an era in which the pace of scientific progress is accelerating more rapidly than ever before. New discoveries often lead to more efficient research tools, which result in a dramatic increase in the rate at which new facts are discovered, and which sometimes permit discoveries to be made that would not have previously been possible. Not surprisingly, the computer has become a central element in this process. It provides both a means of storing vast amounts of information that can be instantly accessed, and powerful methods of analysis that allow comprehension of the otherwise incomprehensible. One has only to think of the World Wide Web, which puts anybody with access to it only a few keystrokes away from a vast body of information ranging from complex scientific data to the means to access resources, for example, that can ease the burden of emotional suffering for patients with non-Hodgkin's lymphoma.

Particularly exciting in recent years in the biological sciences (and, incidentally, heavily dependent upon the computer in a multitude of ways) is the development of new approaches for studying the expression of thousands of genes simultaneously in a variety of cells, including cancer cells. It is the pattern of expression of genes that makes a liver cell a liver cell, and not a brain cell, for example. It is the subtle modification of the pattern of expression of genes in any given cell that can lead to the cell becoming a cancer cell. These altered patterns of gene expression are caused by physical changes to the genes themselves, occurring either by chance, or ultimately, through exposure of the individual to one or more external agents, whether a chemical, or a microorganism such as a bacterium, virus, or other kind of infectious agent.

We can thus envision a time, in the not too distant future, when we shall be able to rapidly examine all aberrations of gene expression in cancer cells, including non-Hodgkin's lymphoma cells, and use this information to hone the precision of the diagnosis as well as to identify patterns that may be associated with a good or poor response to treatment. This new knowledge is also highly likely to lead to novel approaches to treatment. Already it has become possible to create millions of variants of a basic molecule and, in doing so, to fit the molecule to a protein (the product of a gene) in order to inhibit its function. Since some proteins are essential to the existence of the cancer cell, the production of drugs that can selectively target cancer-related proteins represents a new approach to the development of highly specific treatments for cancer—that is, drugs that affect cancer cells and not (or only to a limited extent) normal cells.

At the present time, although highly effective anti-cancer drugs are available, many of which are active in patients with non-Hodgkin's lymphomas, they all affect normal cells to a greater or lesser degree, and have, therefore, a range of side effects. We are at the threshold of a new era in which anti-cancer drugs will eventually be no more toxic than antibiotics used to treat infectious diseases (i.e., produce as few side effects). It will be many years, however, before all the necessary laboratory and clinical studies required to introduce such new and highly specific therapies have been completed.

Researchers who concentrate on the non-Hodgkin's lymphomas have certain advantages compared to research scientists and physicians who deal primarily with other types of cancer. This is because the non-Hodgkin's lymphomas are a type of cancer that affects those cells in the body that mediate our ability to mount immune responses against, for example, microorganisms (germs) that cause infectious diseases, or chemicals present in the environment. As such, they differ in many ways from cancers arising in, say, the breast, bowel, or lung. The cells of the immune system and the nature of immune responses have been of long-standing interest to scientists; in many phenomena unrelated to cancer, including the mechanisms used by the body to fight infectious diseases, the origins of diseases in which the immune system may be in some way overactive (for example, asthma and autoimmune diseases) or the reaction of the body to tissues or organs from another person. This means there is a great deal of information available about the cells of the immune system, as well as the nature of the immune responses directed against microorganisms or substances foreign to the body.

Such information is relevant to an understanding of the non-Hodgkin's lymphomas, since the latter diseases result from the overaccumulation of one or more of the cell types involved in immune responses. This may be a consequence either from the overproduction, or, perhaps more often, from a failure to limit the lifespan of the cells in question. The characteristics of the resulting illness depend upon the characteristics of the cells that are overproduced—for example, whether they proliferate rapidly or slowly, and their pattern of migration throughout the body. Most lymphomas result in swelling of the lymph nodes and other elements of the immune system, such as the liver, spleen, and bone marrow, but others arise in the tissues policed by lymphocytes, including the bowel and skin. In some cases, the lymphoma can be likened to a kind of aberrant immune response. Sometimes, the cause of such an immune response can be identified, for example, a bacterium called *Helicobacter pylori* in a certain type of lymphoma that frequently involves the stomach and may involve other organs. It is not surprising, therefore, that the accumulating cells may include other, normal cells that are attracted by the lymphoma cells, or that systemic effects, such as fever or general lack of well-being, often accompany the lymphoma. These phenomena are caused by the production of molecules that mediate the normal immune response.

Clearly, a detailed knowledge of the mechanisms that control normal immune responses is of great value in understanding the nature of lymphomas (and vice versa). Moreover, such knowledge is likely to lead to a variety of treatment approaches that will apply specifically to lymphomas and not to other types of cancer. Examples may include the use of regulatory molecules produced by normal immune cells to limit the growth of the lymphoma cells, or the use of antibody molecules that bind to so-called receptors on the surface of all lymphoid cells. Receptors are molecules that are the biological equivalent of "locks" that trigger a response in the cell (e.g., cell proliferation or death) when the correct "key" is inserted into them. Of particular interest at the present time are receptors whose key, or ligand as it is correctly referred to, induces the cell to commit suicide. This special form of cell death, known as apoptosis, is a key element in the regulation of the number of immunologically active cells, and understanding how this process is deranged in lymphomas may prove to be a key element in the development of new and better treatment approaches.

One of the functions of the immune system is to protect us against cancer. Consequently, cancer cells (including, interestingly enough, the non-Hodgkin's lymphomas) must devise means of escaping from this normal immunological surveillance mechanism. Identifying the mechanisms whereby cancer cells avoid being recognized and destroyed by the normal immune system may have relevance to the treatment of non-Hodgkin's lymphomas as well as other types of cancer, since it may prove possible to overcome the mechanisms that prevent the tumor from being destroyed by the immune system. Approaches of this kind are known as immunotherapy, and several forms of immunotherapy are being explored in the context of the non-Hodgkin's lymphomas. Of interest in this regard is the use of a vaccine comprised of the receptor that normally recognizes the foreign substance against which the lymphoma cell specifically reacts. This vaccine, remarkably enough, can turn the normal immune system against the abnormal lymphoma cells. Its shows promise in a certain type of slowly progressive lymphoma, known as follicular lymphoma.

As yet, in spite of the extensive research being conducted in the causes and treatment of the non-Hodgkin's lymphomas, no "magic bullet" has been identified that will cure even one type of non-Hodgkin's lymphomas without producing side effects. Indeed, the majority of lymphomas, particularly those that grow more slowly, cannot yet be cured, although control, often for many years, is possible. On the other hand, some types of lymphoma, particularly—paradoxically—those that grow very rapidly (and that comprise the vast majority of non-Hodgkin's lymphomas occurring in children), can be cured, albeit, and depending upon the extent of disease, with rather intensive drug treatment. Indeed, success in treating the very aggressive lymphomas has been of such a degree that the major research emphasis is presently upon using the least amount of treatment possible in order to minimize the immediate and late effects of treatment. Late effects of treatment, which may include impaired fertility, heart disease, and, rarely, second malignancies, are of particular importance in young persons; fortunately, modern treatments have proven to be both successful in eradicating the lymphomas of children and young adults, while producing rather few late effects.

Clearly, the diagnosis and management of the non-Hodgkin's lymphomas is a complex process that requires the participation of expert physicians who specialize, to a greater or lesser extent, in the diagnosis and treatment of these tumors. While physicians do their best to provide the patient with the information they require, the amount of time needed for a sufficiently complete education is much greater than that normally available, at least to the physician. Moreover, such information is often best absorbed at less emotional times than the session in which the physician informs the family of the diagnosis, or during visits for treatment. The comfort of the patient's (or family's) own home is also more conducive to developing an understanding of the disease and its treatment than the physician's office or a hospital room.

The present book provides information in plain English about the nature of the non-Hodgkin's lymphomas, the types of treatments available, and their side effects, as well as the impact the illness is likely to have on the patient's life, and those of his or her family members. Moreover, it should enable the patient and the patient's family to ask better questions of the medical and support staff taking care of them. For the average patient or family, this book is likely to provide far more information than is needed, but even so, it cannot (and is not intended to) cover the medical information with the detail of a textbook meant for the healthcare professional, so some patients may require additional information. Yet for all patients, the book provides a directory of further sources of information, including more detailed medical information as well as listings of organizations involved in lymphoma treatment or research, support groups, and information available on the World Wide Web. It can be dipped into as required, or read from cover to cover.

The diagnosis of cancer of any kind is enough to strike fear into anyone. Yet much of this fear is generated by ignorance of the nature of the disease, its treatment, and knowledge of what can be done to control or cure the disease. The non-Hodgkin's lymphomas are, in some ways, a particularly complex group of cancers, and patients and their families will benefit from access to patient groups and additional sources of information that will help to allay the fear that arises from the unknown. Moreover, the very act of seeking information will provide the patient and the patient's family with ways in which the negative energy generated by fear can be translated into positive energy directed toward working with the entire team of healthcare professionals to bring about the best possible outcome of treatment for the patient, with the greatest degree of comfort for all concerned.

—Ian T. Magrath, MB BS FRCP FRCPath
Chief, Lymphoma Biology Section
Pediatric Branch, National Cancer Institute
Professor of Pediatrics, Uniformed Services
University of the Health Sciences
Bethesda, Maryland

Dr. Magrath's opinions are his own, and should not be taken as an indication that the book is endorsed by the National Cancer Institute.

Preface

He who has begun has half done.

—Quintus Horatius Flaccus

Your decision to read about lymphoma is a mark of courage in the face of fear. There's a great deal of promising information we can share with you about non-Hodgkin's lymphoma, including information about evaluating and choosing treatments; ways to locate and track new treatments being developed; preparatory information about tests and procedures; survivor experiences with keeping or losing friends; handling employers, insurance companies, and the Social Security Administration; and so on. Did you know, for example, that you can find information about the dosage, mode of action, and side effects of medications being recommended for your treatment? And that charitable groups exist expressly to fly you and your family, free of charge, to a distant cancer center where you might plan to be treated? And that if you're being treated away from home, the American Cancer Society's Hope Lodge network can provide you and your loved ones with rooms free of charge?

The medical research underway regarding the non-Hodgkin's lymphomas is vigorous, and progress is heartening. We have a great quantity of solid information to share with you, and much hope and comfort to offer. The information we've collected can increase feelings of control, confidence, and well-being. We aim to bridge the gap in pragmatism between inspirational coping books and medical textbooks.

The chief resources used in developing this book were the journals and texts of Western medicine, which are summarized and presented to you in language understandable by those without a medical background.

Who should read this book

If you've been diagnosed recently with non-Hodgkin's lymphoma (NHL), this guide contains information that will enable you to smooth your path through treatment and long-term recovery. We describe each step of testing, diagnosis, and treatment. We touch on sensitive areas such as how to tell children, other loved ones, employers, and coworkers of your diagnosis. We describe what evolution, both positive and negative, may occur within your friendships as a result of your diagnosis.

If your disease is low-grade and if you've been told that you may have long watch-and-wait periods with intermittent periods of treatment over ten to twelve years, we provide up-to-date information about finding the best treatments with the lowest toxicity, including the newly approved monoclonal antibodies; about how you can follow new, promising drugs still in trials; and how you can enroll in a trial. We'll share with you the strategies and tactics that others have developed for living serenely and well while a cure is being developed by the medical profession. If you have intermediate- or high-grade disease, we'll offer you guidelines for evaluating the treatments available that bring about cure with the lowest toxicity levels.

If you're a long-term survivor of NHL, we provide the information you need to make sense of the possible long-term physical, cognitive, and emotional consequences of disease and treatment that you may be experiencing, such as continued fatigue, as well as the information that some of you may need concerning relapse.

All NHL patients and survivors need to be aware of advances in diagnosis, treatment, and care, as well as long-term effects and insurance- and employment-related complications. All survivors who may be candidates for additional treatment need to be acquainted with the other types of NHL, as low-grade disease can convert to high-grade disease and vice versa.

If you're a caretaker of someone with NHL, the collective and pragmatic wisdom in this guide will enable you to make the most of your caretaking and advocacy efforts, and will assist you in relaxing and staying healthy so that you can best care for your loved one, both emotionally and instrumentally. We can help you understand and respond appropriately to the reactions of your loved one and yourself to the unique stressors that a cancer diagnosis entails.

If you are HIV positive, you are at high risk of developing an NHL, especially if you are unable to maintain adequate levels of T-cells with protease inhibitors or AZT.

Who should not read this book

If you have one or more swollen lymph nodes but have not yet obtained a diagnosis, please pursue a firm diagnosis before reading this guide. Lymph nodes swell for many reasons, and only two or three people out of a hundred with swollen lymph nodes are diagnosed with a malignant tumor.

If you have another cancer that has spread to the lymph nodes, this book contains information that is not correct for your circumstances. Lymphomas are different from cancer that starts in another organ and spreads via the lymphatic system.

How to read this book

We've organized this book carefully to make the best use of what might be the prioritized time and energy of lymphoma survivors and those who love and look after them. The format of this book follows the path of your experience with NHL: symptoms, testing and diagnosis, treatment, long-term effects, and so on. We try to provide you with digestible amounts of information that you'll need at each stage of awareness and treatment. In fact, you might do well to consider reading only the chapters that are meaningful to you at a given point in order to avoid information overload. We believe that this method of organization will enable you to locate the information you need most in a timely manner.

In addition, we've done our best to organize each chapter so that you can find succinct information on a topic within the first two or three paragraphs, and more detailed information in the sections that follow.

A whole chapter (Chapter 11, *Stress and the Immune System*) is devoted to stress and its sometimes surprising effects on the immune system. We offer a variety of ways to cope with stress and insights into making challenging experiences work in your favor. Moreover, in appropriate chapters, we discuss the impact of stress at that stage and its possible effect on your well-being.

Appendix A, *Resources*, discusses references that can be accessed on the Internet, such as Medline, the National Library of Medicine's database of nine million published medical research papers, and the National Cancer Institute's grand-daddy of all cancer information databases. Suggested reading and helpful organizations are also listed here by topic. Additional appendices offer specific technical information in the form of tables. A glossary of medical terms related to lymphoma can be found at the back of the book.

Particular care has been taken to create a truly useful index. If a topic of your interest appears not to be addressed with chapter subheadings, we suggest checking the index.

You might find it upsetting to read about treatment options that don't apply to your situation or to read about the possibility of recurrence or disease progression. Don't feel that you have to read about everything all at once. Not all parts of this book will apply to you. Read only what will be helpful to you at a given stage.

Finally, we encourage you to mix humorous reading and other lighthearted distractions with your serious readings and considerations.

Who wrote this book, anyway?

The hands on the keyboard writing this guide are those of a person whose mother is a twenty-year survivor of non-Hodgkin's lymphoma, and whose husband is a seven-year survivor of Hodgkin's lymphoma. I have a degree in biology, but none of my scientific training prepared me to cope with cancer in my family. I want to share information about non-Hodgkin's lymphoma and empower you to find even more information.

The real voices in this resource guide, however, are the many survivors of non-Hodgkin's lymphoma—those treated for local disease with radiation therapy or surgery, those who are long-term survivors of chemotherapy, more than a few who have had bone marrow transplants, and the pioneers who received the first monoclonal antibodies. This distillation of their experiences is intended to help you know what to expect in advance, to know where to find the best information for your circumstances, and to know that you are not alone.

Some of our contributors have used their real names, but some, in order to preserve their privacy, have chosen aliases or have used first names only. The italicized portions of the text are their thoughts, their feelings, their wisdom, their own words.

Acknowledgments

My first and greatest thanks go to my husband Larry, a lymphoma survivor who possesses a stellar intuition for loving those of us lucky enough to know him, and who without fail provides the framework and love that enable me to use my energy for others.

Special thanks are offered to Karen A., Liz A., Steve A., Bill B., Mary Butler, Nicole D., Steve Dunn, Judy G., Dr. Wendy Harpham, Connie K., Beth L., Deb L., Doug and Janet L., GrannyBarb L., Harry L., Jeannine L., Ron and Sue L., Lou L., Marvin, Janet Nightingale, Robert Scott Pallack (who is list owner of the NHL discussion group), the irrepressible Marilyn Tyler, Charlie Walsh, Louise W., and Barbara Zierten, and to our other contributors who wish to remain anonymous. They agreed readily and eagerly to share their illness experiences so that others will feel less alone and will learn about ways to find help. Their honesty and spontaneity are, I feel, this book's best aspect. Many of them also agreed to review this text in advance, offering a fresh eye and valuable insights that I'd have missed.

To Neeraj A., Nicole D., Deb L., Janet L., and to Nan Suhadolc, M.S.W., L.C.S.W., each of whom gave me more help and guidance than any friend could ever hope for, I give not only my humble gratitude, but my profound admiration, respect, and love. These survivors helped me and others even when their own difficulties made drawing breath arduous for them. They define the word bravery.

I offer many heartfelt thanks to Dr. Alexandre Azevedo, transplantation specialist of Rio de Janeiro, Brazil, and Dr. Richard Miller of Kaiser Permanente, for the irreplaceable time and energy they spent doing very detailed reviews—well beyond the call of duty or goodwill—to make the medical and scientific information in this book as correct and as current as possible. I also gratefully thank Dr. Georgia Vogelsang, Dr. Wendy Harpham, and Dr. Costas Giannakenas for their reviews.

I thank Steven G. Warm, J.D., for his help in analyzing information about employee assistance programs and employee/employer relations.

The team at O'Reilly & Associates that conceived, nurtured, and produced this book and the other patient-centered guides are the finest group of humans I've ever had the opportunity to work with. My editor Linda Lamb's unfailing eye for what the reader will need, her suggestions for handling difficult topics gently, her visionary perspective on cancer care and treatment, and her tact in keeping me on track and motivated are rare gifts among mentors. Carol Wenmoth, editorial assistant, is a kindred spirit in writing who, thank goodness, has the answers before I have the questions, and offers her help and experience with kindness, accuracy, and unassuming good will.

No book written about cancer in the late twentieth century can fail to acknowledge and thank the collection of cancer researchers in the United States and elsewhere who have devoted their lives to caring about our well-being. Thanks to the effort and altruistic collaboration of cancer researchers all over the world, we are witnessing and benefiting from robust progress in the understanding and treatment of cancer.

And finally, I acknowledge and thank each reader who has tapped an inner strength to move against this illness and continue to live a good life.

CHAPTER 1

Symptoms and Diagnosis

*To learn how to treat a disease, one must
learn how to diagnose it. The diagnosis is the
best trump in the scheme of treatment.*

—Jean Martin Charcot

Who among us will forget the moment when we were told we have cancer? Each of us has had a unique experience with symptoms—or the absence of them—and with diagnosis. We may have had either a long-awaited diagnosis after many tests or one out of the blue when we knew nothing at all was amiss.

In this chapter, we'll first look at the symptoms of various non-Hodgkin's lymphomas (NHLs), including local enlargement of lymph nodes and body-wide symptoms. We'll then look at the process of diagnosis, which often happens over some time as the search for the disease narrows.

Before we discuss symptoms and diagnosis in greater depth, it's important to note that the process of discovery of a cancer diagnosis is, by most people's accounts, associated with great emotional upheaval. There may be a few of us who are so highly evolved spiritually or who have lived so full a life that we accept a cancer diagnosis with equanimity, but this is not the case for most of us. We'll discuss the emotional tumult associated with diagnosis and the range of responses people have.

Please note that it may not be useful to read this material if you have not yet received a confirmed diagnosis from your physician, as lymph nodes swell for many reasons, and most often these reasons are not cancer.

Symptoms

Some people are diagnosed with non-Hodgkin's lymphoma as part of a routine exam in the absence of any symptoms, but most people do experience symptoms. Because the experience of lymphoma usually begins with symptoms that you or your doctor may notice, we too begin by describing symptoms. A broader discussion of the lymphatic system and of the non-Hodgkin's lymphomas can be found in Chapter 3, *What Are the Non-Hodgkin's Lymphomas?*

Symptoms of NHL may appear suddenly or may develop gradually over a long period of time. Because lymph nodes and lymphatic tissue occur throughout the body, non-Hodgkin's lymphomas can occur in many places and in many forms, some of which produce no symptoms at all. Nevertheless, about two-thirds of adults diagnosed with non-Hodgkin's lymphoma notice swollen, painless lymph nodes in the armpit, groin, near the collarbone, or in some area of the neck, including the back of the neck. Sometimes a node may rupture and weep. In children, NHLs most commonly develop outside of lymph nodes, such as within the abdomen or jaw.

It's not unusual for two or more nodes in different or distant areas of the body to swell simultaneously. Swollen nodes may appear in the following areas:

- Within the abdomen, where they may or may not be noticed by the patient, but may cause nausea and vomiting, a feeling of fullness after eating even small amounts of food, diarrhea, a feeling of constipation, intestinal blockage, mild or severe back pain, pressure on the bladder, ovaries, or uterus.

- Within the chest, possibly causing shortness of breath, difficulty breathing, coughing, chest pain, pressure under the rib cage, or swelling of the face, neck veins, or arm.

- Within the elbow or knee, most noticeable as a lump that may swell and recede.

- Within bone marrow, causing bone pain, minute fractures, or aberrant blood values. Rarely, NHL may begin within bone as opposed to marrow.

- Within the kidneys, possibly causing headache, high blood pressure, frequent urination, difficult urination, excessive nighttime urination, or back or flank pain.

- Within the central nervous system, causing headache, vision disturbances, dizziness, lightheadedness, true spinning vertigo, numbness,
  tingling, or cognitive disturbances such as memory loss or confusion.

- Within the breast, noticeable as a lump or swelling, or unusual enlargement of one or both breasts, particularly during pregnancy.

- On the skin, manifesting as oozing, scaling, discolored lumps, or unusually easy bruising. For some of the cutaneous NHLs, these symptoms
  may regress and return for years.

- Within a testicle, causing swelling.

- Within the eye, causing a feeling of pressure or a protrusion of the eye.

- Within the liver or spleen, causing aberrations of blood values.

- Within the throat, nose, jaw, or upper chest, causing pain, nasal stuffi-
  ness, ear pain, hearing loss, ringing in the ears, or difficulty breathing or
  swallowing.

In addition, there is a collection of body-wide symptoms that may be
present, such as relentless itching or ongoing fatigue. The following three
symptoms are known as B symptoms or systemic symptoms:

- Drenching night sweats of an intensity that requires changing bedsheets
  in the middle of the night.

- Unexplained loss of more than ten percent of body weight.

- Fever above 100 degrees Fahrenheit (about 38 degrees Centigrade) for
  more than one week.

Finally, some adults report an aching of the affected lymph nodes if they
drink alcohol, although this phenomenon appears not to be recognized by
many authorities.

Survivors' perspectives

As you read the material in this book, the stories of others will be told as
illustrations of the topics in each chapter.

The following story is that of a registered nurse, Nicole, who had a long and
difficult experience obtaining a correct diagnosis. Nicole first describes how
her symptoms were ignored or misinterpreted:

In May of 1997 (I remember feeling pretty awful at our Mother's Day dinner), I started having difficulty breathing. At first I just put it off as a flare-up of my mild asthma. Also, it was spring and could have been my allergies. I tried to self-medicate for about two weeks and finally gave in and went to the doctor. Well, to my dismay, the day I chose to go to the doctor was my regular general practitioner's last day of work before maternity leave. She was only working half a day that day, so I had to see the physician's assistant.

When I saw him, he took all of five minutes with me and brushed me off, saying there was nothing wrong with me, that my lungs sounded fine. This angered me, because I had spent twenty minutes in the waiting room coughing before he saw me. I also had used my asthma inhaler in the parking lot just to be able to walk in the building. He gave me a breathing treatment to placate me, increased my asthma medicines, and sent me on my way.

After this, I waited two weeks before going back, waiting for my doctor's replacement to get settled. I went in to see the doctor and got the same treatment as with the physician's assistant. By this time, I had had friends at work listen to my lungs and they were concerned that I had very decreased breath sounds on the right. I also started noticing that my neck seemed thicker. When I asked the doctor about my neck, she felt it, and said it was fine, it was just my obesity. By now, I'm getting upset. I feel as if I'm being treated like a hypochondriac when in reality I usually wait too long before seeking medical attention, so I end up with pneumonia instead of bronchitis, and so on.

A week later, I went back, begging for some tests, anything. Until now, the only thing done was to listen to my lungs and give me breathing treatments. Also, by this time, my nails were blue, I couldn't walk to work as usual without gasping for air, and my heart rate was 140.

I later found out that I was also really frightening my daughter because I would start coughing uncontrollably and end up gagging, followed by being so out of breath that the only way I could breathe was bent over on all fours on the floor.

After living with pronounced discomfort for too long, Nicole finally was given some basic diagnostic testing. However, her care continued to be mishandled:

I was finally given a chest x-ray after my third visit that month. (I believe more to placate me than anything else.) Well, the radiologist wouldn't let me leave the office until he called my doctor. It turned out that I had pneumonia and fluid in the base of my right lung. I talked with the doctor over the phone, and she said she would call in an antibiotic to my pharmacy. This was Friday evening, and when I went to the pharmacy, they hadn't received a call. I went home thinking she hadn't called yet and checked back after an hour. Still no prescription. Since this doctor was a fill-in, she didn't take calls, so I couldn't call her through the service. I started calling pharmacies and finally found my prescription across town.

When I got the drug, the instructions didn't seem right to me. First, it wasn't a drug commonly used to treat pneumonia. (When I had told her what I was on earlier that year for pneumonia, her only comment was that it was too expensive). Second, the duration wasn't long enough for this drug to act. I remembered this from medical microbiology class in college. Since it was the weekend, I decided to start the drug, thinking I could call the office Monday morning. Sunday I went to work and my condition scared the physician's assistant I was working with. He offered to give me a breathing treatment right then (it's illegal to use state funds and equipment for employees). I was also the only nurse on duty that day, so I couldn't go home. By Monday, I was even worse. I talked with the head pharmacist at work about my prescription and he echoed my concerns. I finally called the office and insisted on getting a referral to someone else. I wasn't going to see this doctor again!

It turns out there had been other complaints about this doctor. They asked me to see someone else in the clinic and got me in right away as a special favor. He started me on a different antibiotic and even gave me enough samples so that I didn't have to buy it. He also put me on prednisone. This seemed to be the magic pill for me (prednisone helps to reduce the size of many lymphomas). When the prednisone stopped, the symptoms got worse. I went back to him a week later because of this. Rather than start me on prednisone again, he put me on a third antibiotic and bed rest for a week. He was going to be out of town the following week, so he gave me a return-to-work slip at that visit.

A week later, I was worse. My family now was very concerned and several times tried to get me to go to the emergency room, but I always refused. I was still blue, especially around my mouth (acrocyanosis), I was still coughing and had trouble breathing. To make matters worse, my head felt like it was about to explode. I was supposed to return to work in one day, my antibiotics were complete (three rounds now), and my doctors were out of town.

Angry and frightened, Nicole realized she must demand proper care:

I decided to make a very bold move. I went up to the clinic, passed a note to the nurse saying I was worse and wanted a plan, blood work, anything—and sat down in the office and waited. No appointment. I was seen within fifteen minutes. This doctor (the fourth in six visits now) did a complete exam. She was very concerned, didn't like the way I looked. She drew blood, sent me for another chest x-ray, and sent me to the hospital to have my blood oxygen measured. After all of this, she called me at home and said she wanted me to see a specialist because my chest x-ray was even worse than before. She considered putting me in the hospital that night, but instead, called a pulmonologist friend at home and made me an appointment for the next day.

I went to see the lung doctor and fifteen minutes later was admitted to the hospital. He did not see the mediastinal tumor on the chest x-ray, but he did see an unusual elevation of my diaphragm on both x-rays. He talked about aggressive testing and joked about insurance companies hating him because he was so expensive. His expensive and aggressive tactics saved my life.

Diagnosis

The most accurate way to diagnose a lymphoma is by whole-node or excisional biopsy, but, as symptoms of non-Hodgkin's lymphoma are so varied and can look like the symptoms for more common conditions, a number of tests or treatments might be suggested before NHL is suspected and definitively diagnosed.

For a detailed description of the tests used to diagnose NHL and to follow the progress of its treatment, see Chapter 5, *Tests and Procedures*.

The early guess

As illustrated in Nicole's story, your family doctor or primary care physician may be the first to suspect a lymphoma, perhaps after treatment for several related conditions have not been successful. Swollen eyes, for example, can be related to an overactive thyroid, allergies, or ocular NHL, among other conditions, but most would argue that thyroid or allergy testing is the sensible first choice. Because doctors are taught, "When you hear hoofbeats, look for horses, not zebras," it's not unusual for several tests and remedies for more common illnesses to be attempted before a series of tests to detect a possible cancer are ordered:

> My husband had increasingly bad back pain for over a year. It was first diagnosed by our primary doctor as a jogging injury. He was given muscle relaxers, and he bought new running shoes and a new office chair with better lumbar support. Several months later he returned to another doctor in the same medical practice and explained that the pain was worse, not better. This time, because the pain had spread from his lower back upward, he was diagnosed as having shingles—a form of chicken pox—even though no blisters were present. A few months later he went to a nearby hospital emergency room in the middle of the night with severe back pain and was diagnosed as having a kidney stone. They sent him home with a sieve to urinate into and discharged him to our primary doctor's care. When no stone passed, our family doctor, whose father had died of lymphoma, ordered a sonogram. The demeanor of the technician who did the sonogram became increasingly serious as the test progressed. It showed a suspicious mass. My husband had a follow-up CT scan that showed, in the words of the radiologist, "a mass most consistent with lymphoma."

> After my husband's CT scan, we were referred to an oncologist and then a surgeon for abdominal surgery. This scheduling of doctor visits, surgery, and recovery took another sixty days. After surgery, the tissue was sent to NCI and took thirty days for analysis. Altogether a tentative diagnosis took over fourteen months, and we waited two more months from the CT scan through full diagnosis to the beginning of treatment.

The narrowing diagnosis

If, following a physical examination, x-ray, sonogram, CT scan, or MRI of a suspicious mass, your doctor has received word that you may have lymphoma, he will discuss choosing an oncologist with you. Initially, you may feel comfortable with whomever he recommends, particularly if his style is simply to recommend instead of discuss and you have been comfortable with this approach in the past, but it is in your best interest to research these choices independently as well. See Chapter 2, *Finding the Right Oncologist*.

Here's another survivor's account of one step in her unfolding diagnosis, one that shows the difficulty of determining clearly what disease process is underway:

> My first and only symptom was an enlarged and growing node in my right groin. I was relatively new to our particular area of the country (we had just moved about eight months prior to this), so I first visited an Ob-Gyn specialist with whom I was not familiar, but who was covered under my health plan. He had a jaded moldiness about him, which was slightly nauseating. I allowed him to finish the examination, during which he dug around and tried to feel as much of the enlarged node as possible, exclaiming, "That's quite a gland you've got there, dear!" The only decent thing he did was to refer me to a local surgeon, who happened to be very competent, both in manner and in execution of the surgery. He must have known that what he removed during the surgery was malignant. I had not really faced that possibility yet. He referred me to the hematologist-oncologist who would deliver the diagnosis and see me through the rest of my treatment.

Definitive diagnosis

After the doctor suspects lymphoma, often after having ruled out more common possibilities, the next step is a biopsy of the area. A biopsy is the most important of diagnostic tests. Types of biopsies are needle biopsies (during which a needle is inserted into the node to aspirate cells from the node which can be tested for cancerous cells) and lymph node biopsies (during which the node is surgically removed and examined by a pathologist).

While needle biopsies are somewhat easier to perform than node biopsies and can spare you some pain, node biopsies are the definitive means for diagnosing a node-based lymphoma. The structure of the entire lymph node, not just the cancerous cells within, is very important in determining the kind of lymphoma that may exist. (Extranodal lymphomas are not diagnosed by node biopsy. The tissue or organ affected is biopsied instead.)

A node can be biopsied relatively easily, and with minimal recovery time, if it can be felt beneath the surface of the skin. At times when the node is located deep beneath the skin, a more extensive, more risky surgery with a longer recovery time is necessary in order to retrieve tissue for a definitive diagnosis. This is more likely if a suspicious mass is noted only within the abdomen, as illustrated by this story:

> When my mother told her gynecologist about a suspicious lump in her abdomen, he dismissed her concern. However, when she returned for her next annual exam and again mentioned this lump, he scheduled an exploratory abdominal surgery. They found a large mass of lymphoma, part of which was biopsied. She was told that the kind of non-Hodgkin's lymphoma she had could be cured in 85 percent of people and that she was not to worry. We were afraid that the doctor was not being honest with her, so I called the doctor myself and was told the same thing, in a tone that implied I was worrying too much. Following chemotherapy and radiation therapy, she has been cancer-free for over twenty years. I know now that she was probably diagnosed with an intermediate- or high-grade non-Hodgkin's lymphoma.

It is critical for the surgeon and the pathologist to coordinate the biopsy effort. The pathologist must be made aware of the suspected diagnosis so that slides and tissue samples can be prepared in special ways for the correct diagnosis of NHL or the elimination of NHL as a possibility.

Subtype and staging

Even after a biopsy is performed and a lymphoma is confirmed, there may be some question about which lymphoma exists, which subtype, and the stage of its progression, levels I through IV. As this information is critical to choosing an effective treatment, all lymphoma diagnoses should be confirmed by specialists called hematopathologists.

Some pathologists and oncologists refer biopsy samples to hematopathologists at the National Cancer Institute for the best possible diagnosis. This review may entail an additional delay in diagnosis. As most lymphomas are generally slow-growing tumors, the delay most likely will not affect the outcome.

Determining the correct stage may entail still more tests to determine if disease is found in the bone marrow, for example. See Chapter 5 for a discussion of tests commonly used to detect and stage NHL.

Final diagnosis may change your treatment plan

Your choice of an oncologist and your first appointment with her may occur before or after the final, highly specific information about your lymphoma is returned from the pathology lab. The oncologist in turn may request additional testing before recommending treatment.

The details of your final diagnosis can affect recommendations for treatment. For example, if you're ultimately diagnosed with a low-grade non-Hodgkin's lymphoma—a lymphoma that is the subject of intense research and evolving treatments—it would be wise to receive treatment or second opinions from a regional cancer center or university hospital with specialists in hematologic cancers. The oncologist you're already seeing may be affiliated with one of these groups, and thus may have the necessary qualifications.

Once the diagnosis is secured, you will discuss with your doctor various options for treatment. The intermediate- and high-grade NHLs are usually treated immediately with several chemotherapy drugs, and perhaps radiation therapy as well, depending on the location and extent of the tumor. Low-grade non-Hodgkin's lymphoma, on the other hand, may be simply watched for a number of years until one or more tumors begin to interfere with the function of other organs, and then treated with a single chemotherapy agent or a monoclonal antibody. Some cancer centers prefer treating the low-grade NHLs immediately with high-dose chemotherapy and stem cell rescue if many organs are involved.

Emotions at this stage

The events from symptoms to final diagnosis, and those that will follow over the next months or years, are very likely to take an emotional toll. There are as many reactions to cancer as there are people, and you can't always be sure how you—or your loved ones—will react in new, frightening circumstances.

Although professional psychologists make fine distinctions among responses, reactions, and coping mechanisms, the emotional happenings described in the following sections are discussed not in clinical terms, but in terms your heart and soul will recognize.

All of the following reactions, and many others, are normal, albeit painful. You may think that these feelings are useless or counterproductive, but like all defensive behaviors, they serve to protect your mind from harm until you can assimilate the experience and begin to build a frame of reference from the facts. You should not berate yourself if you're not feeling like the poster child for mental health week.

If weeks go by and you still feel that your reactions and responses are not serving you well, if you can't eat or sleep, if you can't stop crying, if you've lost a great deal of weight in a short time, or if you feel you are jeopardizing your source of income with suboptimal performance, see your doctor for advice. The newer sleeping pills and antidepressants are very effective in restoring sleep and appetite with minimal side effects, and objective scientific studies have shown that support groups and counseling make a profound difference in one's comfort and ability to deal with cancer. Chapter 11, *Stress and the Immune System*, and Chapter 13, *Getting Support*, describe in more detail methods for dealing with stress and feelings, and offer sources of support.

The physical aspects of fear

If you had any hint that your symptoms might be cancer-related, you are probably already familiar with tremendous, overwhelming feelings of fear and their aftereffects. The physiology of fear is such that your body prepares you very specifically either for battle or retreat when you experience fear. We have evolved to note and react quickly to changing stimuli during a fearful encounter. This may explain why many people, when first diagnosed with cancer, want immediately to start a treatment—any treatment, just so they're doing something to fight back.

Unfortunately, these bodily preparations for action, such as increasing your pulse rate and redirecting blood flow from your limbs to your heart, brain, and other internal organs, are not the ideal biological events to prepare you for understanding and remembering your doctor's explanations. The moment that fear hits and adrenaline pumps, senses become heightened in preparation for life-saving action. However, that sensation that you can somehow see everything around you with remarkable clarity is not necessarily going to help you remember the doctor's description of two tests that need to be done, and a third test only if the first two are inconclusive, and where your doctor said he prefers these tests be done. Instead, you may remember exactly where you were sitting, the color of the doctor's office walls, and that stray hair of the doctor's that wouldn't stay put:

> I remember the still, overheated southwestern summer weather outside, the soft sunlight in the cool examination room in the hematologist-oncologist's office, the chair where my husband was seated, my husband's face as he struggled to remain calm, and the words the doctor used in his moderate Filipino accent.

Numbness, mental slowness

Many cancer patients and their loved ones—intelligent and competent people—report not being able to remember anything of the doctor's explanation after hearing the word cancer. This is sometimes the case even when doctors themselves are diagnosed with cancer. Here's an NHL survivor's account of being numbed by her diagnosis:

> There was this black hole in my ability to reason. I could not link anything to that moment or find a way to transition from it. Nor could I find anything in me to muster up outrage or panic or desperation. It was an otherworldly, emotionally null, intellectually nomadic period of a few minutes. Then, as I looked at my husband and back at my hands (as though they were a sign I still existed), all I could think was, "Well, it's still not my time to go." I have faced tough challenges before and found reserves to draw on. So now I may need to deplete them, but I won't have any of this take me from this great love across the room. And I knew I would need him to get through it. And he would need me to hang tough so his life didn't fall apart either.

Still others report becoming paralytic for days, unable to sleep, rise, eat, or work.

If you will be meeting the doctor in person to discuss test results and treatment choices, be prepared to have difficulty absorbing what is said. For example, you could be prepared to take notes, or take a friend or a tape recorder with you. Tell the doctor that you will be calling back with a list of questions after you have had time to absorb this information. If she expresses impatience or reluctance to help you, consider finding another doctor.

Detachment

Many people note that upon learning of their diagnosis they were completely objective, calm, and felt nothing at all, as if they were outside of their body observing this happening to someone else. This is called dissociation. Dissociation temporarily allows you to absorb information without emotional pain.

Childlike or nonsensical behavior

Some people note that they said and did things that made no sense, sometimes quite childlike things. This can be a seeking of comfort in happier times, technically called regression:

> When my husband phoned to say his CT scan showed what was almost certainly lymphoma, I left my office immediately. Once at home I found that, although I was forty years old, all I wanted to do was reread my old girlhood Nancy Drew books.

Denial

Some people respond to the news of their diagnosis with the belief that there is an error in the laboratory test, or that their results have been confused with someone else's. (While laboratory errors are possible, they are not common.) This reaction, called denial, is a protective reaction to allow you to absorb an onslaught of information more slowly. Denial can be used successfully to help you forget about cancer between treatments, to return to your productive life. Denial may be a dangerous adaptive strategy, however, if you forget medical appointments or become convinced that your health will improve spontaneously with no treatment.

Anger

While many people develop focused feelings of anger some time after their diagnosis, others may feel a generalized anger at the time of diagnosis. They may lash out at the doctor who was the bearer of bad news about the cancer diagnosis, or at loved ones for seemingly meaningless reasons. Sometimes anger is a form of projection, a displacement of painful feelings within the self outward onto others. As such, projection serves to reduce unbearable levels of pain. At other times, the angry person may simply feel overwhelmed by having to face all of the stresses and responsibilities of normal life, plus a cancer diagnosis. Yet others feel that being angry is more socially acceptable than feeling sad. Anger can be a useful emotion if targeted properly and harmlessly, but it can also signal the beginning of depression and can drive away the support of others that you will almost certainly need.

Sadness

Many people report that they cry or otherwise express great sadness, and that they feel better after doing so. Sadness is, of course, an entirely normal reaction to a cancer diagnosis. This change in your awareness of yourself connotes the possibility of great loss: loss of life, possible loss of motility, of career opportunities.

Guilt

If you're feeling guilty about possibly causing your or your loved one's cancer, you need to know that no sure cause of non-Hodgkin's lymphoma has yet been found for most cases: not stress, not environmental agents, not dietary choices.

Blame

Guilt may lead to blame. Like anger, blame can be a form of projection. If someone has been blaming himself for his own or another's cancer, the feelings may become unbearable and he may begin looking elsewhere for an explanation. Unfortunately, some people decide that the best solution is for another person to carry this blame. Those who have been coping with stress in this way for many years sometimes skip self-blame and go directly to blaming others. If someone in your life appears to be blaming you for cancer, you might try discussing this with him. If discussion doesn't improve the relationship, it might be best to remove this person from your immediate circle of activities temporarily and deal with him only when you feel most able.

Withdrawal

Others report that they or their loved ones initially seemed detached, withdrawn, or uncaring. Those who withdraw may do so for many reasons: as a habit formed during earlier stressful experiences, as a means to avoid shameful feelings about expressing emotion, in an attempt to keep emotional levels low so that others won't become upset, as an attempt to reduce exposure to painful ideas, and so on. At times it's almost impossible to know what really motivates you or others, even after serious introspection, or after others tell you what they feel. Your attempts to discuss this with the withdrawn person, or others' attempts to draw you out, may make matters temporarily worse.

Reactions of loved ones

There also seems to be some difference in reaction depending on whether it's you or your loved one who is facing a cancer diagnosis. Many cancer survivors report that, in their opinion, the experience was much harder on their loved ones than on themselves. Clearly this is a topic subject to personal interpretation, as the loving caretaker isn't undergoing treatment that can cause anything from mild discomfort to serious toxicity or even death. A cancer survivor who believes that her loved ones suffer more discomfort than she does, though, may be expressing a useful feeling of immortality, a belief of being in charge of her own fate that will serve her well during treatment.

It might be useful to keep in mind that loved ones face issues that are somewhat different from those faced by the cancer survivor. They may experience guilt that they themselves remain healthy, fear that they will be deprived of the person they love most, and helplessness in the face of cancer, a daunting enemy by anyone's standards.

Summary

We hope that the information we've offered in this opening chapter has helped remove the edge from the fear you're feeling. Knowing that delays you may have experienced obtaining a diagnosis are common; that multiple diagnostic tests are the norm; that the diagnostic process can unfold in stages with increasing levels of certainty, perhaps entailing changes in your treatment plan or your choice of doctors; that you're not alone; that what you're feeling is normal—these are the first steps of the journey.

CHAPTER 2

Finding the Right Oncologist

There are in fact two things, science and
opinion; the former begets knowledge, the
latter ignorance.

—Hippocrates

Choosing the right oncologist to coordinate your treatment is the most important decision you'll make during the early days of your diagnosis. Unless you have been told that your lymphoma is aggressive, generally you can take several weeks to locate the best oncologist for your circumstances without compromising the outcome.

If you're pressed for time, though, or are feeling too anxious just now to pursue this issue with the necessary tenacity, you can limit your search to contacting the nearest university medical school, or to contacting the National Cancer Institute (NCI) at 1-800-4-CANCER and asking for the names of several hematologic oncologists at their institution or in your area.

In this chapter, we first look at the various types of oncologists and how to locate qualified candidates. Then we discuss considerations in deciding on the right oncologist for you, including currentness of medical background, affiliated treatment center, and manner of conducting practice.

Types of oncologists

There are several types of oncologists:

- The medical oncologist, trained in the use of chemotherapy. Almost all NHL survivors utilize the skills of a medical oncologist. The medical oncologist usually is called simply an oncologist. Some medical oncologists specialize, however. For example, a hematologic oncologist is a medical oncologist who specializes in cancers of the blood, such as lymphoma and leukemia.

- The radiation oncologist, trained in the use of radiation therapy. NHL is seldom treated with radiation therapy alone, but small areas of your body may need radiation therapy to reduce tumor bulk or to control symptoms. When this is the case, your radiation oncologist will usually coordinate any treatment you may need with your medical oncologist.

- The surgical oncologist, usually found in subspecialties such as gynecologic oncology. You may need a surgical oncologist if a tumor has invaded pelvic organs or is near the heart.

We recommend that you choose a hematologic oncologist who is a lymphoma specialist as your primary oncologist. Hematologic oncologists specialize in treating lymphoma, and usually are associated with university medical schools. If you cannot find a lymphoma specialist in your area to provide your treatment, you should plan to travel for at least one second opinion from a lymphoma specialist during the course of your treatment. In particular, you should have your biopsy material reviewed by an expert in lymphoma pathology, such as the pathologists found at the National Institutes of Health (NIH).

General considerations

You should search carefully for an oncologist who has a great deal of experience with your illness, and who keeps informed regarding the latest breakthroughs in NHL diagnosis and treatment, because NHL can be a challenge to diagnose, can convert to a different grade, and because treatments are evolving with vigor. It's of course better to make a good choice at first rather than at last; and it's especially important to find the right doctor before you make the decision to start chemotherapy or radiation therapy.

Before deciding on a local oncologist, you should consider traveling for care. Much of the best work being done for lymphoma is done at university medical schools. In Chapter 21, *Traveling for Care,* we'll provide you with more detail, such as charitable groups that will pay travel and lodging costs for you.

A word about managed care: your insurance provider may have restrictions regarding who you may consult or where you may travel for care. Check your policy carefully for such restrictions, and contact the provider before scheduling appointments that might not be covered. Some managed care providers charge only a modestly increased co-payment for out-of-plan doctors; others refuse to pay any of the doctor's fee; still others will pay most or all costs if medical necessity can be proved. If your HMO has a care coordinator, he may work with you to make special reinterpretations of the rules in your case. Often people never challenge their HMO's rules, but frequently those who do win a full settlement or a compromise.

Finding several good oncologists

If you have limited time to get recommendations, you can contact the nearest university medical school or the NCI and ask for the names of several hematologic oncologists at their institution or in your area.

In addition to these two techniques, there are several other ways to search for qualified oncologists:

- The National Cancer Institute designates both Comprehensive Cancer Centers and Clinical Cancer Centers. The former meet rigorous standards of excellence; the latter meet less rigorous but still quite high standards. If you phone the NCI's Cancer Information Service at 1-800-4-CANCER, they can provide you with a list of these centers.

  Be sure to tell them if you're willing to travel for care, otherwise they are inclined to assume that you want only local references. Once you have these lists, you can phone the nearest center and ask for a referral. Note that any institution can simply include in its name the words "clinical cancer center" or "comprehensive cancer center." Be sure that the institution's title is NCI-designated. If you have access to the Web, you can find this information at the NCI's web site: *http://www.nci.nih.gov/cancercenters/*.

- The American Medical Association maintains a list of all licensed doctors, AMA members or not, and can tell you if the doctor you're considering is board-certified in oncology or in an oncologic subspecialty such as gynecologic oncology. They can also furnish information such as year of graduation from medical school, the location of residencies, and type of specialty. The AMA's Physician Select web site is *http://www.ama-assn.org/aps/amahg.html*.

- *The American Medical Directory* and the *Directory of Medical Specialists,* available at your local library, both list doctors by specialty.

- The magazine *U.S. News and World Report*, which can be found in your local library, annually designates hospitals as Centers of Excellence. Usually this "Best Hospitals" issue is published in July. Hospitals ranked best in cancer care are listed by cancer subcategory. With this information, you can phone several of these hospitals and ask to speak with a hematologic oncologist. Ask this doctor for the names of several oncologists in your area or for a referral within her own institution if it's nearby or within your acceptable travel boundaries. You may be able to order a back issue of *U.S. News and World Report*'s "Best Hospitals" edition by calling (202) 955-2000, or by visiting their web site at *http://www.usnews.com/*.

- If your family doctor or primary care physician has recommended an oncologist, ask him why he's recommending this person. Recommendations from another doctor can range from wonderful—"Because she gets such good results"—to lukewarm.

- Phone a reputable nearby hospital, ask for the oncology floor, then ask to speak with the head oncology nurse. Explain that you'd like a recommendation for an oncologist who treats lymphoma and leukemia, and that you'd value the nurse's opinion because he works extensively with so many oncologists.

- Use a computer to access the National Library of Medicine's Medline, or have a friend or relative do so for you. Search on the subject "non-Hodgkin's lymphoma." Scan the last two years' worth of papers and note the authors' names. Some Medline access providers, such as Paper-Chase, show the authors' institutional affiliations; if not, phone the NCI and ask where these doctors can be reached. For more information on using Medline, see Chapter 24, *Researching Your Lymphoma*. The National Library of Medicine's free Pubmed Medline search engine is at *http://www.ncbi.nlm.nih.gov/PubMed/*.

- Contact the Lymphoma Research Foundation of America or the Cure For Lymphoma Society (see Appendix A, *Resources*) for the names of hematologic oncologists who specialize in lymphoma.

Choosing treatment centers

Bear in mind that when you choose a doctor, by default, you also choose a treatment center. Ask the doctors on your short list at which hospitals they have admitting privileges, and which, if any, NCI-designated treatment groups they are associated with.

There are several different types of treatment centers: university hospitals, cooperative lymphoma groups, and community clinical oncology programs.

University hospitals

University hospitals or other research institutions funded by the NCI, such as Memorial Sloan-Kettering Cancer Center in New York, or the Mayo Cancer Center in Rochester, Minnesota, are very likely places to find the latest advances in lymphoma treatment.

When regulatory agencies decide who will be allocated scarce resources or who will be given permission to provide rare services such as PET scanning, the university hospital is a probable choice because the infrastructure, such as skill levels and staffing, is already in place. In addition, the cooperative and collaborative nature of the university hospital tends to attract the most talented medical researchers. In most cases, these same researchers are also expected to provide patient care. This means that the latest treatments are likely to be offered in this setting first, that the accumulated experience level among the staff is high, and that you'll be treated by some of the most talented and knowledgeable people in the country. Some studies have shown that centers that treat more than forty lymphoma patients per year have a higher success rate than centers treating fewer.

University-associated hospitals and cancer centers are the institutions most likely to be designated by the NCI as either Comprehensive Cancer Centers or Clinical Cancer Centers. All NCI-designated centers are nonprofit institutions.

Some people are afraid to receive healthcare at a university or teaching hospital because they fear they will be subjected to unproven or unnecessary treatment by newly graduated medical students who may not know what they're doing. It's true that a training mission incorporated into a hospital's charter means that you may be examined or cared for by more than one doctor, but this can be an advantage as well as a disadvantage. These advantages and disadvantages differ little from having a family doctor who is a member of a large practice: while it's true that you may not always see the same doctor, it's also true that you need not go without help if your doctor is not available.

Newly graduated doctors, called interns, are seldom charged with care or decision-making in the absence of your attending doctor or an oncology resident. You're always free to say that you prefer that a procedure or exam be done by someone with more experience.

In the U.S., unproven treatments are never performed without clear written informed consent if your hospital receives any federal funds or is governed by local laws regarding informed consent. If you are approached to take part in a study of an unproven treatment, called a clinical trial, you always have the right to refuse; if you do decide to enroll, you always have the right to withdraw later.

A most important fact all cancer survivors and their loved ones should be aware of is that, for cancer treatment, a placebo is virtually never used. The new, unproven treatment is offered in clinical trials that compare the new treatment to standard, approved treatment—never to an inactive sugar pill. The rare exception is the watch-and-wait approach suggested for some low-grade NHLs. When there is no standard treatment to which the new treatment can be juxtaposed—such as the very first bone marrow purging procedures in the early days of bone marrow transplantation, or the watch-and-wait procedure—this lack is clearly communicated by those attempting to ensure that consent is indeed informed consent.

Note that a community teaching hospital is not the same as a medical school training hospital, although the community hospital may have residency programs that accommodate certain university medical school training needs, such as emergency room rotations.

Cooperative lymphoma groups

Cooperative lymphoma groups are comprised of university hospitals and cancer treatment centers who take part in administering very large multicenter trials of new treatments. There are about thirteen clinical trial cooperative groups in the U.S. A list of the centers in these groups can be obtained by phoning the NCI's Cancer Information Service.

Community clinical oncology programs

This program links community doctors with the clinical trial cooperative groups described in "Cooperative lymphoma groups." For a list of groups in your area, phone the NCI.

Treatment at no charge

The National Cancer Institute provides free cancer care to those who qualify, but only within clinical trials. A referral from your local oncologist is necessary for entry into a trial. Non-U.S. citizens may be admitted at the discretion of the principal investigator of the trial.

St. Jude Children's Research Hospital in Memphis, Tennessee, provides free treatment for children.

Some university and community hospitals have a policy guaranteeing that they will provide medical care for local residents who cannot pay.

Checking credentials of candidates

If a check on credentials wasn't part of the process you used to come up with a list of candidate oncologists, you can check credentials now. Any doctors recommended by the NCI or a clinical center have undoubtedly already had a thorough check of their backgrounds and qualifications; however, you might want to see them for yourself.

You can check doctors' professional qualifications in some of the same publications listed earlier as aids to locating qualified oncologists.

- The *AMA Directory of Physicians* lists the doctor's name, medical school attended, year licensed, primary and secondary specialty, type of practice, board certification, and physician recognition awards. (Available in libraries or at *http://www.ama-assn.org/*.)

- The official *ABMS Directory of Board Certified Medical Specialties* includes specialty, when certified, medical school and year of degree, place and dates of internship, place and dates of residency, fellowship training, academic and hospital appointments, professional association memberships, type of practice, and current address, telephone, and fax. (Available in libraries or 1-800-776-CERT.)

- Your state medical licensing board should be able to tell you the status of your doctor's license, when the doctor was first licensed by the state, and the status of any misconduct charges or disciplinary actions.

- An easy way to check on your doctor's credentials is to call Medi-Net, a new consumer information service that provides healthcare consumers with a background check on any doctor who is licensed to practice in the United States, including credentials, degrees, training, and board certifications, as well as any disciplinary actions or sanctions taken against the doctor. Each complete Medi-Net physician profile costs $17.00 per doctor (less for subsequent profiles ordered at the same time). Preliminary information is provided on the telephone, with detailed reports mailed or faxed to callers, usually the same day. To order a report, call toll-free (888) ASK-MEDI (275-6334), or find it on the Internet at *http://www.askmedi.com.*

- Another way to reassure yourself about the currency of the candidate doctor's knowledge is to see what he has published. Again, use a computer to access Medline or have a friend or relative do so for you, this time searching by the doctor's last name and first initial. Note that the U.S. National Library of Medicine offers a free Medline search engine at *http://www.ncbi.nlm.nih.gov/PubMed/.* (If you don't have a PC, try your local library. Many have computers for public use.)

In general, if the doctor you're considering has published two or more papers in the last five years on topics that you feel pertain to your condition, she's worth a visit. Keep in mind, though, that many excellent oncologists are involved in research during their training years, then move into private practice and cease publishing. Lack of published material does not mean a doctor is inadequate, nor does the existence of many publications guarantee that he will be a good, caring practitioner. Published papers are just one of many gauges of a doctor's ability.

Choosing the best from a short list

Once you have found one or more board certified oncologists who seem excellent, you can interview them to make sure they're good candidates. No matter how many recommendations you receive or sterling credentials you have uncovered, until you have a candid conversation with the human behind the stethoscope, you won't know if this is a person with whom you'll feel comfortable.

A survivor of low-grade disease describes her perspective on the doctors she considered:

The first oncologist I went to made some attempt to figure out who I was, figuring that he and I would be having a long-term doctor-patient relationship. He asked me to describe the history of the symptoms that led to my diagnosis. He had spoken to my internist. Unfortunately, making judgments based on a one-hour meeting with a newly diagnosed and obviously upset cancer patient can be shaky. He said that there were three options for my low-grade lymphoma: wait and watch for symptoms to appear, mild chemotherapy with oral medication, or more aggressive chemotherapy with a drug that had come to market about a year before. He decided after this one meeting that I was not "psychologically disposed" to sit around doing nothing, and told me I should go ahead with the aggressive chemotherapy because then I would feel that I was "doing something."

Funny, I am the same person who had natural childbirth rather than take medication, who never took a painkiller after my biopsy, who refrained even from taking vitamins to avoid putting something unnecessary into my body.

After seeing two other oncologists, both of whom advised me to delay treatment for as long as possible, I decided to use one of them as my oncologist. The first doctor was surprised that I made this choice—he is local, and I have to travel one hour to see my doctor of choice. But I feel I am "doing something." I feel that I am not using up a chemotherapy option before I really need to. I believe that I have taken charge of my life, even if I cannot control my disease. Most of all, I am appalled that a doctor would suggest using chemotherapy for psychological purposes. There are other ways to treat stress, anxiety, and depression. For these symptoms, I found meditation tapes, music, hot tea, and a good shrink.

Schedule a meeting to ask any questions you have about medical background and about the doctor's attitudes and office policies, such as:

- How many patients with your type of lymphoma has she treated?
- At what hospitals does she have admitting privileges?
- Which clinical trials is she familiar with? It's important to have an oncologist familiar with the latest research in NHL.

- Which institutions is she affiliated with? For instance, does she have a faculty appointment at a medical school in addition to a private oncology practice?

- What treatment does she recommend? After the appointment, evaluate how this recommendation compares with what your reading has taught you.

- What is her policy for handling emergency calls after business hours?

- How will test results be communicated? Will ancillary doctors be given permission to communicate directly with you, the patient? Does the doctor object to leaving information on your answering or fax machine, if that's a method you prefer?

- Are family members welcome to call with questions? Some doctors prefer communicating only with the patient.

- Does the doctor's philosophy about health and life mesh well with your own? For example, does she espouse treatment at all costs over quality of life?

- Use some of this interview time to describe yourself and your expectations, such as how much participation you would like to have in health-care decisions.

Neeraj, a survivor of non-Hodgkins lymphoma (NHL)/acute lymphoblastic leukemia (ALL), describes how angry he felt when an insensitive doctor blurted out his diagnosis, then walked away:

> I was diagnosed with a hybrid of T-cell ALL and non-Hodgkin's lymphoma on Halloween 1994 (was that scary!). I have been in remission since December 1994, and finished high-dose induction followed by twelve months of consolidation chemotherapy in November 1995. I was on low-dose maintenance therapy for two years after.

> It hasn't been roses all the way. My diagnosis was a nightmare. This doctor (not my current hematologist) came in with my CT scan results, asked me what I was studying at school, what and where I was having pain, touched me at my sternum which hurt like hell, and then said in an unconcerned voice, "Okay, I must tell you that you have cancer, and you have it all over, in your chest, spleen…just one big laundry list." Then he said, "We have to do a bone marrow biopsy right away, so follow me," and vanished, leaving me and my brother-in-law behind in a state of

shock. So when I got out of the room, I bumped into a nurse dressed up as a witch for Halloween, and she said, "Did I scare you?" I told her that she didn't, but the doctor sure did.

Even today I have not been able to reduce my resentment for that guy, but the rest of the doctors and nurses have more than made up for that first experience. I can't help but think that I get preferred treatment now that I have established such good relationships.

Overall, you want to make sure that the oncologist you choose has excellent medical credentials, extensive experience with NHL, and is affiliated with a treatment center that offers up-to-date resources. You'll want to weigh in other considerations such as communication skills, personal style, and office location.

Summary

Now that you have information regarding the differences among oncologists, the wisdom of utilizing a hematologic oncologist, and the advantages of care at a well-regarded cancer center or large cooperative lymphoma group, you are equipped to find a good doctor and turn your attention to such issues as the details of your treatment and finding the emotional and instrumental support you will need.

CHAPTER 3

What Are the Non-Hodgkin's Lymphomas?

*Physicians think they do a lot for a patient
when they give his disease a name.*

—Immanuel Kant

There is no single definitive description of the non-Hodgkin's lymphomas because the term NHL encompasses a collection of diseases. How they relate to other lymphomas and leukemias—and if they really are different entities—is still under debate.

There are many theories about potential causes of NHL, but studies are not conclusive. There is much that is not fully understood. There are, however, certain general medical descriptions of NHL that can be made, as well as comparisons to other lymphomas and other cancers. The current state of knowledge about causes, types of NHL, and staging can be described.

In this chapter, we will attempt to categorize information about NHL so that you can begin to build a frame of reference for understanding this disease. First, we will discuss non-Hodgkin's lymphomas in the broader context of all lymphomas. Then we will look at variations in NHL by age, gender, race, geographical location, and other characteristics. Next, we'll look at the various types of NHL and what characterizes them, what is known about the possible causes of NHL, and comparisons of NHL to Hodgkin's, leukemia, and other cancers. Finally, we'll look at identifying and staging individual cases of NHL.

What is the lymphatic system?

The lymphatic system is an infection-fighting circulatory system of body fluids and lymphocytes, traveling in delicate vessels called ducts that collect fluid squeezed from veins during normal metabolism, and bring it back to the veins near the heart. The lymphatic system relies on gravity and muscle compression to propel lymphatic fluid. Lymphatic fluid resembles blood serum—that is, blood fluid containing only lymphocytes—and is returned to the bloodstream at various points in the body so that waste products can be removed by the kidneys.

The lymphatic system also includes various infection-fighting or lymphocyte-producing organs, such as the spleen, tonsils, appendix, thymus, and intestinal Peyer's patch.

A lymph node is a kidney-bean-shaped swelling along a lymphatic duct, responsible for filtering lymphatic fluid of foreign substances. The body has hundreds of lymph nodes. Healthy nodes vary in size from very tiny to almond-size, depending on their position and function near or within various organs.

What is lymphoma?

Lymphomas and leukemias are cancers of white blood cells at various stages of maturation. White blood cells are part of the immune system. They travel through the blood and the lymphatic system and are supposed to protect us from illness and, ironically, from cancer.

As with other cancers, the wayward cells that characterize lymphoma and leukemia do not die as normal cells do, nor do they honor the cycles of orderly cell division as normal cells do: many have no resting phase, instead dividing continuously. What's worse, they divide before they are fully mature, which makes them unable to fight infection as normal white blood cells do. This means that our bodies accumulate nonfunctional white blood cells that, by dividing rapidly or not undergoing normal cell death (apoptosis), crowd out other functioning white blood cells and other nearby normal cells within affected organs. For instance, red blood cells and platelets may be crowded out of the nurturing bone marrow matrix if the white blood cells of lymphoma have affected the bone marrow. The path of lymphatic fluid and its infection-fighting mechanisms may be compromised if lymphoma arises within a lymph node. Lymphomas lodged within the thyroid can cause the secretion of thyroid hormones to go amiss.

Both lymphomas and leukemias can circulate in the bloodstream or lodge in lymph nodes or other organs. Some researchers feel that, because of this and other similarities, such as the existence of viruses that can cause both lymphoma and leukemia, separating lymphomas from leukemias is an out-moded idea. They believe that lymphoma and leukemia are different mani-festations of the same malignant cell, and this is partly reflected in the new Revised European American Lymphoma (REAL) classification system of hematologic cancers. The REAL classification system is described in Appendix D, *Classification Systems*.

Many lymphomas arise within a lymph node, perhaps suggesting an error in cell division or maturation during the calling forth of white blood cells from the lymph node following an infection or other stimulation of the immune system. Others arise within the bone marrow, within other immune system organs such as the spleen or thymus, or within areas of the intestine called Peyer's patches that are rich in lymphocytes. Despite their predilection for lymph nodes and other lymphocyte-rich sites, lymphomas can arise essen-tially anywhere. Some rare NHLs arise within the bone itself, as opposed to the bone marrow.

What is NHL?

The following sections discuss the unique aspects of the non-Hodgkin's lym-phomas.

The name "non-Hodgkin's lymphoma" might lead you to believe it's a single lymphoma type that just isn't quite one of the Hodgkin's lymphomas, about which more is said below. NHL is actually a collection of many varied lym-phomas. There are many more types of NHL than there are types of Hodgkin's lymphomas.

Incidence

NHL is a disease of increasingly serious proportions. Industrialized nations experience a higher incidence of NHL than do developing countries, and the highest incidence rate in the world is seen in the United States and Canada, with forty to fifty thousand new cases per year in the U.S. According to the National Cancer Institute's Surveillance, Epidemiology, and End Results (SEER) statistics, NHL is the sixth most common cancer and the sixth most common cause of cancer death, accounting for 4 percent of all cancers and 4 percent of cancer deaths. As SEER statistics sample only about nineteen loca-tions within the U.S., and because there is no comprehensive national tumor registry in the U.S., the true incidence of NHL may be much higher. Some estimates range as high as 80,000 cases a year.

The rate of follicular NHL—that is, NHL arising from lymphoid follicles within a lymph node—is higher in the U.S. than in other parts of the world. Follicular NHL represents 20 percent of NHLs in developed countries, but is rare in developing countries.

Trends

In the U.S., NHL exhibits the frightening characteristic of having occurred more often in recent years. Even after numbers are adjusted to account for increased rates of NHL among those in the U.S. with AIDS, 40 percent of the overall increase is unexplained. For all ages, genders, and races in the U.S., the rate of increase of newly diagnosed cases of NHL from 1973 to 1991 was 73 percent. For the same group from 1946 to 1988, the rate of increase was 150 percent. This compares to a worldwide rate of increase during the same time frame of 43 percent. The annual rate of increase of NHL—3.3 percent—is comparable to that of melanoma and prostate cancer and, if it proceeds at the same rate unchecked, will double the number of people being diagnosed with NHL by the year 2021. If this trend continues, NHL soon will rival colon, lung, breast, and prostate cancers as a leading cause of illness and death in the U.S.

In the United States, the incidence of high-grade NHL is increasing more rapidly than low-grade NHL, and the incidence of extranodal presentations—NHL arising outside a lymph node—is increasing more rapidly than nodular presentations.

Types of non-Hodgkin's lymphomas

There is a confusing array of NHLs. If you attempt to compare yourself to others who appear to have the same diagnosis, bear in mind that their diagnosis may have been made using criteria that are different, perhaps in subtle ways, from those used by your own diagnosticians. This means that treatment decisions from one person to the next may differ as well.

Most NHLs arise within a lymph node, but a significant and increasing number arise in areas other than nodes, such as the jaw or brain, especially among children and those with AIDS. The range from low-grade, indolent disease to aggressive, high-grade disease does not fall into discrete categories, but is instead a continuum. Mixed grades, as determined by the appearance of the tumor cells or other criteria, sometimes are found in the same patient at the same time—in the same node, in different nodes, or in both nodes and marrow. When mixed grades are present in the same patient, this may represent the progression of disease.

Why are so many of these cancers, some quite different from the others, clustered under one name? Until recently, science was not able to make fine distinctions among these subtypes. Advances in molecular genetics have shown, though, that NHL is actually many diseases.

With these improved diagnostic techniques and advances in microbiology and genetics, it is becoming increasingly common for subtypes of NHL to emerge from a background of confusing similarities. The mucosa-related lymphoid tissue (MALT) lymphomas, viral T-cell leukemia/lymphoma, cutaneous T-cell lymphoma, as well as primary central nervous system lymphoma so frequently seen among AIDS survivors, are examples of the divergence of NHLs.

Some of the NHLs more closely resemble leukemias than they do the Hodgkin's lymphomas. As more becomes known, some lymphomas that were categorized as NHLs may be reclassified with other cancers.

It is beyond the scope of this book to describe each cellular and behavioral difference among the many types of NHL. To do so would require about a thousand additional pages and would duplicate the fine efforts of others. A superb source of detailed information on these differences is the 1997 edition of *The Non-Hodgkin's Lymphomas*, edited by Ian Magrath.

A listing of all NHL types and subtypes as delineated by the various classifications systems can be found in Appendix D.

How is NHL different from Hodgkin's?

While NHL is characterized by many different cell types, and may arise in many different locations, sometimes simultaneously and via unknown paths, Hodgkin's lymphoma (HL) consists of just four subtypes and in many cases is a more orderly cancer. It is more likely to occur entirely within nodes and to spread into adjacent, contiguous nodes, probably spreading through lymphatic ducts.

NHL is more frequently diagnosed in older people, whereas, in the U.S., HL most often arises during the second and third decades of life.

One subtype of NHL, anaplastic large-cell lymphoma (ALCL), resembles one subtype of Hodgkin's lymphoma, lymphocyte-depleted Hodgkin's lymphoma (LDHL). Care must be taken when diagnosing these subtypes, as their treatments differ.

Although many of the same drugs are used for both NHL and HL, treatments that are successful for NHL are less so for HL and vice versa.

Epstein-Barr virus (EBV) seldom is found in B-cell NHL tumors unless they arise in an immune-suppressed person or in cases of Burkitt's lymphoma in Africa, whereas about 40 percent of HL tumor samples test positive for Epstein-Barr virus.

The appearance of NHL cells under the microscope is different from most types of HL, and the non-Hodgkin's cell surface antigens, which are markers on the outside of the cell membrane, are different from those for most, but not all, HLs.

How is NHL different from some leukemias?

Some NHLs resemble certain leukemias known as lymphoid leukemias. Nonetheless, there are differences as well.

Most NHLs arise within a lymph node or solid organ and do not release large numbers of easily detectable cancerous cells into the bloodstream, whereas most leukemias arise in the bone marrow and circulate readily in the bloodstream.

In spite of these differences, the lymphoblastic and small lymphocytic NHLs are very similar to acute lymphoblastic leukemia (ALL) and to chronic lymphocytic leukemia (CLL). At times, diagnostic efforts are unable to differentiate these illnesses, and the patient is described as having NHL/ALL or NHL/CLL. Indeed, the new REAL classification system of lymphomas includes some leukemias such as CLL, lymphoblastic leukemia, and plasma-cell multiple myeloma (MM) as neoplasms related to NHL.

How is NHL different from other cancers?

The foremost difference between NHL and other cancers is that, as a cancer of the white blood cells, NHL is a cancer of the body system that is supposed to protect us from cancer. While upon first thought this betrayal may seem a cruel hoax, it may also account for the great success seen in treating some lymphomas. The ongoing research done for curing NHL and other lymphomas—efforts involving therapeutic vaccines derived from tumor samples, and antibody therapy, for example—tend to become bellwether strategies for improving progress against other cancers.

For many cancers, detection while the cancer still has not spread outside the original organ greatly improves one's chances of survival. While it is generally true that NHL caught early may be more successfully treated than that caught late, it is not unusual nor is it a hopeless prognostic sign for NHL to arise in multiple locations at the same time. Metastases, even to bone marrow, are not always of the same dire significance that they may be for some other cancers, because frequently these NHLs continue to respond to treatment and to cease spreading.

Likewise, aggressive NHLs can at times be more successfully treated than low-grade or indolent tumors. This is discussed more fully in Chapter 4, *Prognoses*.

NHL is more likely to arise in certain organs and not in others, specifically but not always the organs of the immune system such as the lymph nodes, spleen, tonsils, and thymus. It is rare, however, to find a primary NHL in certain organs such as the pancreas or muscle.

Perhaps owing to the hormonal connections between the central nervous system and white blood cells (see Chapter 11, *Stress and the Immune System*), lymphomas can arise first in the brain or central nervous system, not necessarily as a result of spread from elsewhere.

Who gets NHL?

You would be a most unusual person if you didn't wonder why you developed NHL and where you are in the spectrum of others with the same disease. In this section, we discuss the demographics of NHL; possible causes are discussed in the section, "What causes NHL?"

Gender

Young males are diagnosed more frequently with NHL than are young females, but this difference decreases with increasing age.

Race

Whites are diagnosed with NHL 50 percent more often than Blacks, Asians, and Hispanics combined. This trend is exhibited worldwide.

Age

Those under age 65 develop NHL less often than those over age 65. For those under age 65, the incidence is 8.5 per 100,000 people; for those over age 65, the incidence is 68.8 per 100,000. Among those over age 75 diagnosed with NHL, the proportion of NHLs affecting only the follicles of the lymph node is 400 percent greater than NHLs diffused throughout the lymph node. This is meaningful because follicular presentations are usually of lower grade than diffuse NHLs, requiring different treatment.

Immune status

People with suppressed immune systems are in some cases more likely to develop NHL than others. They fall into three categories:

- Those with HIV/AIDS
- Those who have had solid organ transplants, but this risk decreases significantly by twelve months after the transplant
- Those with certain inherited immune deficiencies

NHL cases related to immune suppression are much more common than instances of the Hodgkin's lymphomas among the immune-suppressed.

Eight to 27 percent of NHLs being diagnosed today are AIDS-related. Many arise as primary cancers of the brain or central nervous system, ocular disease, gastrointestinal tract, body cavity, head, neck, or nasal passages, but they often are characterized by unusual presentations such as the pancreas or esophagus. For children with AIDS, the rate of developing NHL is about ten times higher than that of adults with AIDS.

Among the immune-compromised, NHL normally appears as an aggressive, diffuse, high-grade disease with a rapid course.

Children

Differences in presentation between children and adults are striking and puzzling. Children more frequently manifest disease outside the node (extra-nodal sites)—that is, follicular lymphomas are rare among children. The most common types of NHL found in children are high-grade lymphoblastic or small noncleaved NHL of Burkitt's subtype. Childhood NHLs have very good prognoses with aggressive chemotherapy, with a cure rate of 70 to 90 percent.

Although childhood cancer is rare, and childhood NHL even more rare, NHL is the third most common pediatric cancer and accounts for 6 percent of childhood cancers.

As with the Hodgkin's lymphomas, NHLs among children and adolescents occur most often in the second decade of life. Often, juvenile NHL resembles acute lymphoblastic leukemia, and the treatments for both are similar.

What causes NHL?

Many people try to determine what gave cancer a foothold, sometimes from intellectual curiosity and sometimes from a determination not to suffer a relapse.

Only two causes of NHL have been proven, but there are several circumstances and substances which are suspected to play a part in the development of at least some NHLs. It's probable that you'll never know the exact cause of your illness, but the following sections offer possible explanations.

Before a clear discussion of the causes of NHL can ensue, you need to know a bit about what causes cancers in general.

How cancer develops

Human DNA is stored on forty-six paired chromosomes. With a couple of exceptions, each cell in our body has one copy of all forty-six chromosomes, coiled tightly in a ball, stored in the cell nucleus. Each chromosome is composed of two long strings of genes held together like a ladder, with rungs consisting of electrochemical bonds.

Many if not all instances of cancer are accompanied by changes in the tumor cell's DNA. At times, a gene is entirely missing, or has been half-spliced with another gene after DNA strands from two entirely different chromosomes accidentally overlap, break apart, and rejoin. Such chromosomal inversions and transpositions are well known among the NHLs and other cancers. Translocations between chromosomes 14 and 18, for example, are common among the follicular lymphomas. In some cases, an entire chromosome may be missing, as with some acute leukemias.

All of the body's work is accomplished using proteins. Our bodies build proteins from genes by reading the base pairs of DNA in groups of three, until special repeating sequences recognized as terminators are encountered. Each triplet encodes for one amino acid, and the complete string of amino acids comprises a protein. The string of amino acids that accumulates—that is, the protein built as the DNA is transcribed—is unique to that gene.

If the gene is damaged by the crossing-over of two chromosomes, a protein built from it will be based half on one gene and half on another, and most likely will be completely nonfunctional or even toxic.

If one base pair is deleted from DNA, the transcription of the three base pairs into one amino acid is shifted off by one, almost exactly like placing one's fingers on a piano or computer keyboard in the wrong starting position: every subsequent movement up and down the keyboard will produce wrong notes or wrong letters when the starting point is wrong. Thus, when one or more base pairs are missing, the resulting protein will be entirely different from that which the body is expecting to accomplish some metabolic task.

When these aberrant changes occur in, or very near, genes that regulate cell growth, trigger orderly cell death (apoptosis), or regulate maturation or cell division and reproduction, cancer may result.

Two known viral causes of NHL

Two viruses have been linked to some cases of NHL:

- Epstein-Barr virus (EBV)
- Human T-cell lymphoma/leukemia virus (HTLV-I)

It is known with certainty that 1 to 2 percent of those who are immunosuppressed shortly after solid organ transplantation, or owing to HIV/AIDS, develop NHL that is linked to the presence of Epstein-Barr virus, a human herpesvirus present in more than 90 percent of humans by adulthood. These virally induced NHLs can regress if immunosuppression is reduced, and clearly are linked to the suppression of functioning white blood T-cells. Unlike other cancers, which are monoclonal, indicating growth from only one precursor cell, these NHLs can be polyclonal, more closely resembling a process of white blood cell growth similar to that following infection.

Moreover, virtually all cases of Burkitt's lymphoma found among children in Africa test positive for the Epstein-Barr virus, although this is not always the case among Burkitt's lymphoma found elsewhere in the world.

For those with transplanted organs, reducing immunosuppression involves lowering doses of immunosuppressive medications. For those with AIDS, reducing immunosuppression currently involves raising the count of white blood T-cells by using AZT and protease inhibitors.

It is also known that those who are infected early in life with the human T-cell lymphoma/leukemia virus I (HTLV-I) have about a 3 percent chance of developing aggressive T-cell lymphomas or leukemias, as well as other health problems such as illnesses of the central nervous system. Although present worldwide in small pockets, HTLV-I is found in highest concentrations in parts of the Caribbean, parts of Japan, and in lower concentrations in the southeastern U.S. Very intimate exposure is required for transmission, such as sexual contact or the ingestion of breast milk from an infected woman.

Unproven, possible causes of NHL

As mentioned earlier, there are a number of possible causes of NHL that have yet to be proven scientifically. Some have stronger evidence than others, and some have produced conflicting results in studies, but all have at least some validity.

Nitrates in drinking water

One very strong candidate for at least those cases of NHL that arise in the American Midwest that are not explained by other risk factors is the ingestion of high levels of nitrates from drinking water. Nitrates are thought to find their way into drinking water from runoff following the use of nitrogen fertilizer by the farming industry. One study has shown a dose effect among those who were exposed to nitrates in drinking water; that is, as levels of nitrates in drinking water sources rose, more cases of NHL were found among those using that source. Demonstration of a dose effect between exposure to a substance and the development of cancer, while not a guarantee of causality, is nevertheless a compelling piece of evidence.

Pesticides, including Agent Orange

Pesticides, consisting of insecticides and herbicides, have been examined as a possible cause of NHL.

The higher incidence of NHL among Midwestern farmers may support the theory of increased risk associated with pesticide exposure, as may the lower incidence of NHL among those in the same or similar professions who wear protective clothing and masks. Particularly interesting is the demonstration of higher rates of NHL among those exposed to pesticides, even when rates of other cancers in these groups remain level or decrease. Some studies have shown a fifty to two-hundred-fold increase in risk among those exposed to the herbicide 2,4-D.

As home use of pesticides contributes five to ten times more contaminant to the environment than does farming, we are wise to continue to study this possibility, to protect ourselves if we must use pesticides, and to use only the safest products available. Some or most pesticides can be absorbed directly through the skin and often are inadvertently inhaled, thus making questionable the safety studies performed by the industry which rely on oral dosing to prove that some pesticides do not cause cancer in laboratory animals.

The herbicide dioxin, also known as Agent Orange, has received a great deal of scrutiny. Some studies have shown no clear connection between exposure to dioxin in Southeast Asia and the development of lymphomas, but other studies have. The U.S. Veterans Administration acknowledges a link between dioxin and certain cancers, however, and will pay disability benefits to those who have developed certain lymphomas (including NHL) if they can document exposure to dioxin based on the geography of their military assignments in Southeast Asia.

Hair dye use

Some studies have shown that those who use dark hair dye are more likely than the general population to develop NHL, but other studies have not supported this.

Foods

Some studies have shown that those who drink a great deal of milk are more likely than the general population to develop NHL, but not all studies examining the connection between NHL and milk consumption have supported this conclusion.

High consumption of meat has been linked in some studies to an increased risk of NHL, but other studies show no connection.

On the other hand, studies have shown that those eating a diet rich in carotenes, vitamin C, carrots, dark green vegetables, citrus fruits, whole-grain breads, and pasta have a lower incidence of NHL.

Drug, alcohol, and tobacco use

Amphetamines, quaaludes, lysergic acid diethylamide (LSD), and especially cocaine use have been linked to the development of NHL in men by one recent study, as was prescription amphetamine use in a second recent study that did not specify gender. Other studies suggest that the long-term illegal use of narcotic drugs may also increase NHL incidence. More research is needed to confirm these associations.

Phenytoin, or Dilantin, used for control of seizures, has been shown to increase the rate of a lymphoproliferative syndrome that resembles NHL.

Alcohol and tobacco use have been shown by several studies to have no effect on the rate of NHL.

Other infectious suspects

As mentioned earlier in the section, "Two known viral causes of NHL," Epstein-Barr virus and HTLV-I are implicated in some cases of NHL. Other infectious agents are suspected as well.

The higher incidence of NHL among slaughterhouse workers and farmer-breeders also hints at possibly a third, as yet unknown, viral association.

Those who have chronic liver disease caused by infection with the hepatitis C viruses early in life are more likely to develop primary splenic and liver (hepatic) NHL.

AIDS-associated NHL, usually an aggressive NHL with a diffuse appearance, has in some cases been linked to human herpesvirus 8 (HHV-8) based on traces of viral protein found within the tumor, but less research on this link has been done than on that between Epstein-Barr virus and NHL in the immune-suppressed. Nonetheless, HHV-8 is a reasonable suspect, as it's known to cause Kaposi's sarcoma, a skin tumor, among those with AIDS, and also has been linked to aggressive body-cavity or primary-effusion NHL.

In recent years, it has become clear that some cases of gastric lymphoma of the mucosa-associated lymphoid tissue (MALT) is linked to infections of *Helicobacter pylori*, a bacterium capable of surviving in the acidic stomach environment. When *H. pylori* is treated with antibiotics, in many cases the lymphoma recedes. Not all grades of gastric MALT lymphoma recede when *H. pylori* is treated with antibiotics, however. The effect of antibiotic treatment on other MALT lymphomas has not been closely studied to date, but a few studies have shown a possible link between *H. pylori* and MALT lymphoma in the lungs.

Genetic predisposition

Many people diagnosed with NHL become concerned that their siblings or children also may face a risk of developing NHL. Unfortunately, the familial aspect of NHL remains unclear. For example, a family history of leukemia or lymphoma increases the risk for NHL to two to three times the risk of the general population, but cases occurring within the same family account for less than 5 percent of all cases.

It is most important to bear in mind that, as the cause of NHL is still the subject of research, "familial" may imply an inherited genetic error, a shared exposure to an infectious cause, or a shared lifestyle. That is, the risk might come from inherited genes that predispose someone to develop NHL, just as there are genes that affect other aspects of our body's appearance and function; the risk might be that family members tend to be exposed to the same viruses or bacteria; or the risk might turn out to be that families that live together are drinking the same water or living next to the same toxic dump.

Attempts to understand any increased risk among family members may be made even more difficult if the way that many research studies use the word "genetic" is not understood. We who are not involved in research tend to use the word "genetic" interchangeably with "heritable" or "inherited," but the study of genetics encompasses a broader meaning, and researchers usually are not referring to the heritable sense when they use the word "genetics."

Many genetic changes occur within cancerous cells, but only genetic changes or errors that arise and persist in sperm or ova can be inherited.

Predisposition to a certain illness can arise when there are natural variations in genes. Such multiple versions of genes are called alleles, and many such exist. For example, it is highly likely that you have two alleles for every gene in your body, having inherited one allele for each from your father and one from your mother.

Genes are translated into proteins to accomplish their metabolic goals; proteins always fold into a specific shape dictated by their chemical makeup. Even a small difference in only one location of a gene can cause a protein string to fold differently, and this final shape dictates how or if the protein will function. Proteins that are created from the differing alleles, then, may have different structures and shapes, and may behave differently in metabolic reactions. Thus, researchers have begun to note that those who have specific versions of the HLA-DR gene on chromosome 6, for example—a gene controlling some of the behavior of white blood cells—appear in some cases to be more likely to develop certain diseases.

In fact, throughout this discussion of potentially causative factors, you can see that most of these factors could be explained using predisposition, heritability, or infection as the scientific model.

Immune disorders

Familial immunodeficiency appears to predispose certain families to more than the expected incidence of NHL. The following list of inherited immune deficiencies has been adapted from Chapters 19, 21, 45, and 47 of Magrath's 1997 text, *The Non-Hodgkin's Lymphomas*:

- X-linked severe combined immunodeficiency (SCID)
- Omenn's syndrome
- Purine nucleoside phosphorylase deficiency
- X-linked agammaglobulinemia
- Ig-A deficiency
- Common variable immune deficiency
- X-linked hyper-IgM syndrome
- IgG subclass deficiency

- Wiskott-Aldrich syndrome
- Ataxia telangiectasia
- DiGeorge anomalad
- Hyper-IgE syndrome
- X-linked lymphoproliferative syndrome
- Chediak-Higashi syndrome
- Bloom's syndrome
- Enteropathy-associated T-cell lymphoma among northern Europeans
- Hashimoto's thyroiditis (for MALT lymphomas)

Blood transfusions

There is a low but present risk of developing NHL following blood transfusions, especially among the elderly. This might indicate an infectious process or a derangement of the regulatory efforts of the immune system when coping with alien blood products.

Occupational risk

An increased incidence of NHL has been noted among those in the following professions: farming, livestock breeding, rubber workers, chemists, chemical workers, dry cleaners, metal workers, funeral directors and embalmers, petroleum refinery workers, printing workers, those exposed to ethylene oxide, beauticians/cosmetologists, woodworkers (including those in sawmills and pulp mills), and those exposed to certain chemicals such as ammonia or to organic solvents such as benzene.

Risk associated with other illness

A small increased risk is seen among those with asthma, allergies, arthritis, rheumatic fever, nontropical celiac sprue, tuberculosis, and infectious mononucleosis (Epstein-Barr virus is considered to be the cause of infectious mononucleosis.) Asthma, allergies, nontropical celiac disease, and some forms of arthritis are illnesses caused by the inappropriate or misdirected activity of white blood cells. As NHL is also a disorder of white blood cell production and maturation, and can in some cases be triggered by over-activity of white blood cells, some researchers speculate that there may be a connection between these disorders and NHL.

Continuous antigenic stimulation

Many of the possible causes of NHL that we have discussed in the preceding paragraphs may act by soliciting an ongoing reaction from our immune system. Some researchers believe that chemicals, infections, or allergic or autoimmune reactions are all capable of producing an ongoing immune system reaction that triggers NHL and other related illnesses. This is sometimes called continuous antigenic stimulation.

The substance or infectious agent itself may not be causing the cancer, but the immune system reacting to the substance might. For example, some B-cell lymphomas such as gastric MALT lymphomas appear unable to grow unless white blood cells specific for killing *Helicobacter pylori* bacteria are also present. This growth of cancer only following action by part of the immune system also is seen in the failure of growth of grafted B-cell tumors in severe combined immunodeficiency (SCID) mice, which are bred without immune systems for research purposes. But when missing T-cells are injected, the tumors begin to grow.

Currently, the best place for this theory remains within the laboratory. It is of little practical import whether a substance, or the immune system's reaction to it, is to blame for cancer if simply avoiding a substance can reduce your risk.

The possibility for dangerous continuous antigenic stimulation is also the basis for the FDA ruling requiring warning labels on some nutritional supplements, such as melatonin, sold as immune boosters.

The aging immune system

In opposition to continuous antigenic stimulation discussed above, some researchers feel that the greatly increased rate not only of NHL, but of most other cancers among those over age 65, hints at a general weakening of the immune system with age. Others feel that this more likely may be a product of the modern world we live in: that genetic damage from substances in an industrialized environment accumulates over time and first becomes apparent among the oldest.

Grading and staging NHL

It is most important that your disease be correctly identified, graded, and staged so that the best treatment can be planned. All biopsies of tumor tissue should be reviewed by an experienced hematopathologist to be certain that subtype and grade are correctly identified.

Brief definitions of stage and grade are:

- Staging describes how far disease has spread from its original site. Staging for many, but not all, cancers consists of stages I through IV.

- Grading describes how aggressive the tumor is. Grades for the NHLs are low-, intermediate-, or high-grade, although many researchers combine intermediate- and high-grade diseases in discussion of treatment.

Please see Chapter 4 for important deviations in what these characteristics mean to success of treatment. It is not always true, for instance, that a stage IV, high-grade patient has fewer hopes for cure than a stage IV, low-grade patient.

For years, the Rappaport and Ann Arbor systems used for Hodgkin's lymphoma, and the Working Group and Kiel systems, were adapted to describe NHL in a way that attempted to reflect tumor characteristics, and thus to some degree prognosis, but none was entirely satisfactory. Most recently, the Revised European American Lymphoma (REAL) classification system was proposed by an international cooperative group of researchers to more correctly identify lymphomas based on immunologic characteristics.

The lack of fully acceptable staging and grading systems for NHL has resulted in many universities and cancer treatment centers devising their own systems. Each system attempts to correlate cellular or disease characteristics to treatment outcome. An excellent discussion of these staging controversies can be found in Magrath's *The Non-Hodgkin's Lymphomas*.

One consequence of this variety of descriptive systems is that you may become confused when talking to other survivors who state that they have the same subtype, grade, and stage as you do, but who are receiving different treatment with perhaps different results.

Some cases of NHL have characteristics of two or more known entities. In these cases, identity or staging decisions can be difficult to make. The following sections describe efforts to grade and stage NHLs for choosing the best treatment.

Grade

A tumor can be graded as indolent, intermediate, or highly aggressive by several measures. All NHL tumors are graded on their appearance under the microscope, known as histologic grade; some are graded on behaviors that leave traces of tumor activity in the bloodstream or other body tissues.

Histologic grade

The grade of a tumor often can be correlated to the cell's appearance under the microscope. The description of this appearance is known as histology. While some characteristics of cell appearance for some subtypes of NHL do indeed correlate to the stage of disease, such as increasing tumor cell size in low-grade disease converting to a higher grade, for other subtypes this is not so. Nevertheless, at one time, histological staging of NHL was the best that could be done.

Other factors affecting grade

Recent progress in research has shown that there are additional characteristics, not related to cell appearance, that bear on grade. For example, proteins called immunoglobulins created by damaged genes within cancerous white cells and circulating in the bloodstream may be meaningful to the aggressiveness of disease by virtue of their unusual quantity or shape.

Stage

Staging is a measure of how much of the body is affected by NHL.

Often, the Ann Arbor staging system is used for staging NHL patients, but it was developed to describe Hodgkin's lymphoma, not non-Hodgkin's lymphoma. As a result, it is not an entirely satisfactory measure of the effect of NHL on the patient's body. Many oncologists and institutions incorporate other clinical measures—age, ability to do normal everyday things, tumor size, lactate dehydrogenase (LDH) blood levels—to discuss more accurately the effect of disease. Ask your oncologist what standard was used to assess the spread and effects of your disease.

The divisions of the Ann Arbor staging system are:

Stage I

Stage I designates disease in a single lymph node or lymph node region, or localized involvement of just one extranodal site, such as the spleen, which is designated as stage IE.

Stage II

Stage II designates disease in two or more lymph node regions on the same side of the diaphragm.

Stage IIE is local disease in a single extranodal site, such as the lung, including its regional lymph nodes, with or without affecting other lymph node regions on the same side of the diaphragm. The number of nearby lymph node regions affected may be indicated by an appended number, such as II3.

Stage III

Stage III means that lymph node regions on both sides of the diaphragm are affected. Disease also may be accompanied by local involvement of an extranodal organ or site, such as the liver, or by involvement of the spleen (IIIS), or both (IIIS+E).

Stage IV

Stage IV means widely spread, multiple involvement at one or more extra-lymphatic sites such as the bone marrow, with or without associated lymph node involvement, or involvement of an isolated extranodal organ with distant nodal involvement.

Extranodal sites

Extranodal sites are identified by the following notation:

    N = lymph nodes
    H = liver (hepatic)
    L = lung
    M = bone marrow
    S = spleen

P = pleura (lung)

O = bone

D = skin (dermis)

Restaging

Staging may be clinical staging (CS), based only on a physical examination, or pathologic staging (PS), based on the later findings of node biopsy and other diagnostic procedures such as bone marrow aspiration or abdominal surgery.

This means that you might initially be staged at level II, based on your oncologist's first physical exam detecting just a few swollen lymph nodes in your neck, armpit, or groin, but after bone marrow biopsy and a bronchoscopy, you might be restaged at level IIE, III, or IV.

Recurrent disease

Often you'll find in the medical literature that patients who have relapsed are no longer discussed by stage, but are instead described as having recurrent disease. In some cases, recurrent disease may be the equivalent of stage I, such as is seen in the relapse of certain patients with limited low-grade disease. For intermediate- and high-grade disease, though, recurrent disease often is considered to be the equivalent of stage III or IV.

Immunophenotype

One of the most important strides that has been made in understanding not only NHL, but the behavior of all cells, was the discovery that all cells have on their surface bits of protein that extend outward and interact with other cells and proteins, somewhat like businesspeople trading business cards. These tags, or cell surface antigens, have been analyzed, and it has been found that tumors have antigens that differ from those on healthy cells. It has been found that different types of cancer and—most important for our purposes—different subtypes of NHL have differences in types and quantities of cell surface antigens.

Immunophenotyping is the categorization of cells based on these cell surface antigens. Moreover, it is known that these antigens, which dictate cellular immunity, change in tandem with corresponding changes in the cell's DNA.

But what is phenotype? By definition, one's phenotype is the outward, visible, or demonstrable expression of one's genes or genotype. For example, blue eyes are the phenotypic expression of the genotype for blue eyes. Thus, any outward or visible cellular characteristic related to immune function that changes with genetic change is an immunophenotypic characteristic.

An example of immunophenotyping that you are probably familiar with is the red blood cell antigen system, ABO. Most of us learn eventually whether we have blood type A, B, AB, or O, where type O indicates the absence of any such marker. This information is critical to those needing whole blood transfusions, because receiving the wrong blood type can cause a fatal immunologic war within, as incoming alien blood cells are targeted for destruction by our own white blood cells and vice versa. (The ABO system, while meaningful to NHL survivors who must have transfusions, is used in this paragraph only as an example of phenotype; that is, the ABO system has no bearing on the type or outcome of NHL treatment.)

Cell surface antigens have become very important in the categorization and treatment of NHL. Cancerous cells produce different cell surface antigens, or a great deal more of them, than do healthy cells. Tumors may express in turn different cell surface antigens at different levels of disease progression. They may express more than one abnormal cell surface antigen or may express the abnormal antigens along with normal antigens.

The REAL lymphoma classification system relies heavily on these immunophenotypic markers exhibited by lymphoma and leukemia cells (as well as on unusual proteins secreted by cancerous white blood cells), rather than on cell appearance, to separate the various subtypes of NHL. Because categorization by immune marker is a completely new way to identify lymphomas, the REAL system includes not only NHL, but also other hematologic cancers that share these markers, such as the Hodgkin's lymphomas, plasma cell myeloma, and chronic lymphocytic leukemia (CLL). As you can see, the REAL classifications system has breached significant traditional boundaries in the thinking about differences among lymphomas and leukemias.

In its initial form, REAL has not met with complete acceptance by all researchers and clinicians, some of whom would prefer a classification system more meaningful to the everyday treatment of NHL. Proposed modifications to REAL are being evaluated. See Appendix D for the details of this and other staging systems.

New treatments have been designed that exploit the fact that tumors have different markers on their cell surface that our bodies seem to ignore, instead of sensing and attacking. Monoclonal antibodies (abbreviated as mabs or moabs) are perhaps the most widely known new treatment exploiting this characteristic. Monoclonal antibodies are molecules secreted by white blood cells that attach to foreign bodies such as viruses. Attachment is a signal to other classes of white blood cells to attack and kill the intruder. Because cancerous cells express more or different cell surface antigens than do normal cells, monoclonal antibodies can be designed and manufactured to recognize and attach to these tumor cells, thus tagging them for destruction. Monoclonal antibodies have been used for years in laboratory medicine to identify different cell types, but the first monoclonal antibody for cancer therapy was not approved by the FDA until 1997, when Rituxan for NHLs expressing the CD20 antigen was approved.

Another example of immunophenotyping is the broad categorization of white blood cells into B cells and T cells. B cells are white blood cells that originate in bone marrow; T cells, broadly speaking, are those that originate in marrow and travel to the thymus where they are trained (differentiation) to recognize specific enemies. B- and T-cell development, though, is far more complex than one would believe based on this brief description. Both B-cells and T-cells spend time within lymph nodes, either resting, maturing, or differentiating, and each fulfills different but complementary roles in immune surveillance. NHLs are divided somewhat successfully into T-cell or B-cell lymphomas; however, there are cases of NHL that are T-cell–rich B-cell lymphomas.

In the future, immunotyping may supplement or eclipse Ann Arbor staging and histologic grading as the means by which tumors are identified and assessed for their effect on the patient and the outcome of disease.

Summary

The preceding pages have attempted to categorize information about NHL so that you may begin to build a frame of reference for understanding this disease.

The most important points we should bear in mind are that the classification of this disease is the subject of ongoing discussion, as are the causes, that the rate of NHL incidence in the U.S. is increasing, and that all biopsies of tumor tissue should be reviewed by an experienced hematopathologist to be certain that subtype and grade are correctly identified.

If you attempt to compare yourself to others who appear to have the same diagnosis, bear in mind that their diagnosis may have been made using criteria that are different, perhaps in subtle ways, from those used by your own diagnosticians. This means that treatment decisions from one person to the next may differ as well.

As you can see from the discussion of possible causes of NHL, concerns you have about what may have caused your illness are probably premature, because in most instances the cause of NHL is unknown.

With a framework for understanding symptoms, diagnosis, and various characteristics of NHL, we are now ready to discuss treatments.

CHAPTER 4

Prognoses

*Because of the multiplicity of histologic
subtypes and of the possible manifestations of
a lymphoma, it is impossible to predict
the outcome of therapy accurately
in individual patients.*

—Coiffier, Salles, and Bastion
The Non-Hodgkin's Lymphomas

Almost everyone wants to know how serious his or her cancer is and what the prospects are for survival. This questioning is completely normal.

In this chapter, we do not provide you with simple answers, because there aren't any. We first review factors that limit the ability of this book—or any printed resource—to predict outcomes for NHL. The last half of the chapter describes what risk factors have been studied, and what factors matter the least and the most. It is important to grasp that several poorly understood circumstances limit one's ability to say that events will happen in a certain way for a person diagnosed with NHL.

When you've finished the chapter, you won't have an absolute, unchanging answer about your prognosis. However, you'll have an idea of factors that might influence your prognosis, a respect for the complexity of the topic, and an awareness of the dangers of predictions.

Limitations on accurate prognoses

The limitations on our ability to predict the course of NHL include the general limitations of all medical studies and statistics; that is, there are still many unknowns, and not all unknowns can be predicted from what we do know. There are also limitations specific to NHL, such as rapidly improving treatments, differences between blood and other cancers, and differences in NHL classifications. The following are factors to keep in mind when reading any discussion of prognosis for NHL, no matter how recent.

Improving treatments

First, owing to robust research, treatments for NHL are evolving so rapidly that information regarding prognoses stated unequivocally today may be obsolete tomorrow. The recent FDA approval of certain monoclonal antibodies—white blood cell proteins designed to attack only tumors—is one example. The increasing use of bone marrow transplantation is another; the tremendous gains made in supportive care, such as new antifungals and antinausea drugs, are others. As always, your doctor, a well-trained and skilled person who most likely you chose carefully as outlined in Chapter 2, *Finding the Right Oncologist*, is your best resource for the most current information. You may choose to follow the progress of new treatments on your own. Ways to do this are discussed in Chapter 24, *Researching Your Lymphoma*.

Do not treat what is written about prognoses in this book as definitive information about your condition.

Difficult classifications

The difficulty of categorizing NHL makes discussing research results equally difficult. Chapter 3, *What Are the Non-Hodgkin's Lymphomas?*, and Appendix D, *Classification Systems*, discuss and delineate the systems used to categorize NHL and the problems encountered when trying to do so. Many major cancer centers have developed their own categories in order to tackle NHL in a consistent manner to effect a cure. This means that multiple studies from different institutions that yield conflicting results from the same treatment regimen may not compare readily to each other, and, most importantly, may not apply to you regarding fundamentals such as tumor cell type. Some NHL survivors, for example, in casual conversation might refer to having had lymphoma in the abdomen. There are several types of NHL that can occur in the abdomen, and they are sufficiently different to make comparisons about their response to treatment fruitless.

Do not become confused and worried because others with cancers that sound similar to yours appear to be doing better or worse than you.

Limitations of statistics

Survival statistics are developed using groups of people, many of whom are not very much like you, even if they appear to have the same disease, categorized using the same system or by a single research center. Your chances may be considerably better, for instance, than those of someone who has several chronic illnesses such as heart disease or lupus along with NHL. In addition, many of those whose cases find their way into medical journals, and who become the basis for statistics regarding the success of one technique versus another, are those who have had many different treatments and who may have one or more organ systems compromised owing to repeated toxic treatments.

Those of you who studied statistics in school are aware that many different statistical methods exist to manipulate data, any two of which may in some cases give differing results. Statistical analysis is really just a method for making sense of large amounts of otherwise incomprehensible data. Consequently, sometimes the statistical model chosen represents science's closest guess regarding how to analyze the outcome of treatment; some statistical models chosen may not be a good fit for some collections of data. In spite of the best faith on the part of researchers and statisticians, these inconsistencies may creep into research papers. For more information on this topic, we recommend reading Steven Jay Gould's essay, "The Median Isn't the Message." Steven Jay Gould is a popular evolutionary biologist, and a survivor of a rare form of cancer called abdominal mesothelioma. His essay appeared in the June 1985 issue of *Discover* magazine, and can also be found on the Cancerguide web site at *http://www.cancerguide.org/median_not_msg.html*.

You and your disease may not fit any statistical category.

Correlation is not causation

Everyone who has ever entered my office has had a nose. Thus, you could say that there is a correlation between being able to walk into my office and having a nose, but one cannot say that having a nose causes one to walk into my office or that walking into my office causes a nose to grow. For example, some say that increasing age correlates to a poorer outcome among those with NHL, but other researchers believe that the actual determining factor appears to be the other illnesses of aging that a patient may have which affect outcome, not age per se. Beware of correlations. They are not necessarily causative.

Complexity of the immune response

Humans and their capacity to withstand stressors are, thank goodness, always confounding medical theory. Everyone knows of someone who was told he had only three months to live, but was alive twenty years later. People can argue that these cases represent misdiagnoses, but this explanation is not likely to cover all such instances, and gives no credit for variables such as the many immune-system factors that are still unknown.

We have a great deal to learn about the immune system and are learning great amounts quickly owing to well-financed cancer research and the sharing of knowledge across scientific disciplines.

Blood cancers are unlike other cancers

Lymphomas and leukemias are hematopoietic cancers—that is, cancers of white blood cells, the disseminated body products responsible for protecting you from injury and disease, including cancer. Thus, some of the facts that apply to other cancers do not apply to lymphomas and leukemias. For example, various alternative treatments which purport to enhance the immune response against cancer may in theory make lymphomas or leukemias worse by stimulating growth of diseased white blood cells. Some alternative products such as melatonin carry printed warnings about this.

In addition, the spread (metastasis) of non-Hodgkin's lymphomas to multiple sites within the body does not necessarily mean that a successful outcome will be less assured. The idea of having cancer spread frightens many people because they have heard of people with cancer who could not be helped because their cancer had "spread to lymph nodes," "spread to the bone," or "spread to the brain." Although the involvement of certain organs may imply a worse outcome if they are found to contain NHL, and although a very large tumor burden spread to many sites is not a good sign, it is not universally true that any spreading of NHL to other organs is necessarily predictive of a poor outcome. Spread to the spleen, for instance, generally can be managed quite well by removal of the spleen, called splenectomy. Spread to bone marrow can be handled by high-dose chemotherapy and bone marrow rescue, or by the newer monoclonal antibodies. Spread to the central nervous system, including the brain, can be managed with radiation therapy or chemotherapy injected within the spine.

For reasons that are not fully understood, spread of cancers of the immune system are more manageable than the dissemination of cancers from a single organ, such as lung cancer. Thus, general statements that are true for other cancers may not apply to NHL.

Physical characteristics of patients in studies

As mentioned earlier, many NHL patients who enter clinical trials are "heavily pretreated," to use the phrase found in research papers. The practice of admitting to trials only those who have failed several standard treatments is considered the most ethical approach when the outcome of a new treatment cannot be guaranteed. To deny a patient standard treatment that might work better than the new treatment being tested is, in almost anyone's ethical scheme, immoral. Thus, often, but not always, only those who are perceived to have no other chance for a good outcome are entered into clinical trials. This means that the percentages of survival found in studies of new substances using heavily pretreated patients may be lower than the survival rates that will be found as the treatment moves into general use as first-line therapy, that is, therapy used on those who have never before been treated for NHL.

The same treatments used on any one person may produce better results; the same treatment used on the general population of NHL patients may produce better results than were seen in clinical trials with heavily pretreated patients.

Long natural history

Some subtypes of NHL have very long and evolving courses. It is not unusual for patients to pass years in watch-and-wait mode before treatment is needed, then for treatment to yield a remission of three years, and upon relapse to be followed by another treatment which yields another remission of three more years, and so on. Statistically, half of the people with these indolent subtypes survive for twelve years or longer, during which time new treatments are unfolding. Golda Meir survived for almost 20 years, including her years as Prime Minister of Israel, with a type of leukemia that's closely related to low-grade NHL.

At the time this book is being written, there are about 190 clinical trials underway for NHL funded by the National Cancer Institute, and this number does not include trials funded solely by pharmaceutical companies. For a better understanding of what this may mean for those who are diagnosed today, consider that only twelve years ago we did not have:

- Granulocyte colony stimulating factor, G-CSF, approved in 1991 for growing new white blood cells to prevent you from catching infections if chemotherapy wiped out your white blood cells.

- Erythropoietin, or Epoietin, for growing new red blood cells when bone marrow has been suppressed by chemotherapy or radiation therapy.

- Interferon alfa, a manmade copy of a blood product that can suppress NHL.

- IL-2, another manmade copy of a blood product that is active against melanoma, leukemias, kidney cancer—all cancers once considered hopeless unless caught very early.

- Monoclonal antibodies, white blood cell proteins that are grown outside the body where they are taught to travel to and attack tumors. They are almost unique in their ability to avoid damaging healthy tissue, and thus are less likely to cause serious side effects.

- Safer bone marrow or stem-cell transplants. Twelve years ago, bone marrow transplants (BMTs) were far more dangerous, done only with donor marrow because the medical community did not know for certain how to clean (purge) the cancer patient's marrow of cancer cells and reuse it. Moreover, BMTs were done only on relatively young people. Since 1993, the age of patients considered acceptable for bone marrow or stem cell rescue using their own marrow has risen from forty to sixty and, in some cases, the seventies if the patient is otherwise healthy.

- Magnetic resonance imaging (MRI) for finding very small tumors and NHL that have spread to the brain and spine, something not readily available until about eleven years ago.

Thus, bear in mind that the future holds great promise.

The aging of printed material

This phenomenon is akin to the robust research mentioned at the start of this chapter. Owing to the amount of time it takes to enroll patients into trials, perform research, analyze results, write the research paper, peer-review the research paper, print the results in a medical journal, and summarize many such papers in a textbook, there can be a lag of at least one year, and usually much more, between the completion of research and the results being disseminated among doctors and the concerned public. During this interval, research has continued and better information may have become available. For this reason, we encourage you to become familiar with medical journals that report progress in the treatment of lymphomas. Three such journals are *Leukemia and Lymphoma, Blood*, and *Transplantation*. Methods for finding and understanding the basics of research papers are discussed in Chapter 24.

Remember that what you read about survival and treatment success here, and in all but the newest texts, will never be as current as the information you can receive from a well-trained oncologist active in his specialty who has access to medical journals and to other researchers.

Which factors matter least and most

With all of the previous information of this chapter in mind, please read the following sections for a summary of the features of NHL—and of the patients who have NHL—that seem to matter (or not) regarding outcome of treatment. This summary was prepared using Chapter 35 of the 1997 edition of Magrath's *The Non-Hodgkin's Lymphomas,* and the U.S. National Cancer Institute's PDQ *State-of-the-Art Physicians' Treatment Statements* for the non-Hodgkin's lymphomas. The chapter within the Magrath text references 233 research papers, of which most span the mid-1980s through 1994, with two papers dated 1995, and two dated 1996. Additional Medline and journal references were used to revisit the issue for possible prognostic factors examined and published after 1996.

Even with the following list of risk factors, nobody will be able to speak in absolute terms about your overall prognosis. You undoubtedly will have at least one risk factor for a poorer prognosis, and you will undoubtedly have several factors that point to a better prognosis.

The most important point to remember is that what are used today as reliable prognostic indicators may become meaningless when new treatments that surmount old difficulties are engaged. You might find it encouraging to read Chapter 23, *The Future of Therapy*, after you have read this chapter.

The order of the sections that follow does not imply a greater or lesser effect on outcome.

High-dose therapy with bone marrow transplantation

This subject, a mode of treatment, is being discussed first, because its use may significantly change the body of statistics for many subtypes of NHL in favor of longer survival.

High-dose therapy with bone marrow transplantation is common terminology used to described several related procedures, namely marrow or stem cell transplantation, or marrow or stem cell rescue.

For all of the non-Hodgkin's lymphomas, bone marrow transplantation appears to offer longer survival or cure if treatment-related side effects can be controlled, but a longer period of follow-up is necessary to be certain that the longer remissions are statistically significant for low-grade disease. Some studies indicate a better chance of relapse-free survival with donor marrow—allogeneic transplantation—than with one's own marrow. Another study has found that achieving remission during induction therapy for transplantation is a "powerful prognostic indicator" for long-term survival.[1]

There are serious advantages and disadvantages to each type of transplant with respect to side effects and outcome, for which see Chapter 20, *Transplantation*.

Tumor grade

In general, treatments other than bone marrow transplantation or rescue for low-grade non-Hodgkin's lymphoma are not considered cures at the time this book is being written. Very long remissions, however, provide an opportunity for survival until a cure is found. In other words, the word "incurable" does not necessarily translate as fatal. The newly approved monoclonal antibody treatments may provide a repeating treatment regimen with very low toxicity for the low-grade NHLs.

Intermediate- and high-grade non-Hodgkin's lymphomas are considered curable in many instances, depending on various factors.

Note that a low-grade NHL can convert to a higher grade, and that high-grade disease can retain some characteristics of low-grade disease, even as it is progressing.

Histology

Histology is the medical term for how your body's cells look under a microscope. This includes cell parts (organelles) such as mitochondria, which burn oxygen to power the cell—but histology cannot examine DNA and its composite genes in fine detail.

As we mentioned earlier in the chapter, the histologic naming classifications of NHL are very complex. There has been controversy about which naming classifications might correlate with overall prognosis. Confusion can be caused by the presence of two conflicting histologic features within the same tumor, for example.

The following histologic naming conventions have *not* been found to have a consistent bearing on long-term survival. We're explicitly listing them here because these naming conventions may be cited in an older study or book as a possible risk factor in prognosis.

- **Follicular.** Not all patients with follicular disease have indolent, slow-growing disease that requires no initial treatment. Up to 50 percent have abnormalities that must be addressed immediately.

- **Follicular large-cell.** Some follicular presentations have only small cells, some only large cells, some both. Large cells within follicular nodes sometimes are correlated with a more aggressive disease, but this is not consistent across all studies.

- **Diffuse large-cell.** The diagnosis and categorization of this group are so complex and so subject to overlaps with other types that predictions about the success of treatment based on differing naming conventions *alone* are not useful.

- **Small lymphocytic/lymphoplasmacytoid (immunocytomas).** The diagnosis and categorization of this group are so complex, and so subject to overlaps with each other, that predictions about the success of treatment based on differing names alone are not useful.

- **Noncutaneous T-cell.** Differences in survival between small- and large-cell subtypes make generalizations about noncutaneous T-cell lymphoma difficult. Those that express the CD30 cell surface antigen seem to have a better prognosis.

- **Cutaneous T-cell.** Other factors, such as spread of disease, are more meaningful than the naming category of this subtype.

- **Adult Burkitt's.** Other factors, such as LDH levels, are more meaningful in predicting outcome. LDH is discussed later in the chapter.

These histologic categories, however, appear to have a consistent correlation with outcome:

- **Anaplastic large-cell.** Seems to have longer survival than other noncutaneous T-cell lymphomas.

- **Mucosa-associated lymphoid tissue (MALT).** Most patients have limited disease outside of any lymph node and have a good prognosis. Those with gastric MALT having a diffuse large-cell component of 1 to 10 percent appear to have a worse 10-year prognosis than those without a diffuse large-cell component.

- **Mantle cell.** Patients with mantle cell disease may have very widely spread disease and consequently may face a poorer outcome.

- **Mantle zone.** True mantle zone disease appears to have a better prognosis than mantle cell.

- **Childhood Burkitt's.** Most children with Burkitt's will have long survival, unless bone marrow or the central nervous system is involved, which would confer a slightly worse prognosis.

Immunophenotype

Immunophenotyping is a way of identifying how certain genes within a tumor manifest in the tumor's appearance or immune-response behavior. The tumor cell's genotype is its collection of genes; its phenotype is the collection of physical characteristics that result from having one set of genes versus another. Thus far, immunophenotyping has concentrated mainly on identifying cell surface antigens, that is, proteins that protrude from the cell's surface and act as identifying signals and attractants to other cells and to other molecules.

The science of immunophenotyping, or immunotyping, is a rapidly advancing subfield of cancer research. Some researchers say that advances in this method of analyzing tumor cells will provide us with the most meaningful information possible for designing patient-specific anticancer products.

- **B-cell versus T-cell.** White blood cells can be divided into B cells, arising from the bone marrow, and T cells, which also arise from marrow but mature in the thymus gland or descend from early T cells of the thymus. Some studies show that T-cell non-Hodgkin's lymphomas are harder to treat successfully than B-cell NHLs; other studies do not support this. Keep in mind that some tumors have both B-cell and T-cell characteristics (composite lymphoma), and some tumors have neither.

- **Cell surface antigens.** This very new method of categorizing cancer cells may prove useful for targeting tumor cells only. All white blood cells have proteins protruding from them, called cell surface antigens, which cancer cells produce in greater abundance or in different quality from normal cells. This allows cancerous white blood cells to be targeted instead of healthy cells. Examples of cell surface antigens are CD20, CD5, CD19, CD30 (Ki-1), and so on.

- **p80 antigen.** In anaplastic large-cell lymphoma (ALCL), expression of the p80 antigen has been associated with a good outcome in one study.[2] Additional studies are necessary to confirm this.

Genetic characteristics

A normal white blood cell has forty-four paired chromosomes, plus two X chromosomes (female) or one X and one Y chromosome (male). Tumors are often, but not always, tested for genetic abnormalities, since some abnormalities have been shown to impact prognosis and may make a difference in the treatment recommended.

Some genetic abnormalities may be present in all tumor samples from the same patient, some are present in one sample but not in others, and some are present at diagnosis, but others accumulate as time progresses.

The significance of many individual genetic aberrations is not yet clear, although there is some consensus that a high number of genetic abnormalities may confer a poorer outcome. For instance, a tumor showing deletion of both chromosomes 5 and 7, extra copies of chromosomes 8 and 12, and transpositions of two or more other chromosomes would be considered to have a high number of abnormalities.

There have been some studies that indicate a statistical correlation between certain kinds of genetic damage and outcome:

- Damaged or missing material for chromosomes 7 and 17 have been correlated with a worse prognosis.

- Damage to the cell-death gene (tumor suppressor gene), p53, which resides on chromosome 17, appears to affect negatively the outcome of many cancers, including the NHLs, but at least one study has found that it does not affect prognosis in the NHLs.[3]

- Excessive material (three copies) of chromosomes 7 and 14 have been correlated with a worse prognosis.

In other studies, some aberrations are found in or appear to affect the outcome of only specific subtypes of NHL:

- In intermediate- and low-grade lymphomas, aberrations in chromosome 1 have been correlated with a poor outcome.

- For low-grade lymphomas, three copies of chromosome 12 (trisomy 12) have been associated with a worse outcome, and a small study has shown that trisomy 5, 6, or 8, chromosome 5 abnormalities, and damage to parts of chromosome 14 confer a worse prognosis.

- For large-cell lymphoma, a study of 205 tumors showed a correlation between damage to chromosome 1 and a shortened survival.

- For follicular disease transforming to diffuse disease, loss of chromosome 6, aberrations of chromosomes 17 and 8 and others, and swapping of chromosomal parts between chromosomes 14 and 18 have been found, implying that these chromosomal aberrations may be related to the less favorable prognosis of some diffuse tumors.

- For nonlymphoblastic T-cell lymphomas, one study has found that the presence of Epstein-Barr virus (EBV) in the tumor's DNA is a predictor of poor outcome.[4]

Patient characteristics

Many cancer survivors wonder if their ethnic background or gender, for example, have a bearing on successfully fighting the disease. These are the factors that appear to matter most for NHL:

- Age. There is disagreement in the medical community regarding the influence of age on outcome of treatment. Several studies indicate that general health status or tumor bulk is more important than age in predicting the success of treatment. Other studies show that increasing age greater than 65 is indeed a poor prognostic factor, independent of other characteristics. Patients of any age in good health who can withstand full doses of chemotherapy with few delays fare better than those who must accept repeated reduced doses on a schedule significantly delayed by recovery from adverse side effects.

- **HIV infection.** Individuals whose HIV positive status has progressed to full AIDS and who are not able to maintain CD4+ white blood cell counts greater than 100/microlitre using protease inhibitors or other antiviral therapy have a poorer prognosis. Those who are able to maintain higher CD4+ counts have a prognosis similar to those without HIV, if good supportive care is available to withstand infection.

Tumor mass

It is generally true for most cancers that early detection is desirable. Here are the specifics for NHL:

- The tumor burden the body is carrying is directly related to outcome, with higher tumor burden within many organs related to poorer outcome than disease spread only to one organ.

- The number of nodal sites, however, is no longer considered relevant to outcome.

- In large-cell and follicular lymphomas, an increasing number of extranodal sites (spleen, liver, marrow, brain) is correlated to poorer outcome, but extranodal disease is in itself not riskier than nodal disease.

- Bone marrow involvement confers a worse prognosis only for Burkitt's and lymphoblastic lymphoma. The outcome for follicular cell lymphoma, immunocytoma, and mantle cell lymphoma with bone marrow involvement, however, appears no worse than these same subtypes without bone marrow involvement.

- One study has found that abnormal results from the magnetic resonance imaging (MRI) of the femoral (thigh bone) marrow "is associated with a significantly poorer survival in patients with malignant lymphoma, regardless of histologic findings in the marrow."[5]

- Pleural effusion, a collection of fluid in the lungs, is associated with a poorer outcome.

Blood-borne products of metabolism

Increasingly fine biochemical tools provide a means to assess tumor progression or the success of treatment by detecting substances secreted by tumors in the bloodstream:

- **LDH, lactic dehydrogenase.** This is an enzyme associated with the breaking down of cells for any reason, is directly correlated to tumor burden and thus to outcome, with higher LDH levels indicating more disease. This is true for almost all NHL subtypes excepting some large cell lymphomas (LCLs). It's not a foolproof indicator, though, because other things that cause cells to burst, such as recent strenuous exercise or the administration of G-CSF or GM-CSF, can temporarily raise LDH.

- **Beta-2 microglobulin.** This is a newer measure of tumor burden, and higher levels have been shown to be directly related to poorer outcome for large-cell and follicular lymphomas. This measure has not been tested in large studies, however.

- **Other blood-borne products.** This includes compounds such as tumor necrosis factor (TNF) and various cytokines such as the interleukins 6 and 10 (IL-6, IL-10) that are thought to be a measure of the body's response to the tumor as opposed to clearly meaningful prognostic tools, although some of these products appear to mirror tumor burden. Several of these blood values—sICAM-1, erythrocyte sedimentation rate (ESR), serum thymidine kinase (sTK), albumin, and orosomucoid—rise and fall along with LDH, so their value as independent predictors is questioned. At this time, these substances are not commonly used as diagnostic or follow-up tools.

Other tumor-related substances

Many new biochemical tools, such as polymerase chain reaction (PCR), fluorescence in situ hybridization (FISH), and immunoperoxidase staining, can detect tumor products that reflect tumor activity.

bcl-2 is a rearranged gene that some people with NHL are tested for. What these levels mean for prognosis is not clear. One study has found that bcl-2 levels do not correlate to prognosis.[6] Another has found that bcl-2 does predict poor outcome, even among those who achieve full remission on treatment.[7] A third study has found that expression of the bcl-2 protein correlates to a poorer outcome in large-cell lymphomas.[8]

Patient's response to tumor

Different patients respond differently to being ill and to treatments. These patient characteristics appear meaningful in predicting outcome.

- **B symptoms.** Unexplained loss of 10 percent or more of body weight, drenching night sweats, fever of 38°C (about 100°F) or higher for more than one week. Today, only unexplained weight loss appears to be related to the amount of disease.

- **Performance status (Karnovsky or ECOG).** Measures the patient's ability to do everyday things. The lower the performance status at diagnosis, the poorer the outcome. This measure does not apply to temporary setbacks while coping with the side effects of chemotherapy.

- **Serum albumin level.** Lower levels correlate with a worse prognosis.

- **Hemoglobin level.** Untreated anemia is correlated with a worse prognosis.

- For mediastinal (thymic) NHL, poor performance status, pericardial effusion, bulky or residual mediastinal abnormality, or inadequate response after front-line treatment predict poor response and later relapse. These patients may be candidates for high-dose treatment.

Patient's response to chemotherapy

A recent study found that long-term survival could be predicted for those with follicular lymphomas based on the tumor's response to chemotherapy, with an initial complete remission giving the best prognosis.[9]

Dose intensity of chemotherapy

The necessity to reduce dose intensity owing to patient characteristics is correlated with a poorer outcome.

Emotional issues

Although there are often similarities in how people with NHL feel about the effect of their disease on their future, and in how they choose to adapt to it, differences exist as well. Each person tends to find his or her own way along the path. The following survivor stories illustrate varied perceptions of living with NHL.

Acceptance

A seven-year survivor of low-grade NHL describes her comfortable outlook on the watch-and-wait approach to low-grade disease:

> It's now six years since my diagnosis with NHL, and a bit over two years since my relapse from first remission. Looks like the disease is holding steady. Here are the latest reasons I believe that to be true:
>
> A breast lump last month had to be biopsied and proved to be yet another swollen lymph node. The biopsy showed the histology to be the same as at my diagnosis, follicular small cleaved cell lymphoma. In other words, there is no sign of the disease transforming to a more aggressive type.
>
> I had a CT scan this week, and the results are just in: "Some minimal, probably insignificant, growth of the same nodes that were visible last time." And no symptoms have ever occurred. The doctor didn't even think I needed to come in and talk to him about it. He just said, "Make an appointment for sometime in the next two months."
>
> So! Watch-and-wait continues.

Denial

This snapshot of feelings is offered by Nicole, a registered nurse diagnosed with aggressive NHL:

> I still haven't accepted my mortality yet. Despite my diagnosis, I haven't made out my will, much to my parents' dismay. I started my durable power of attorney papers, but never completed them. I never completed my living will either. I have never asked my doctor my prognosis, and she has never really offered. No one pushes the issue. I guess I'm simply not willing to accept it yet. I've talked briefly with my daughter

Courtney about who she would want to live with if I died, but she's uncomfortable with the conversation also. I figure if I relapse, then I'll get my affairs in order. I don't know.

Happiness in spite of reality

Harry has decided that he has too far to go to dwell on the end of the journey:

> I think that I have been through two or three mental stages since my diagnosis and chemotherapy. At first it was panic. Then it was fear of the unknown. Now? I know that in the end I will lose the war, but you can bet I will win a few battles and put up one heck of a fight.
>
> We took care of our legal things, and I gave Mary power of attorney here at home and at the veterans' hospital where I am being treated. As for the big projects, the biggest project that I have been able to do is to build an electric swinging hoist for the back of our Dodge Caravan. It works great. Even I can load and unload my electric scooter (on a good day) by myself.
>
> The electric scooter has improved my life and attitude tremendously. For me, wheelchairs are worthless on gravel, in the grass, or on any slope, except downhill. I just don't have the strength to push one very far. With the scooter, I can browse the flea markets, navigate the largest mall, and participate in any cookout or outside activity. It just gave me back my freedom.
>
> I guess the point I am trying to make is that once you are comfortable with your state of affairs, big projects, and honey-do's, you are left drinking your tea or coffee and burning up a few smokes…and waiting. At some point in time I decided, "To heck with it. I have things that I want to do." And I just started doing them.
>
> From the time I was a little kid, I always wanted a radio-controlled airplane. I never did it [before] because of the cost and other responsibilities with the kids at home. [Recently] I joined a R/C airplane club, bought a couple of radios and couple of airplane kits, and did it. I don't have any trouble getting help at the R/C (radio-control) airstrip. All of us kids like to play with our toys. (The youngest is 31.)

I was expected to have had another round of chemotherapy over a year ago. My oncologist says that he didn't expect me to do nearly as well as I have. I just told him that I have too many things I want to do and too many places to go. I didn't have time for all of these medical problems. Nearly every visit he remarks that attitude makes a difference.

I really believe that.

Gifts and obligations

Marvin feels that he has life as a gift from God, and that with it come certain obligations:

I just think that we owe it to our God and to ourselves to live life while we can. I don't think we should delude ourselves we will last forever, but I also feel that everyone knows he'll die someday, yet everyone doesn't have the right to give up living because of the inevitable end.

When my ability to focus on living weakens (and it does weaken sometimes), I think of the utter waste that giving up would be, and it pulls me back.

Summary

This chapter has reviewed most of the known factors that may influence the outcome of the NHLs and their treatment. As stated at the beginning of this chapter, however, these factors are only relevant to treatments in use at the time this book was written. Newer treatments may rise above current limitations such as genetic damage or tumor burden. Your doctor is always your best source of up-to-date information.

CHAPTER 5

Tests and Procedures

X-rays: their moral is this—that
a right way of looking at things
will see through almost anything.

—Samuel Butler

When your doctor suspects that you have an illness that may be lymphoma, she will order one or more tests in an effort to arrive at a firm diagnosis. After diagnosis, several of these tests may be repeated throughout your treatment in order to gauge how well you are responding to treatment, and several after your treatment to confirm that you are still in remission.

This chapter begins with a description of general preparations to keep in mind for all procedures; then we list tests and procedures alphabetically. For each test, we state whether it is inpatient or outpatient, describe what the test or procedure accomplishes, tell how to prepare for the test, detail how it is administered, relay how most people rank the test regarding pain, discuss recovery issues, and outline any risks.

General information

It's most important that a correct diagnosis of lymphoma type and subtype be made before treatment starts. Some of the tests performed are necessary to determine exactly the kind of lymphoma you may have. One subtype of non-Hodgkin's lymphoma, for example, resembles Hodgkin's lymphoma, and another shares characteristics with chronic lymphocytic leukemia. As certain lymphomas and lymphoma subtypes are treated very differently from others, some oncologists have all lymph node tissue samples reviewed by expert hematopathologists such as those at the National Cancer Institute or the Armed Forces Institute of Pathology to ensure that the lymphoma is correctly identified.

A biopsy procedure must be coordinated between your surgeon, your oncologist, and the pathologist at the hospital in order for the necessary diagnostic tests to be performed correctly. This includes the doctors agreeing in advance how the tissue samples should be prepared: perhaps by freezing as well as by fixation within a paraffin block, for example.

Request in writing that the hospital keep your preserved tissue samples essentially forever. Some cancer survivors have discovered that hospital policy specifies that tissue samples be kept for only a number of years. This may become a problem if your lymphoma converts to another form or grade and your oncologist needs to compare a newer tissue sample to the original, if there should arise some question regarding the original diagnosis years afterward, or because some of the newest treatments now emerging require analysis of tumor cells. Unless your lymphoma is also detectable in the bloodstream—which is uncommon—having access to samples of the original tumor is important and, with a few exceptions discussed in Chapter 18, *Relapse*, may spare you a second biopsy.

You have the right to ask for and receive pain medication before the test is administered. It is not unusual to feel nervous about tests. If you are an adult patient, you may have some idea regarding your sense of pain, but if you are an adolescent, a very young adult, or the caretaker of a child with lymphoma, you have the right to know how painful a test may be and to ask in advance about options for controlling pain. Various pain-controlling medications can be requested in advance, such as the injected relaxant Demerol, the brief amnesiac Versed, also injected, the topical cream EMLA (which contains the drug Xylocaine familiar to us from dental care), or the short-acting anti-anxiety tablet Ativan.

If you are the caretaker of a child with lymphoma, pay special attention to the control of pain. Lobby for pain relievers and become informed about less invasive procedures. Communicate as honestly as possible with your child about the details of upcoming tests. Nancy Keene's books, *Your Child in the Hospital* and *Childhood Leukemia*, do an excellent job of describing ways to help children cope by explaining tests in advance, play-acting with toys, and using pain-killing medications such as EMLA. One point she makes most clearly is that communicating the details to children is mandatory because the child's anxiety decreases and trust increases when he knows what to expect.

Become aware of alternatives. For tests about which you feel unaware or uneasy, ask the following:

- Why is this procedure or test necessary? Will it change my treatment plan?

- Is there a safer or more comfortable alternative?

- What are the risks and side effects?

- How will pain be controlled?

- Will you explain this procedure to me or provide me with literature that describes it thoroughly?

- How experienced is the technician or doctor performing this procedure?

To spare yourself agonized waiting, you should discuss in advance with your oncologist how test results will be communicated. Some patients mistakenly assume that their doctor will take the initiative and contact them, when in fact the doctor's policy may be that the patient should take the initiative and call for results. If you know that your best method of coping includes acquiring as much information as possible as quickly as possible, tell your oncologist that you appreciate timely communication, and offer to expedite communication by making yourself available. Be aware that some oncologists are reluctant to leave test results on an answering machine without assurance from you that this is not a violation of your privacy. In addition, many ancillary doctors involved in your testing may choose for ethical reasons to communicate only with your primary oncologist unless instructed otherwise. Discussing these issues in advance with your oncologist is wise.

Never assume that the hospital staff administering the test are fully aware of your circumstances. Always tell the technicians doing the test that you are a non-Hodgkin's lymphoma survivor. Always tell them of any other health problems or allergies you have—such as previous allergic reactions to the iodine in shrimp—and of any prescribed or over-the-counter medications you are taking.

Make comfort a priority. Many of the tests done today require that you lay on a table for extended periods while cameras and x-ray machines do imaging. Get comfortable for this opportunity to nap by asking for extra blankets and finding a position that you can maintain pain-free for long periods. Ask for pillows to support your back and knees if you suffer from back pain.

The tests that are described in this chapter are those most commonly used for lymphomas. As non-Hodgkin's lymphoma can occur almost anywhere in the body, however, your doctor may order additional tests not described here. An excellent resource for finding information about other tests is *Everything You Need to Know About Medical Tests*, published by Springhouse, written by more than seventy medical experts, and having in sixteen chapters and 690 pages descriptions of more than four hundred tests. See Appendix A, *Resources*, for other recommendations.

A patient's story

This NHL survivor's story illustrates that, at times, several tests must be performed to obtain a correct diagnosis:

> When I was admitted to the hospital, we weren't sure what was going on. There were several things to rule out; cancer was never one of them. The first test I had done was a V-Q Scan. This nuclear medicine test checked both the blood flow to my lungs as well as the airflow. First you breathe in a nuclear mist for about ten minutes. It burns a little, I think because the particles are suspended in an alcohol solution. Then you get pictures taken, a nuclear dye is injected, and the same thing happens again. The whole process takes about thirty minutes. This test is often done to check for the possibility of a blood clot in the lungs.
>
> My test results were awful. I basically had no blood flow to my right lung. Hmmm…sounds like a blood clot. But even more strange was the fact that I had very little airflow to that lung either. This would indicate a blockage of some type.
>
> The next day, I was to have a chest CT and a bronchoscopy. The CT scan was done in the morning, and those results changed my life. After the CT scan, the doctor came in and said they found a mass in the center of my chest, and would need to biopsy it. When I heard the word biopsy, I asked him if it was a tumor, and he said yes.
>
> Everything after that seemed to go into fast-forward. Just the day before, I had a stubborn pneumonia, and now I have a tumor. I have surgeons and anesthesiologists coming in. I found myself thinking, "Wait. Stop. This isn't supposed to be happening to me. I'm only 32. I don't smoke. I'm obese, but otherwise I'm healthy. I live above my means for

my middle-income job, I take care of others, I don't show my feelings, and I have a teenager I'm trying to raise."

Then the surgeon came in to see me. He was very sweet, very gentle, if somewhat somber. He held my hand and explained the surgery, and told me he thought it was most likely a lymphoma, probably Hodgkin's disease.

After the surgeon left, I called my mom. I couldn't even get the words out. She and my step-dad came right to the hospital. By then I was crying. I was so embarrassed. I don't show my feelings. After all, I'm a nurse, I know what's going on. I was so overwhelmed by the evening that I asked the nurse to come back in the room so I could repeat what I thought the doctor had said to me. I wanted to be sure I heard him right. This conversation lasted about two hours.

During surgery they ended up only having to make a simple incision at the base of my neck. Originally I was told a T-flap (a more complex chest surgery) would have to be done, and possibly even the removal of part of my first rib. I don't know how long I was in surgery, although I remember flashes of waking up in the recovery room. I remember them starting really painful IVs in my feet. I remember the sound of the heart/ oxygen monitors. I remember being given morphine for pain and asking for something for my dry lips. My daughter was at my bedside, holding my hand, when I woke up in my room. I could taste the anesthesia gas in my throat and eventually it made me throw up. My neck really hurt, I couldn't move my head. I knew I needed to get up and walk to the bathroom, but I really felt hung over from the morphine. I was given more in my room after vomiting, as well as a Compazine suppository for the nausea. My daughter and mother sat in my room and fed me ice chips as I drifted in and out of sleep. Later that night, I finally woke up and was able to keep a sandwich and some Jell-O down. I got to go home the next morning.

I went back to the lung doctor on Tuesday. It was a very anticlimactic appointment since the biopsy results weren't back yet. All we had was the surgeon's gut feeling that it was nodular sclerosing Hodgkin's disease.

He did explain, however, that my breathing difficulties were in part due to the phrenic nerve being paralyzed. The phrenic nerve serves the diaphragm, so on the right side where most of my tumor was, the diaphragm didn't work. This caused my right lung not to be able to expand normally. He didn't know if this was permanent or not. The other difficulty came from the tumor cutting off both the blood supply and the bronchi to my right lung.

At this time, he also took the time to discuss oncologists with me. I told him that I prefer female doctors as a general rule and had heard there was a new one. He agreed that he thought we would get along well, and took the time to call her and explain my case as well as set up an appointment with her, ordering my staging CT scans. He also signed papers for me to be off work for another three months.

Between doctor appointments, I started scouring the Web. I joined a Hodgkin's disease Internet discussion group and started asking questions. I looked at home pages of survivors, NCI pages—anything I could get my hands on. During my nursing-school rotation in oncology, we only had one patient with lymphoma, a young man in his twenties with Hodgkin's disease. My textbooks had very little on lymphomas. Research gave me solace. Even if the news wasn't good, I thrived on information.

On Thursday, July 3rd, I met with my oncologist. She was a young, petite woman who was very caring. She was new to oncology, but I felt this was a benefit because she was more apt to research things and ask questions. I was right. She apologized for not having the results yet of the biopsy—it had to be sent out of town for a special staining procedure— and told me that I should bring as many people as I wanted to the next visit for questions and answers.

At the first visit, blood was drawn and more appointments were made for staging, as well as for a central line to be placed. I knew in advance that I wanted one, because intravenous lines (IVs) were so troublesome for me. I was all bruised from the IVs I had received in the hospital. From what I knew about chemotherapy, there was no way I was going to have a peripheral IV (an IV in the arm vein).

On the 4th of July, I received a call from my oncologist. The lab called, and had preliminary results of my biopsy. I had non-Hodgkin's lymphoma, intermediate grade, B-cell. She said that I would receive chemotherapy called CHOP four times, and then they would do a CT scan again to see if I needed more; that they could do a maximum of eight rounds. She also said I would have radiation following chemotherapy. This was it: this made it real. First I called my mom with the news, then I conference-called both my dad and his sister.

The first test I had that really frightened me was the bone marrow biopsy. I had bilateral tests done (i.e., in both hips). Back when I worked in oncology, I had assisted with these tests. I remembered the huge needles that were used and the pain that people went through. We did them in patients' rooms at the bedside back then and only used a little Lidocaine at the [injection] site. My mother had gone through a biopsy a few years earlier and kept trying to reassure me that it was nothing. I didn't believe her. I was so nervous about the procedure that I had diarrhea and had to keep leaving the waiting room to use the bathroom.

When all was said and done, it was quite comical. My mother and my daughter were allowed to stay in the room with me. The procedure was done in one of the emergency room exam rooms by the pathologist at the hospital. I was told ahead of time that I wouldn't be able to drive because of the medication they would give me. First a lab assistant came in and had me sign consent forms. She explained the procedure to me, and what would be necessary for care afterward to my family. Then a nurse anesthetist came down to start my IV and to administer drugs called Versed and Fentanyl. This produces a twilight or conscious sedation. I remembered Versed as a drug that "loosened lips"—people would often tell their doctors how cute they were or let out rather bawdy comments while under Versed. The best, or worst, part of it was that you didn't remember what you had said afterwards.

I don't remember how long before I fell asleep. My daughter said I was soon snoring so the doctor said they could proceed then. She was thrilled with watching the procedure. According to her, they used lots of Lidocaine. Whenever I groaned, they gave me more medication. I felt nothing! Apparently the procedure was quite funny to watch, the doctor had a difficult time obtaining the core samples and was rocking me back and forth, sweating and grunting. Apparently all this woke me up because I remember saying something about drinking milk (you know: strong bones and all). I guess I said this repeatedly and the doctor finally told me to stop drinking milk!

The next test done was the CT scan of the abdomen and pelvis for staging the tumor. Since the chest CT had been done in the hospital two weeks earlier, there was no need to repeat it. The biggest lesson to learn here is to check with the radiology department to make sure your preparation instructions are correct. By not drinking the dye the night before the procedure, I lost three days on staging time. The CT is painless; the only problem I had was in drinking the dye. I already felt nauseous, and it took me close to two hours to drink sixteen ounces of liquid.

With the bone marrow biopsies and CT scans done, I was ready for my second oncologist appointment. She admitted to being disappointed that I didn't have my central line placed yet because she wanted to start chemotherapy that day. My heart felt like it fell to my feet at that statement. I wasn't emotionally prepared for chemotherapy that day, so that was the last thing I wanted to hear. Instead we talked about my stage. I learned that my bone marrow was clean, but that I had tumors in both kidneys and in my left lung. Since there was no marrow involvement, I thought I was stage III, but the doctor informed me I was actually stage IV. We also reviewed my lab work at that time. My LDH (lactate dehydrogenase) was elevated, often a sign of lymphoma.

According to what I had read at the National Cancer Institute web site, this was bad news for me. I now had two strikes against me, prognostically: staging at level IV and the LDH level. I still never asked what my "chances" were. I was also given all of my chemotherapy prescriptions at that time: Prednisone as part of the chemotherapy, Ativan to help me sleep with the Prednisone, Zantac to protect my stomach from the Prednisone, Compazine for nausea, and Allopurinol to protect my kidneys from the onslaught of dead tumor cells they were about to experience.

The following week I had a Hickman catheter placed in my chest. I knew about central lines already from my experience in oncology. I always thought that if I ever had cancer I would get an Infusaport. Well, I discussed pros and cons of catheters versus ports with the IV nurses every time I went to the hospital. The nurses felt I should get a catheter instead because of my weight. They said they had had problems with ports tipping or flipping on bigger people. Frankly, at this time I liked the idea of no needle sticks, and if I couldn't do catheter care at home, who could? I asked my oncologist if she minded, and she said no. I also discussed it with the surgeon, and while he disagreed about the tipping problem (he said he could make a pocket for it to prevent this) he did think a catheter was a better idea, since it could be removed in the emergency room if it got infected instead of going back to surgery.

When I finally had the surgery, it was done in an outpatient setting, using Versed again as the anesthesia source. According to my mom, the procedure lasted about an hour. The surgeon came out and talked with them afterward, explaining that there had been some difficulty putting it in because the tumor kept pushing on the catheter.

When I awoke in recovery, I was also dismayed to find out they had used Betadine on me despite my repeatedly telling them that I was allergic to it. The recovery room nurse changed my soiled bandages and cleaned all the Betadine off of me and the catheter. I went home with a very sore shoulder and my prescription for Vicodin.

Specific tests

The descriptions that follow list tests and procedures alphabetically, state whether they are inpatient or outpatient, describe what the tests and procedures accomplish, tell how to prepare for these tests, detail how they are administered, relay how most people rank them regarding pain, discuss recovery issues, and outline risks.

Abdominal surgery (laparotomy)

Laparotomy is the medical name for any incision into the abdomen. While laparotomies are no longer routinely performed for diagnosing lymphoma, it may be necessary if your only evidence of disease is within the abdomen. The only way to get a sound diagnosis is by removing and examining lymph nodes or other suspicious tissue. Imaging tools such as CT scans cannot depict tumors in enough detail for your doctor to use the results as a basis for planning effective treatment, and fine-needle biopsies sometimes fail to retrieve enough tissue for a diagnosis.

Use of the laparoscope (a camera-guided surgical tool containing a microscope) for this surgery is still uncommon, but is becoming more common in some major cancer centers. When a laparoscope is used, the procedure is called laparoscopy instead of laparotomy, the incision is smaller, and healing time is shorter. Some disadvantages of laparoscopy are the relative inability of the surgeon to have a clear view of the entire internal abdomen, and the possibility that tumorous tissue will break apart and remain within while the surgeon is trying to remove it using only camera-guided instruments.

Laparotomy is an inpatient procedure; laparoscopy can be either an inpatient or outpatient procedure.

Preparation

Prior to scheduling this surgery, you may need to submit in writing to your insurance company evidence of the necessity of surgery. You should verify with your insurance company how long a hospital stay they will approve and whether home aftercare is provided. You should consider filling out a durable power of attorney so that your loved ones can make decisions for you while you are recovering. Pre-operative tests such as a chest x-ray, electrocardiogram, or blood testing may be necessary.

You will be asked to fast for twelve to eighteen hours before surgery. You may be instructed to use enemas or laxatives beforehand. The risks associated with this surgery will be explained to you, and you will be asked to sign a consent form. If in the past anesthesia has made you nauseous during recovery, tell the anesthesiologist. She will give you antinausea medication.

Method

A local anesthetic is injected in the skin near the vein that will be used for the general anesthetic, and an intravenous line (IV) is inserted once the area is numbed. An oxygen mask may be fitted over your face while you are still awake. A general anesthetic to make you fall asleep will be injected into the IV line; afterward, you may be kept asleep with either gas anesthesia or an IV sedative.

While you are asleep, the surgeon, in coordination with the pathologist, will remove a few lymph nodes, as well as small pieces of other tissue if they look suspicious, for examination in the pathology laboratory. The surgeon will carefully examine all surrounding tissue for signs of cancer. The incision is then closed layer by layer. Surgical staples or stitches will be used to close both internal and external layers of tissue. Dissolving synthetic fabric layers may be used internally to prevent a form of internal scarring called adhesion.

Recovery

When you wake, you will still have the IV line, now supplying you with saline, nutrients, and pain killer. As you become less sleepy, you may notice that additional equipment was added during your surgery: you may, for example, have a temporary catheter in the urethra to collect urine, a temporary tube in your nose that passes to your stomach to keep it empty, or a respirator to help you breathe. These temporary assists are removed when the nurses become aware that you can function without them. In general, the sooner you are able to rise from bed and walk, the sooner you will regain full function of all body organs, as movement aids the healing process.

Hospitalization times vary based on the patient's condition and the type of insurance in effect. If you feel you need to stay longer in the hospital, but your insurance policy limits your stay unless the doctor requests otherwise, be sure to make your needs known to your doctor and the nursing staff.

When you are discharged, you may be restricted from driving for several weeks, depending on the location of your incision. Certain activities such as climbing stairs may also be restricted. Full recovery may take as long as six weeks and may include pronounced fatigue.

Pain

Directly after surgery, you will be given by IV a pain medication that most likely will be morphine. Sometimes the hospital staff looks for signs that you have awakened from general anesthesia before administering pain medication which will once again make you sleepy. This precaution is taken to ensure that you are not overdosed. Be sure to make clear your need for pain medication as soon as you are awake and are experiencing pain, as excessive pain can interfere with healing. Most patients report pain at the incision site, perhaps a sore throat from the breathing tube that was inserted and removed while they were asleep, and perhaps hip pain if a bone marrow biopsy was performed. A few report pain at the IV site.

Additional pain medication beyond day one will be given freely if you ask. Many hospitals now use patient-controlled infusion (PCI) pumps for morphine dosing, as they yield a more even dose—about twenty microdoses per hour—than pain medication given by tablet or IV. PCI pumps also will yield a limited amount of additional morphine if the patient pushes a button on the pump for this purpose. The minicomputer within the pump counts the number of patient pushes so that the staff will have a good idea of your need for pain medication. Most patients find they need a minimum of three days of morphine for abdominal surgery.

When you are discharged, you will be given a prescription for oral pain medicine. Many patients report a lingering dull ache in the area beneath the incision for months afterward.

Risks

There are varying risks associated with surgery done under general anesthesia, including excessive bleeding from the incision site and a very small risk from the anesthesia itself. Your doctor and the hospital staff will explain fully the risks that apply most closely to your surgery.

Barium enema

See "X-rays."

Blood product transfusion

This outpatient procedure is a means of replenishing your red blood cell and platelet blood supply if chemotherapy or radiation therapy have significantly lowered them, or have limited your bone marrow's ability to produce new blood cells.

Preparation

You should check the blood product brought to you for infusion to be sure it matches your ABO blood type. Platelet matching on ABO may also become necessary after many platelet transfusions, as the body gradually becomes sensitized to and attacks donated platelets.

Be sure to tell the nursing staff if you have ever before had an allergic reaction to donor platelets.

Method

An intravenous (IV) line is inserted into a vein in your forearm or into your central catheter if you have one that can be used for transfusions. The blood product to be transfused is hung from an IV pole and is dripped into you over a period of about four hours.

If you have chills, fever, or difficulty breathing during a transfusion, notify the nursing staff immediately. This may be the beginning of an allergic reaction.

Pain

If you have no catheter and an IV line is inserted into your vein, you may feel mild pain during its insertion.

Recovery

There are no recovery issues following transfusion. On the contrary, you can expect to feel much less tired almost immediately after red blood cells are infused.

Risks

There is a risk of serious allergic reaction if donated blood products are not properly matched to yours. There is a slight risk of infection at the site of IV insertion.

Blood tests

Various blood tests detect various conditions. Each blood test's purpose is discussed following the name of the test. All are outpatient procedures.

Preparation

Most blood tests require no preparation; however, some may require an overnight fasting diet or the cessation of certain medications for a few days. Always tell your doctor and the staff administering the test of any drugs you are taking, prescription or over-the-counter. Zantac (Ranitidine), for example, can suppress platelet production and could cause an inaccurate result in a complete blood count.

Method

Most blood tests are performed by drawing blood into a syringe from the vein just inside the elbow. If your veins have been damaged by chemotherapy, if they are hard to find, or if they roll—more common in muscular people—the technician (phlebotomist) may use a vein on the back of the hand or on the back of the lower forearm. Some implanted catheters can be used for blood draws (see "Catheter insertion").

You can make your veins easier to access as follows:

- Lay a wet, warm cloth on the vein just before blood is drawn, or ask to use a restroom to soak the forearm in warm water.

- Vigorously pump the muscles in that arm just before the draw.

- Hang the arm lower than the rest of the body for a few minutes just before the draw.

- Drink lots of fluids starting four hours before blood is to be drawn.

Once a vein is accessed successfully, a blood draw takes less than three minutes.

Pain

Most people report minor pain or no pain during a blood draw. If, however, you are afraid of needles, of the pain of needles, or of the sight of blood, you are not alone. A policeman describes his fear of needles:

> When a piece of metal lodged in my eye, my eye doctor called in a surgeon from Baltimore. It turned out that the metal was already gone, but they had to remove the rust that was still in the fluid part of my eye. The surgery was done in a dark room while I was awake and lying on a table. It didn't hurt, and everything was okay until I realized they were using a needle. I thought they were going to use a laser! They finished what they had to do, but I was not happy about the needle. Good thing I was already lying down!

Here are a few tips for reducing fear and pain during a blood draw:

- Slap or rub the injection site just before the draw so that you will be less likely to feel the insertion.

- Ask for EMLA cream to use two hours before your appointment. Keep the site covered with an airtight bandage until your draw.

- Ask the phlebotomist, most of whom are quite skilled at reducing pain, to stretch the skin at the injection site.

- Look away while the blood is drawn.

- Think of someone who delights you and makes you smile.

- Ask the phlebotomist about his or her life, photos, liking for the job, and so on. "So, how's business?" can be a good opener.

For some children, blood draws can be an especially difficult ordeal. It might be possible for the technician to use a finger-prick or the earlobe if only a small amount of the child's blood is needed, after the area has been numbed with EMLA cream.

Recovery

Most blood draws entail no recovery, but you may have slight, painless bruising at the injection site the following day. Stretching the skin to make the blood draw less painful may increase this chance of bruising. Steady pressure on the injection site for sixty seconds or more directly after the needle is withdrawn facilitates clotting and can reduce the chance of bruising.

Risks

Unless you have blood that won't clot normally, there are only minor risks associated with a blood draw, such as the possibility of painless bruising.

Specific blood tests

Blood tests are listed alphabetically. Normal values for these blood tests are described in Appendix B, *Blood and Marrow Test Values*.

Alkaline phosphatase
> This product's value may be abnormal if liver function is affected by the tumor or if bone is being dissolved, for example, when calcium levels are out of balance.

Bcl-2 or bcl-6 gene rearrangements
> Gene rearrangements are detected using sophisticated tools that analyze the DNA in our chromosomes. Patented procedures such as polymerase chain reaction (PCR) may be performed first to provide a sample large enough for analysis. Bcl-2 gene rearrangements might be detected in either blood or bone marrow.

Beta-2 microglobulin (B2M)
> This product of white blood cells is detected using a test that is fairly new as of this writing. Like LDH, B2M is a surrogate for tracking tumor burden and is thought to be a measure of how successfully NHL tumors are responding or will respond to the treatments in use today.

Bilirubin
> As with other liver products, the level of this substance is a reflection of the tumor's effect on liver function.

Complete blood count (CBC)

This test measures the three blood cell types and reports on their proportions, age, and other important parameters. During chemotherapy and radiation therapy, white counts in particular can drop and make the patient susceptible to infections. See Appendix B for more detail on complete blood counts.

Creatinine (serum creatinine)

This substance is an indication of how well your kidneys are working. NHL can press on the ureter—the tube leading from kidney to bladder—and can impair kidney function. Creatinine may also reflect the amount of dangerous toxins being released by the tumor as it breaks down. This is called tumor lysis syndrome.

Electrolytes

Levels of various minerals in the blood are sometimes a reflection of problems related to tumor metabolism or to chemotherapy. Levels of calcium, potassium, magnesium, iron, and other electrolytes can be modified by disease or by its treatment.

Erythrocyte sedimentation rate (sed rate)

This test measures how quickly red blood cells sediment. Red blood cells that sediment quickly indicate an inflammation within the body. Although alone it is not reliable for diagnosing NHL, it is a surrogate for tracking tumor burden in those already diagnosed by other means.

FISH (fluorescence in situ hybridization)

This test of the DNA contained in blood cells or other tissue uses fluorescent chemicals to mark damaged genes. The chemical consists of molecules constructed to match exactly the gene being sought, so FISH is not practical for broad screening for DNA damage. The probe untwists (denatures) the two strands of DNA and, when a match exists between the chemical probe and a gene, attaches itself to the one piece of DNA being sought, thus the term hybridization. Using a special microscope, the pathologist or geneticist can visualize the gene, its breakpoint, any crossing over with other genes on the same or other chromosomes, and so on, by viewing the fluorescence it produces. This is an exquisitely sensitive technique for differentiating certain lymphomas and leukemias.

Flow cytometry

This method of examining tissue exploits two principles. First, cancer cells can be tagged with chemicals and thus be made to look different from normal cells. Second, these cells can be forced to flow single-file through a narrow tube so they can be counted one at a time, much like children returning from recess. The tagged cancer cells are counted as they pass through a light beam or other tool for detecting whatever tagging agent was used. In this manner, bone marrow cells and blood cells can be examined for very specific features indicating cancer, such as abnormal surface antigens.

Immunoglobulin studies (IgM, IgA, IgD, IgG, IgH, IgE)

Immunoglobulins are one weapon in the arsenal of the immune system, part of the seek-and-destroy repertoire of white blood cells. These tests measure the amounts of products called immunoglobulins secreted by special white blood cells called plasma cells. The tests are done to rule out illnesses related to NHL, such as multiple myeloma, Waldenstrom's macroglobulinemia, or inherited immune system disorders.

Lactate dehydrogenase (LDH)

Testing for high levels of LDH in non-Hodgkin's lymphoma survivors is useful because LDH is released when body tissues break down for any reason. Although alone it is not reliable for diagnosing NHL, it is a surrogate for tracking tumor burden in those already diagnosed by other means.

Liver enzymes (SGOT, SGPT, ALT, AST)

Unusual amounts of liver enzymes correlate loosely with the presence and extent of disease.

Polymerase chain reaction (PCR)

PCR can use many different source tissues as long as they contain genes and chromosomes (DNA). Blood and bone marrow are two such likely sources, particularly for the lymphomas and leukemias. PCR is a method, not a test or substance. It involves taking a very small amount of genetic material and replicating it over and over so that enough exists to run tests that will require large amounts of genetic material. PCR is used primarily to detect minimal residual disease in patients with lymphomas and leukemias.

Uric acid

> As with creatinine, this substance reflects kidney function and possible effects of the tumor on the kidney, such as tumor lysis syndrome.

Bone marrow aspiration/biopsy

By examining the liquid marrow or the solid core of marrow/bone structure under a microscope, a pathologist can determine if lymphoma has spread into the marrow or if chemotherapy or radiation therapy have affected the marrow's ability to function. Bone marrow aspiration involves drawing a small amount of liquid bone marrow into a narrow needle; bone marrow biopsy involves drawing a piece of bone and its attached marrow into a larger needle called a trephine. Although in most people all bones are capable of producing marrow, for these tests the large bone of the hip is usually used. Bone marrow aspiration and biopsy is usually, but not always, an outpatient procedure.

Preparation

A sedative and/or an amnesiac may be given to you in advance—see "Pain." Bring a heating pad with you, and ask the staff if you can place it over the hip area for ten minutes or so beforehand, as some patients report this reduces pain afterward. If you have had biopsies in the past and prefer the technique of a particular staff member, try to obtain an appointment that matches his or her schedule. Be sure your sedative or local anesthetic has become fully effective before allowing the staff to proceed.

Method

A local anesthetic is injected over the back of the hipbone and a very small incision is made. Into this incision the needle or trephine, or each in turn if both aspiration and biopsy are being done, is inserted to penetrate the bone. For a marrow aspiration, the liquid marrow is drawn into the needle and the needle is removed. For a biopsy, the trephine is pushed through the bone to collect a core of bone and its attached marrow, and is removed. If not enough marrow can be obtained, a second insertion through the same incision but into a different area of bone will be tried. Pressure is applied over the insertion point for a few minutes to stop bleeding. A small bandage is applied.

Pain

Many patients report moderate to severe pain during this procedure. Be sure to ask for a sedative or an amnesiac such as Versed if you know from past experience that you prefer being very much unaware of pain. You may feel unpleasant pressure as the needle is pushed through the bone, especially if your bones are very dense. You may feel a unique unpleasant sensation as the marrow is drawn into the needle. You may feel pain if the needle slips across the bone surface as it is being inserted.

Recovery

Unlike a bone marrow harvest for transplantation, for aspiration or biopsy very little marrow is removed, so subsequent lightheadedness and fatigue are rare. Afterward, your hip may feel sore for a few days. This can usually be relieved with Tylenol-type medications.

Risks

There is a slight risk of infection at the incision site.

Bone marrow harvest

A bone marrow harvest usually is an inpatient procedure with specific preparation and recovery. It's covered thoroughly in Chapter 20, *Transplantation*.

Bone scan (scintigraphy)

This outpatient test exploits the fact that some bone irregularities will absorb more of a substance than will healthy bone tissue. Your doctor will choose a scintigraphic agent that works best with the type of tumor you have and its location.

Preparation

For a bone density scan, no contrast agent is injected. For imaging of suspected tumors, a mild radioactive agent, usually Technetium-99, will be injected and you will be asked to return later, perhaps in three hours, for scanning. You will be encouraged to drink copious amounts of water to spread the agent from soft tissue into bone. Get comfortable after lying down on the table for the scan, because you must hold this position for up to an hour.

Method

Scanning is done by having the fully clothed patient lie on a table that has, above and below it, a camera that is sensitive to the energy emitted by the agent injected. It is important to hold still for duration of the film exposure. The table is fully open, not enclosed like an MRI machine, and you'll see the arm of the camera passing over your body starting with your head and going toward your feet. The arm is about six inches wide and about as long as the table is wide. It moves slowly; a whole-body scan can take thirty or forty minutes.

Pain

A slight sting may be felt when the scintigraphic agent is injected.

Recovery

There are no recovery issues associated with this test.

Risks

As with other imaging techniques, there are risks of false-positive and false-negative readings.

Bronchoscopy

See "Endoscopy."

Catheter insertion (central catheter, central line)

This procedure can be inpatient or outpatient. A central catheter or line is a flexible tube that is threaded into a very large vein near your heart. Its presence in a large vein dilutes chemotherapy drugs amidst a large volume of blood and thus makes chemotherapy safer. Moreover, depositing chemotherapy drugs near your heart will distribute them more quickly and more evenly to all parts of your body than is possible when chemotherapy is infused directly into an arm vein. Using a central catheter can eliminate damage to arm veins during chemotherapy, and can eliminate somewhat painful penetration of arm veins for blood testing and for administering other drugs.

Preparation

You need to decide whether a catheter is the right choice for you. You will also need to decide whether to get an external catheter (with tubing emerging from the skin) or a subcutaneous catheter (under the skin). Your oncologist may have very strong opinions on this topic.

Some advantages of catheter use are:

- Chemotherapy is safer when diluted by lots of blood.

- Chemotherapy is spread throughout the body more quickly and evenly with a central catheter.

- Vein damage is minimal or nonexistent.

- Some models can be used for blood transfusions.

- Some models can be used for hemapheresis, the collecting of stem cells for a stem cell transplant.

Note that, with an external catheter, there are no needle sticks that hurt, but with an internal catheter, no periodic cleaning is necessary.

Some drawbacks of catheter use are:

- Surgery is required to install a central catheter.

- External catheters must be cleaned and flushed daily or tri-weekly, and kept dry.

- Infections can lodge in a catheter. Their treatment may entail use of very strong antibiotics with risky side effects such as permanent vertigo, or may require surgical removal with a third surgery for reinsertion at a later date.

- The external types that emerge from the skin of the neck or chest can make the patient feel unsightly.

- The types that do not emerge from the skin still require somewhat painful skin penetration to access the port.

- Central catheters can break and travel through the vein to your heart.

- Central catheters can kink and make drug infusion difficult.

You may be given the choice of a local or a general anesthetic. If you choose a general anesthetic, preparation for and recovery from this procedure may be more complex. On the other hand, some who choose a local anesthetic report that they can feel deep pain during the procedure.

See "Abdominal surgery" for a description of preparation for general anesthesia. See "Node biopsy" for a description of preparation for local anesthesia.

You will be asked to dress in a hospital gown and will be taken to a surgical suite. After the anesthetic has taken effect, two areas, both on the chest, or one on the chest and one on the neck, will be cleansed and two incisions will be made. The surgeon will access the large vein near the heart through one of these incisions. The central line will be threaded through the large vein until it rests near your heart. The other end will be threaded beneath your skin and, for an internal port, secured there. For an external port, it will be threaded through the surface of the skin with an anchor just below the surface.

Recovery

See "Abdominal surgery" for recovery issues after general anesthesia. See "Node biopsy" for recovery issues after local anesthesia.

You will be taught how to clean and flush your port if you have chosen an external catheter. Redness, swelling, or bleeding that persists at the incision site should be reported to your doctor.

Pain

Some who have had a central line implanted report pain when moving their arms or when lying in a certain position. This pain may continue for several weeks following implantation. Some who elect local anesthesia report feeling deep pain during the procedure:

> I had a Groshong catheter implanted in anticipation of many different needs for vascular access. That was a tough thing to accommodate without feeling like an alien. The same surgeon who had done such a good job removing the malignant node seemed to turn into Conan the Barbarian for this procedure. I had no general anesthetic to relax me, nor was I aware I could ask for one. He inserted a needle several times into my chest to administer a local, and I quietly wept both from shock and pain. A nurse stroked my head and patted my shoulder, whispering that it would not last long.

Risks

Refer to the list of drawbacks under "Preparation." In addition, surgery entails risks such as accidental penetration of a major vein, uncontrolled bleeding, and slight risks associated with anesthesia.

Colonoscopy

See "Endoscopy."

CT scan (computed tomography, "CAT" scan)

An outpatient procedure, computed tomography is a series of many very narrow x-rays taken at many varying depths of tissue and from different angles around your body. These x-ray images are then analyzed and reassembled by a computer into an image of your internal organs. CT scans differ from traditional x-ray imaging in that x-ray imaging can't readily distinguish organs that are lying behind other organs. Imagine looking at several veils hanging one behind the other, each painted with a different design. You can imagine how difficult it might be to discern the design on the farthest veil. CT scans, on the other hand, are able to delineate even those organs that are obscured by other tissue.

Preparation

You may be asked to fast overnight, to use a laxative, or to purchase and drink a contrast agent if a CT scan of your abdomen and/or pelvis is planned.

Your studies may require an iodine-based contrast agent. Be sure to tell your doctor and the staff doing the test if you have thyroid disease or are allergic to iodine in seafood or other sources. A non-iodine version of the contrast agent can be substituted.

Because the iodine contrast agent used may cause a sensation of heat, skin flushing, or rapid heartbeat, be sure to tell the technician if you have heart disease, high blood pressure, or any other health concerns in addition to being a lymphoma survivor.

If you have internal staples from a previous surgery or pieces of metal embedded in your body from a previous injury, tell the technician. They represent no danger to you during the scan, but may appear on the film as unexplained phenomena.

CT scanners are open, doughnut-shaped machines that generally do not cause patients to feel claustrophobic.

Method

CT scans are performed while you are lying in a carefully chosen position that has been aligned with the machine. It is important to maintain the position that was chosen until the technician says you can relax. Most CT scan sessions include a fast, initial pass with no contrast agent, followed by a second, slower scan with a contrast agent. The first scan images the entire body to use as a frame of reference for the rest of the scanning. During the first scan, you'll feel the table you're lying on move smoothly through the doughnut-hole of the machine, without stopping and starting.

While the second, slower scan is underway, you may be asked to hold your breath briefly over and over. Some scanning machines take ten to twenty minutes to scan, depending how much of the body is being scanned. During this time, the contrast agent is slowly dripped into your vein. The part of you being scanned is positioned inside the doughnut-hole, which is about twelve inches thick. You'll feel the table you're lying on move slowly through the machine a few centimeters at a time, stopping and starting. Some people enjoy taking a nap at this point.

Newer scanners can do the entire scan very quickly, in about twenty seconds. For these machines, you may have to hold your breath for the entire twenty seconds, and if a contrast agent is injected, it will be pushed rapidly into your vein instead of slowly dripped. This quick administration of the contrast agent may cause stronger feelings of heat and faster heartbeat, sensations that are not considered an allergic reaction. You will feel the table you're lying on move smoothly through the doughnut-hole of the machine without stopping and starting.

For some studies of the stomach or bowels, you may be required to drink a contrast agent just before the scan is taken.

Pain

CT scans are painless. However, when a contrast agent is used, it is injected into a vein, perhaps causing minor discomfort (see "Blood tests"). As mentioned under "Preparation," the iodine contrast agent used may cause a sensation of heat, skin flushing, or rapid heartbeat.

Recovery

If you have had a study that required drinking a contrast agent, you may experience gas, diarrhea, or constipation for one to three days afterward. Drinking large amounts of water will hasten the removal of the contrast agent from the digestive tract. If you have had a contrast agent injected, you may have a harmless and temporary discoloration of the urine or skin for several days afterward. If you are sensitive to iodine or have a thyroid condition, you may feel fatigue for several days after receiving an iodine-based contrast agent.

Risks

A CT scan, if repeated over and over for many years, may deliver enough radiation to body tissue to cause health problems later in life, such as lung, thyroid, or breast cancers. However, as CT scanning technology has improved, the amount of radiation delivered has lowered.

Endoscopy (colonoscopy, bronchoscopy, gastroscopy, sigmoidoscopy)

This outpatient test uses a microscope and light source on a narrow flexible tube to examine and sample parts of the body that would otherwise require open surgery to access. For the non-Hodgkin's lymphomas, the organs most often examined are the larynx, bronchial tubes and lungs, stomach, complete colon, or sigmoid (lower) colon.

Preparation

Depending on the part of the body being examined, you may be asked to restrict your diet, to use a laxative or an enema, or to forego certain medications such as aspirin for a day or more. You may be asked to bring someone with you to drive afterward. If a colonoscopy is planned, discuss sedation with your doctor, as some but not all patients report pain with this procedure.

Method

First, a sedative may be injected into a vein of your forearm to relax you. It may be administered with a syringe or by an IV that will remain in place until you are ready to go home. A self-inflating blood pressure cuff may be used on your upper arm, and a rubber thimble for monitoring oxygen levels may be placed on your finger.

Once the sedative has taken effect, the endoscope will be inserted and a painless, quick examination will ensue. Very small pieces of tissue may be collected painlessly and sent to the pathology lab for testing. While the scope is being used, you may be asleep or you may be vaguely aware that the procedure is underway. You may retch if the scope's tube is inserted in your throat, but the sedative will make you feel as if it is happening to someone else.

Recovery

If a sedative was used, it may take about a half hour to awaken. For several hours after having a sedative, it is unwise to drive, even if you feel able to do so.

Pain

Some patients report pain during colonoscopy. Some report a panicked feeling of being unable to breathe during bronchoscopy.

Risks

There are a few low risks associated with endoscopy, such as the risk of puncture of the esophagus or intestine. There is a very small risk of the sedative injection site becoming infected.

FISH (fluorescence in situ hybridization)

See "Blood tests."

Flow cytometry

See "Blood tests."

Gallium scan (scintigraphy, gallium scintigram)

This outpatient test exploits the fact that some lymphoma tumors will absorb more of a substance than will surrounding tissue or healthy lymphatic tissue. Your doctor will choose a scintigraphic agent that works best for the type of tumor you have and its location. Circumstances when different scintigraphic agents may be used include:

- Low-grade non-Hodgkin's lymphoma sometimes absorbs thallium more readily than gallium.

- T-cell tumors may absorb gallium more readily than B-cell tumors do.

- Abdominal tumors of several types may be hard to distinguish from normal tissue with either gallium or thallium.

- Especially in children, a normal but enlarged thymus gland may appear malignant in a gallium scan following chemotherapy.

When a tumor absorbs gallium well, it is called gallium-avid. If a tumor is suspected not to absorb gallium well, any one of a variety of other agents, such as technetium-99m or Indium-111, may be used instead. Tumors that are not gallium-avid may be so because the lymphatic ducts are blocked, because internal tumor pressure is too great to allow the substance to enter, or because surrounding tissue is inflamed and takes up just as much gallium, thus reducing contrast.

Sometimes this procedure is repeated using a camera that is sensitive to the emission of a single positron (a positron is a piece of an atom). This is called a SPECT or SPET scan, and works on a similar principle, that is, the gallium makes your tissue more visible to the camera. The gamma camera, if it is used, is not a doughnut-shaped solid thing like a CT scanner. It's more like a shield that moves back and forth in half circles starting at the top of the body and working down. It moves close to the body, but does not touch it.

Preparation

An enema or laxative may be necessary the day before the test. After lying down on the camera table, get comfortable, because you must hold this position for about one hour.

Method

An injection of gallium-67 is made into a vein in the forearm and the needle is withdrawn. Depending on the agent used, the patient may be scanned repeatedly in two, four, twenty-four, forty-eight, or seventy-two hours, or a combination of these times. For the repeated tests, the patient must return to the hospital. No second injection is required before the second scan. Scanning is done by having the fully clothed patient lie on a camera table that is sensitive to the energy emitted by the agent injected. It is important to hold still for the duration of the film exposure. Some patients are embarrassed to note that, although they are fully clothed, the computer-assembled image on the screen is of the naked body.

Pain

A slight sting may be felt when the scintigraphic agent is injected. You won't have to stay away from others later to avoid exposing them to radioactivity, as is necessary after receiving injections of some other isotopes. Allergic reactions are extremely rare.

Recovery

There are no recovery issues associated with this test.

Risks

As with other imaging techniques, there are risks of false-positive and false-negative readings with gallium.

GI series

See "X-rays."

Intravenous pyelogram

See "X-rays."

Laparotomy

See "Abdominal surgery."

Lumbar puncture

See "Spinal tap."

Lymphangiogram (bipedal lymphangiography, lymphography)

This outpatient test, which is rarely used these days because better tests exist, allows the oncology team to view lymph nodes within the lower body. The nodes will absorb an iodine dye that causes them to be visible on x-ray film. Cancerous nodes sometimes will be different in appearance from normal nodes and other body parts. This test does not always illuminate all cancerous nodes in the lower body, especially if the spread of lymphoma blocks a lymphatic vessel or destroys the structure of a lymph node, but this is also true of other imaging tests that use contrast agents such as dye.

Preparation

This is an outpatient procedure. You may be asked to restrict your diet to clear liquids for one day prior to the test. Because this procedure can be a painful one, you should determine several days in advance how experienced the technician is. Ask your oncologist if the procedure can be done elsewhere if the technician does not do lymphangiograms more than five times a year.

Tell the technician if you are allergic to iodine, have ever had trouble breathing or an outbreak of hives after eating shellfish, have thyroid disease, or are pregnant.

Empty your bladder before the test, because its timing ranges from ninety minutes to six hours.

Method

A small amount of blue-green dye is injected into the top of the foot between the toes in order to highlight the lymphatic vessels. When one or more lymphatic channels becomes visible, a local anesthetic is injected and a small incision is made above the vessel. Into each incision a very small needle is placed to inject iodine dye that will trace through the lower lymphatic system. Sometimes the needle must be repositioned in order to enter the lymphatic vessel. The dye is injected slowly via automatic pump over an hour or more. While the dye is being injected, a fluoroscope, which is a type of x-ray machine, is used to trace the progress of the dye through the lymphatic system.

While the dye is being injected, the patient must sit or lie quietly, so be sure you are warm and comfortable at the outset of this lengthy procedure. Pay particular attention to the position and relaxation of your feet, as they must stay in this position for several hours, so an awkward position quickly will become a weary one.

After the dye has been injected, the incisions are stitched and the patient is x-rayed. The dye will remain in the body for up to a month and repeated imaging can be done. Most likely you will have x-ray sessions scheduled over two or more days to capture increasingly fine detail as the dye travels well into the nodes.

Pain

This procedure ranges from minor to severe with respect to pain. Some patients report severe pain if needles must be repositioned to find a lymphatic vessel, because the procedure can stretch from the normal ninety minutes to five or more hours. Discuss in advance the possibility that the local anesthetic may wear off if lymphatic vessels are not found on the first try, and ask what they will do to keep you pain-free. Others report that the pain of recovery lasts a week owing to the incisions that must heal, and report that walking is difficult and that wearing shoes is impossible. The iodine dye can cause a mild warmth, burning, or pressure sensation as it travels through the lower body, especially in the feet, behind the knees, or in the groin.

Recovery

Recovery lasts from three days to one week while incisions heal. Urine, feces, skin, and vision may have a blue-green discoloration for a few days. Stitches must be kept dry, and a return visit to remove stitches is necessary.

Risks

There is some discussion in the medical literature whether thyroid dysfunction may occur in those who have had both lymphangiogram and radiation therapy. Infection at the incision site is possible. Some people, especially those who are allergic to iodine, have an allergic reaction to the dye, such as difficulty breathing. Some people develop a fever and swollen lymph nodes from the dye.

Mammogram (mammography, breast x-ray)

An x-ray of the breast is called a mammogram. Certain lymphomas can lodge in the breast and must be distinguished from benign cysts and other cancers of the breast. If you are a male or female survivor of NHL and notice a lump in the breast, contact your doctor immediately.

Preparation

If you are female and are still having menstrual periods, schedule your mammogram for somewhere in the ten days following the first day of your period. This will lessen the chance that your breasts will be tender and will give a more accurate x-ray result. Avoid caffeine, chocolate, and other foods that may contribute to breast tenderness for several days prior to your mammogram.

Request an appointment that includes a patient/doctor consultation directly following the x-ray session, so that you can discuss immediately with the doctor any unusual results, and have repeat x-rays or ultrasound if warranted. Otherwise, if the results are questionable, you may have to wait several highly stressful days, or even longer, for the staff to find an opening in their schedule for repeat testing or for the doctor's availability.

Tell the technicians and the radiologist that you are a non-Hodgkin's lymphoma survivor.

Before the mammogram, remove all aluminum-based antiperspirants and all metallic jewelry. Be sure the technician is aware of moles, scars, or other skin characteristics that may appear questionable on the films.

You will be asked to remove all clothing from the waist up and to replace them with a gown. While the mammograms are being performed, however, the gown must be partially removed to facilitate placing the breast above the photographic plate.

Method

Mammography is usually done while the woman is standing with the breast resting against a warmed, flat surface that contains a photographic plate. The technician will measure the density of the breast tissue and slowly lower a matching plate from above until the breast is somewhat compressed. While you are holding that position carefully, she will step behind a radiation shield and activate the x-ray machine for about three seconds.

Usually, two x-rays of each breast are taken, each from a different angle, to maximize the amount and location of tissue imaged. It is particularly important to capture the tissue high against the chest wall, approaching the collarbone, because in fact breast tissue extends beyond what we traditionally refer to as the breast. Using equipment commonly available today, tissue compression remains necessary to ensure good visualization of all breast tissue.

You will be asked to wait, wearing the gown, until the films are developed to ensure that films of high clarity were obtained. If unclear, the studies must be repeated. If unusual features are present on one of the films, the x-ray may be redone using a small compression paddle to highlight a particular area of breast tissue. Alternately, ultrasound may be used to re-image the breast in an attempt to distinguish benign fluid-filled cysts from other lesions.

If the radiologist should ask to immediately aspirate a suspicious cyst or to immediately biopsy a suspicious lump, decline such on-the-spot procedures unless your oncologist has told you that this radiologist is experienced with handling lymphoma biopsies. It is, of course, wisest to do an assessment of the radiologist's capabilities before making your mammography appointment so that no extra delays are encountered if you do need an aspiration or biopsy.

Pain

Many women report discomfort, minor pain, or moderate pain during breast compression. Some women report a great deal of pain. If you have had previous breast surgery or breast implants, you may experience pain that is qualitatively or quantitatively different from that experienced by other women.

Recovery

Many women report a bruise-like pain or a discharge from the nipple for a day or two. Report these after-effects to your oncologist and your primary care doctor.

Risks

Some researchers believe that the accumulated dose of radiation delivered to breast tissue over a lifetime may increase a woman's risk of getting breast cancer. This, of course, must be weighed against the risk of failing to detect a breast cancer or breast MALT lymphoma. The risk associated with bruising or discharge from the nipple is thought to be minor or absent.

MRI (magnetic resonance imaging)

This outpatient test uses large magnets and radio waves to cause the different atoms that make up our cells to vibrate at different speeds. The different speeds are then mapped by a computer into an image of the body part being examined. MRI is better than a CT scan for imaging soft tissue, such as cartilage or the brain.

Preparation

You will be asked to lie on a table that moves in and out of the tunnel-shaped MRI machine. The body part being scanned may be positioned within a basket-like brace to help keep the position chosen by the technician.

MRI machines make hammering noises because the magnets are being repositioned constantly while the images are being generated. The technician will supply you with disposable earplugs.

A contrast agent may be injected for imaging certain organs. Imaging the brain, for example, is sometimes facilitated by injecting a very safe agent called gadolinium. Ask the technician about the risk associated with the agent being used, and tell her if you have any allergies or problems with blood clotting.

Some people find the enclosed models of MRI machines claustrophobic. Certain MRI machines have an open gazebo-like design to reduce claustrophobia, with the magnets overhead supported on pillars; others are made of clear plastic. While images from open models may be distinct enough for diagnosing knee problems, for example, they might not be detailed enough for mapping the brain.

If you're claustrophobic, there are several things that will help, such as knowing that there is a two-way speaker inside the machine so that the technician can hear you if you ask for help, and that you, in turn, can hear him. There is also a hand-held beeping summons that you can press if you feel tense. Most facilities have a sound system and will let you choose the music. You may also notice that relaxing photographs have been taped to the inside of the machine. Fans circulate fresh air into the tunnel at all times. It's also possible that, unless your head is being imaged, only part of your body will be within the machine and your head may not. Most relaxing of all may be the thought that this is seventeen million dollars of technology, and for one hour, it's all yours.

Some people, on the other hand, report that the MRI experience is comforting, like a return to the womb. In fact, a friend reports that he likes to have an MRI because it's the only place where nobody can interrupt him.

If you still feel that claustrophobia will be a serious problem, ask your doctor whether a sedative would interfere with the imaging process.

Method

An initial scan to set benchmarks is done rapidly using no contrast agent. A second scan for finer detail is then repeated at slower speed. If a contrast agent is to be used, it is injected into a vein in the arm before the second scan. Although sound is muted by earplugs, you will hear hammering noises that vary in speed and pitch. While being scanned, one must remain as still as possible, but breathing is not restricted as it sometimes is during a CT scan.

A scan of the knee or brain, for example, takes about forty minutes. After scanning is complete, there is a five- to ten-minute wait while the computer analyzes and maps the signals generated by the magnets. The technician will check the resulting images to be sure they are readable.

Pain

The imaging process is painless, although you may feel a slight sting or warmth during injection if a contrast agent is used.

Recovery

If a contrast agent is used, temporary changes in the color of skin, urine, or feces are possible.

Risks

There may be risks of an allergic reaction associated with specific contrast agents; ask your doctor or the technician. As always, there is a very slight risk of infection or minor, painless bruising at the injection site.

MUGA scan (multiple gated acquisition scan, gated blood pool scan, radionuclide ventriculography [RNV])

This outpatient test is used following certain chemotherapies to determine if the heart has been damaged so that an assessment can be made regarding how much additional chemotherapy can be administered safely. It is done both before and after cancer treatment to assess pre- and post-chemotherapy heart function.

Preparation

You may be asked to restrict food or caffeine intake for about three hours prior to the test. Wear comfortable clothing, because you may be walking on a treadmill or riding a stationary bicycle for about fifteen minutes.

Method

A safe, mildly radioactive contrast agent such as technetium-99 or thallium is injected into your forearm and subsequently collects in the heart, arteries, and veins. Sometimes a binding agent for the contrast agent is injected first. Alternately, a small amount of blood may be drawn, and the contrast and binding agents mixed with this blood and reinjected. You may be resting, exercising for fifteen minutes, or both while this test is performed. The scanning camera will be placed above your chest if you are lying down or in front of your chest if you are exercising. For the resting scan you must hold quite still.

An electrocardiograph machine may be used at the same time. Its electrodes will be attached to about six areas of your rib cage using sticky bandages.

> *Two weeks after my first chemotherapy, I had a MUGA scan done to check the health of my heart since the Adriamycin in the CHOP can be very damaging to the heart. There was nothing to this test, but I was disappointed that they couldn't use my catheter and instead had to inject the dye in my arm. A small amount of blood was drawn from my arm and then mixed with a radioactive tracer. This sat for thirty minutes and then was reinjected into my arm for the pictures. All in all, the procedure took about sixty minutes total: thirty minutes of waiting and thirty minutes of pictures, once without the dye and then again with.*

Pain

Minimal pain is possible at the injection site. If you experience chest pain during this test, tell the technician immediately.

Risks

There is a very slight risk of developing cancer associated with the very small amount of radioactive material used—more so if you have had many previous x-rays, CT scans, radiation therapy, or other procedures that use radioactive agents, as radiation dose is cumulative. There is a slight risk of infection at the injection site.

Needle biopsy (fine-needle aspiration, CT-guided needle biopsy, percutaneous biopsy)

This outpatient test is a means for diagnosing non-Hodgkin's lymphomas that are not contained within a lymph node or that may have affected other organs such as the liver. Biopsies of suspected lymphomas are sometimes done with a needle instead of an incision. Organs commonly examined using needle biopsy are the thyroid, kidney, liver, lung, breast, uterine cervix, pancreas, salivary gland, spinal fluid, and bone marrow. Bone marrow biopsies and spinal taps will be discussed separately.

This test is not considered a good choice for identifying lymphoma within a node. The architecture of the entire lymph node contributes important information for the diagnosis; needle biopsy cannot retrieve the entire node. Indeed, at times needle biopsy retrieves no cancerous tissue. Instead, a healthy part of the cancerous node is mistakenly sampled, or no tissue at all can be sampled because malignant nodes can be dense, inaspirable tissue.

This procedure can be helpful, however, to determine the recurrence of a lymphoma, and in these cases, flow cytometry and morphological studies often are done to evaluate the suspected recurrence.

Preparation

You may be asked to fast for twelve hours before the procedure if a sedative or general anesthetic will be used, or if the tissue being biopsied is part of the digestive system. Prior to biopsy of the uterine cervix, you should not have sexual intercourse for twenty-four hours. Blood or urine samples may be collected prior to the biopsy. For children, ask the doctor if the procedure can be done under sedation or general anesthesia, or if EMLA cream can be applied at the site of the puncture two hours before surgery. Bring comfortable clothing to wear afterward, and plan on not being able to walk or drive alone after a sedative or general anesthetic is used.

Method

You will be lying flat on a table for most such biopsies, although lung biopsies may be done while you're either lying flat or seated. The skin will be cleaned. A local anesthetic will be injected, or a sedative or general anesthetic may be given by injection or by inhalation, or, if a fine-needle biopsy is planned, no anesthetic may be used. Directly before the biopsy, the area of interest may be imaged by CT scan or x-ray, and the skin above may be targeted with ink or dye. Depending on the organ being examined, you may be asked to regulate your breathing or to hold quite still during the biopsy. A tiny incision is made and the biopsy needle is inserted through the incision. For kidney biopsies, a guide needle may be used first. A small amount of tissue is drawn (aspirated) into the syringe. The needle is withdrawn, pressure is applied to halt bleeding, a bandage is applied—no stitches are required—and the tissue is sent to the pathology lab for analysis.

For breast biopsies, stereotactic needle biopsies, which are computer-guided and very rapid, are sometimes performed. While you are lying face-down on a table equipped with an area to accommodate the breast, the tissue of interest is mapped from several angles. The automated biopsy needle enters and exits the breast within seconds.

Pain

A slight sting from injected anesthetic or fine-needle biopsy is common. Depending on which organ is being biopsied, you may feel pressure, a brief, sharp pain, a dull, deep ache, or cramping. For liver or other digestive tract biopsies, you may feel pain in the shoulder. Tenderness or bruising may exist at the site of the biopsy and within any intervening muscle tissue for three to seven days. Some physicians prescribe Tylenol or Tylenol/codeine combinations for the aftereffects.

Recovery

After biopsy of the uterine cervix, you may be asked to forego sexual intercourse for seven days. Following kidney biopsies, you may be asked to lie on your back for twelve to twenty-four hours, and you may note blood in your urine for twenty-four hours.

Risks

Risks of organ failure while under general anesthesia, of infection, of bleeding, internal or external, at the site of the puncture, or of injury to adjacent organs exist. For lung biopsies, risk of a collapsed lung exists, and any difficulty breathing should be reported immediately to your doctor. For kidney biopsies, blood in the urine may persist beyond twenty-four hours and should be reported to your doctor.

Node biopsy (excisional biopsy)

This test is the best means for the diagnosis of nodal non-Hodgkin's lymphomas. It is usually, but not always, an outpatient procedure. An inpatient stay usually is necessary if the node being biopsied is in the abdomen (see "Abdominal surgery").

Preparation

No physical preparations are necessary. For children, however, ask the doctor if EMLA cream can be applied at the site of the incision two hours before surgery.

Method

While lying flat on a table, the area above the node will be cleaned and a local anesthetic will be injected. At times a general anesthetic is given by injection or by inhalation, but this is uncommon. An incision is made, the entire node is removed, and the incision is stitched. The node is sent to the pathology lab for analysis.

The surgeon and the pathologist must coordinate the preparation of the node for pathology after its removal.

Pain

A slight sting from the local anesthetic is common. Tenderness may exist at the site of the biopsy for three to seven days.

Recovery

You may be instructed to keep the incision dry until the stitches are removed. Stitches usually are removed in seven to ten days.

Risks

A slight risk of organ failure while under general anesthesia exists. A slight risk of infection or bleeding at the site of the incision exists.

PCR (polymerase chain reaction)

See "Blood tests."

Sigmoidoscopy

See "Endoscopy."

Sonogram (ultrasound, sonography)

An outpatient procedure, sonography creates a map of how your body structures appear when sound waves echo from them. The sonography equipment includes a wand that generates sound waves and a microphone for sensing the echoes the sound waves generate. The wave signal is passed to a computer that reformats the signals into a picture of body organs on a screen.

Bone interferes with sonography, so scanning the brain with this equipment is not successful using the equipment readily available today.

Color Doppler ultrasound is specialized sonography that can detect the speed and direction of blood flow within the body. The differences appear as different colors. This is useful because some tumors commandeer a large blood supply, and this excessive blood supply may be visible and meaningful using color Doppler ultrasound. A common use today is visualization of the ovaries and breasts to distinguish fluid-filled cysts from solid tumors.

Preparation

For a pelvic sonogram, you may be asked to drink large quantities of water, because the bladder acts as a window for sound waves when it is very full.

Method

You will be lying on a table while the technician gently presses the wand over your body. Depending on what body part is being imaged, you may be asked to remove certain items of clothing and to wear a sheet in their place. The technician will first apply warmed gel to your skin to make the wand move smoothly. She may ask you to tilt your body and to maintain the tilt with your muscles, or she may place pillows under you.

For a transvaginal ultrasound, she will apply warm gel to a special wand and ask you to insert it comfortably into your vagina. Once in place, she will guide it from side to side to visualize the uterus and ovaries. This specialized wand is quite long, which means that the technician's hands are not very close to your private body parts, and, being covered by a sheet, you probably won't feel that your body is overly exposed to a stranger.

If you are having pelvic sonography along with a second sonographic scan, ask the technician to do the pelvic scan first so that you can empty your bladder.

Many sonography facilities have an overhead screen so that you can see the same image the technician is seeing.

Pain

Sonography is not painful. Having to maintain a very full bladder for a pelvic sonogram is uncomfortable.

Risks

There are no known risks associated with sonography.

Recovery

There are no recovery issues following sonography.

SPECT or SPET (single positron emission computed tomography)

See "Gallium scan."

Spinal tap (lumbar puncture)

This outpatient test collects a sample of cerebrospinal fluid (CSF) that surrounds the spine and brain. For the non-Hodgkin's lymphomas, CSF usually is examined for the presence of cancer cells, but it also may be collected for many other reasons, such as identifying opportunistic organisms that may gain a foothold during chemotherapy.

Preparation

No physical preparation is necessary.

Method

You will be asked to lie on your side with your knees pulled up to your chest and your chin down on your collarbone during the drawing of the fluid, which takes only a few minutes. The area around your lower spine will be cleaned and a local anesthetic will be injected. After the anesthetic has taken effect, a needle will be inserted between two bones of your backbone (lumbar vertebrae) to tap the fluid that lies under the membrane that surrounds your spinal column. Once the needle is inserted, you must hold very still in the curved position to avoid spinal damage. The spinal fluid is drawn into the syringe, the needle is removed, brief pressure is applied to stop bleeding, and a small bandage is applied.

Immediately after I was admitted to the hospital for my first high-dose chemotherapy session, I underwent a spinal tap. I had never had a spinal tap before, but I recalled the procedure from my student nursing days. Without that experience, I think I would have surmised that this is just about as barbaric as the practice of medicine could get…but of course subsequent elements of my treatment would far surpass the spinal tap in that category.

The physician who must have pulled the short straw came in with a terse introduction and sat right down to begin, instructing me to relax. As if it's that simple: a man with a long needle positioned where you cannot see it is telling you to relax.

Lying on my side was unsuccessful—when I felt the skin punctured, my natural reflex was to snap my spine straight, closing the space between the vertebrae and therefore any opportunity to insert the needle into the spinal fluid. So I sat up and bent over and tried to think of other things—and somehow that worked, even though it took two tries. It wasn't all that painful, just frustrating.

Surely there is better preparation for patients prior to receiving these types of tests. (I wanted to know everything, and after that I made sure the hospital staff knew as well.) I was tempted to ask my lucky physician to come back so I could try one on him.

Pain

Some people report a brief, sharp pain as the needle enters the membrane. Others report pronounced pressure until the needle is properly positioned. Some people report severe headache after the procedure, especially if they were not able to lie flat afterward for the six or eight hours recommended.

Recovery

You must lie flat for six to eight hours after this procedure to allow your body to replace and redistribute spinal fluid surrounding the spine and the brain. This posture prevents headache.

Risks

A serious risk of spinal damage or paralysis exists if movement during the procedure displaces the needle. Slight risks of infection at the injection sites or of bleeding into the spinal column exist. Risk of headache exists, especially if the patient does not lie flat for several hours after the procedure.

Thallium scan

A thallium scan for studying the heart is very similar to a MUGA scan, described in its own section. A thallium scan for locating lymphoma tumors is very similar to a gallium scan, also described in its own section.

Ultrasound (ultrasonography, sonogram)

See "Sonography."

X-rays (radiographic studies)

X-ray imaging may be used early in the diagnostic process to detect unusual masses and determine the extent of disease in the chest, although chest x-ray studies in the absence of a biopsied lymph node cannot positively diagnose a lymphoma. During treatment, x-rays can be used to locate intestinal blockages caused by certain chemotherapies and to detect other secondary conditions. X-ray imaging is diagnostic and is different from x-radiation therapy in that it delivers much lower doses of radiation to tissue.

X-ray studies are an outpatient procedure.

Preparation

You may be asked to fast overnight, to use a laxative, to purchase and drink a contrast agent, or to drink copious amounts of water if x-ray imaging studies of your colon or kidneys are planned.

If your studies will require an iodine-based contrast agent, as is used for certain x-ray studies of the kidneys, be sure to tell your doctor and the staff doing the test if you have thyroid disease or are allergic to iodine in seafood or other sources. A non-ionizing version of the contrast agent can be substituted.

If you have internal staples from a previous surgery or pieces of metal embedded in your body from a previous injury, tell the technician. They represent no danger to you during the x-ray session, but may appear on the film as unexplained phenomena.

Method

X-rays are taken while you are sitting, standing, or lying in a carefully chosen position that has been aligned with the x-ray machine. It is important to maintain the position that was chosen and to remain very still until the technician says you can relax.

For some studies of the stomach or bowels, you may be required to drink a contrast agent while the x-rays are being taken.

For some bowel studies, an enema may be administered to fill the lower bowel with a contrast agent. Hospitals with the latest equipment will help you retain the fluid with an inflatable bulb that is part of the enema package and is inserted just inside the rectum and painlessly inflated when correctly positioned. If this newer equipment is not available, you will be expected to retain the contrast agent using rectal muscles alone for up to ten or fifteen minutes. While not painful, this may be uncomfortable, because in these circumstances the urge to empty the bowel is quite strong.

Pain

X-ray studies are painless. However, if a contrast agent such as dye is needed, it may be injected into a vein, causing minor discomfort (see "Blood tests"). Some studies require positioning of the body that may be temporarily uncomfortable if, for example, you suffer from back pain. If you are having a barium enema, ask the technician to let you remove the nozzle of the enema yourself when the test is complete to reduce the chance of rectal discomfort.

Recovery

If you have had a study that required a contrast agent in the stomach, small intestine, or large intestine, you may experience gas, diarrhea, or constipation for one to three days afterward. Drinking large amounts of water will hasten the removal of the contrast agent from the digestive tract. If you have had a contrast agent injected, you may have a harmless and temporary discoloration of the urine or skin for several days afterward. If you are sensitive to iodine or have a thyroid condition, you may feel fatigue for several days after receiving an iodine-based contrast agent.

Risks

X-ray studies, if repeated over and over, may deliver enough radiation to body tissue to cause health problems later in life, such as lung, thyroid, or breast cancers.

CHAPTER 6

How the NHLs Are Treated

There are no such things as incurable,
there are only things for which
man has not found a cure.

—Bernard Baruch

The non-Hodgkin's lymphomas are a collection of diseases. How they are treated depends on what type of NHL is found; the location of the tumor or tumors; the number of tumors; how rapidly the tumors are progressing; the health of the patient, including HIV status; and her willingness to undergo certain therapies, including promising experimental therapies in clinical trials.

In this chapter, we will discuss the theories behind chemotherapy, radiation therapy, marrow transplantation, and biological treatments. (Marrow transplantation is discussed fully in Chapter 20, *Transplantation.*) Typical treatments used today against many of the various types of NHL will be outlined. However, full details of all treatments for all subtypes of NHL cannot be covered in a chapter of this length. Several excellent references for additional information are listed in Appendix A, *Resources.*

This chapter will not outline which treatment is best for you, as such information changes continually with treatment, research, and time. Nor will this chapter discuss rare treatments used outside the U.S. and Canada or treatments classified as alternative. Rather, we list generally accepted standards of care for broad classes of NHL at the time this book was written. These descriptions are provided to give you an overview of treatments and a starting point to find out more about the treatments your doctors recommend for you.

The experiences of receiving treatment are described in Chapters 7 and 8, *What to Expect During Chemotherapy* and *What to Expect During Radiotherapy*.

The information in this chapter is drawn from the National Cancer Institute's NHL *State-of-the-Art Treatment Statements* for physicians, and is supplemented from various sources, such as the second edition of Magrath's *The Non-Hodgkin's Lymphomas*, as well as current research papers.

A word of caution

Most medical writers approach a chapter such as this one with great caution, and so should the reader. The reason is this: no single publication of this type can possibly reflect current progress in cancer research.

Few formal vehicles of communication, printed or otherwise, can reflect the continually evolving judgment of the finest researchers in the field. None is permitted to publish very early results from promising clinical trials until the results are vetted by peer review. The best any medium can hope to capture is a snapshot of theories and findings as understood at the moment.

For your needs in battling NHL, that's not good enough.

As you read this chapter, you must keep in mind that, no matter how recent the copyright date in the opening pages of this or any other medical book, you will always get the latest information on the best way to treat your disease from the medical doctors and researchers in the trenches. Your oncologist, who knows how to tailor your treatment and schedule to suit your circumstances, may recommend treatment options that are different from those you'll read here or elsewhere. You should always verify treatment information with your doctor, and you should attempt to find the very latest information on treatment using reliable sources such as peer-reviewed medical journals. How to find this information is discussed in Chapter 24, *Researching Your Lymphoma*.

Please note that cell histology (cell appearance), which is currently heavily used to distinguish subtypes of NHL, may be eclipsed by the evolving discipline of immunogenetics for the identification and treatment of the non-Hodgkin's lymphomas. The design and function of monoclonal antibodies, for example, are based on genetic characteristics of cancer cells and their resulting physical characteristics and immunologic behavior. This means that current attempts to describe treatments based on terms such as "indolent," "aggressive," or "diffuse" may become outdated and misleading if treatments are designed that work equally well on both indolent and aggressive sub-types of NHL.

Currently, there are about forty multi-drug chemotherapy regimens used to treat the NHLs. New combinations and agents arise almost daily, so don't be concerned if you don't see your regimen mentioned in this chapter. Instead, ask your doctor for a breakdown of the drugs used in your regimen, and for an explanation of its superiority over other approaches and its appropriate-ness for your case. For translations of combination chemotherapies described as acronyms, such as CHOP or CVP, and for common single drugs and their abbreviations, see Appendix E, *Common Chemotherapies*.

Theories of treatment

Chemotherapy and radiotherapy regimens currently used against NHL work by interfering with a cancer cell's ability to sustain and reproduce itself.

Surgery, with a few exceptions, generally is a means to remove a badly dis-eased organ or to supply biopsy material rather than a method to achieve a cure.

Biological therapies work in a variety of ways, usually by mimicking or emphasizing a natural body process.

Marrow or stem cell transplantation or rescue allow very high, marrow-killing doses of chemotherapy and radiation therapy to be used.

In order to understand how each of these cancer treatments work, we first need to understand a bit about cell division and genetics.

DNA and cancer

Chemotherapy and radiation are often described as effective at killing rap-idly dividing cells. This section describes the events that take place as cells divide, and describes some of the points in a cancer cell's division when it is most vulnerable to cancer therapies.

Human DNA is stored on 46 paired chromosomes. With a few exceptions, each cell in our body has one copy of all 46 chromosomes, coiled tightly in a ball, stored in the cell nucleus.

Each chromosome is composed of two long strings of genes held together like a ladder, with rungs consisting of electrochemical bonds. Because the rungs and sides of the ladder are not symmetrical, the ladder twists along its length. Owing to this configuration, a strand of DNA often is referred to as a double helix.

When a cell begins dividing, DNA relaxes out of its balled shape. On each strand of DNA (chromosome), the ladder rungs break, giving two separate strings of genes. These gene strings are processed by polymerase enzymes that are present in the nucleus for creating and lengthening DNA strings. When this process is complete, an exact replica of each chromosome exists, the cell has 92 chromosomes—double its usual number—and can commence dividing in two.

In a normal cell, the process of replication and division is a scheduled, orderly process. In a cancer cell, it's a continual, dictatorial annexing of bodily resources, nutrition, and space.

During the process of replication, when DNA is uncoiled and separated, it is vulnerable to damage. A large proportion of each cell's time and energy is devoted to making sure our DNA is repaired, intact, functional, and correctly copied.

In most tumors, and especially in high-grade NHLs, cancer cells divide rapidly, so their DNA is untwisted and separated—naked—more often than that of a healthy cell. Naked DNA is more vulnerable to damage induced by many substances, including chemotherapy and radiation. When the DNA of a cancer cell is damaged, it may die, or, at the very least, cease being able to replicate. This immobilization deprives it of the essence of cancer: continuous, uncontrolled cell division and growth.

Most cancer treatments used today exploit the vulnerability of a cancer cell's naked DNA, and the fact that cancer cells divide more rapidly than most normal cells.

Newer treatments that exploit other cellular characteristics and other bodily processes, such as the growth of new blood vessels, are described later in this chapter in the section "How biological therapies work," and in Chapter 23, *The Future of Therapy.*

How NHL chemotherapies work

There are five categories of chemotherapy drugs used for NHL: topo-isomerase inhibitors, tubulin binding agents, alkylating agents, antimetabo-lites, and immune suppressants. In addition, there are several drugs used against NHL that don't fit well into any of these five categories, and several that are used to offset the dangerous effects of chemotherapy.

Topoisomerase inhibitors

Topoisomerases are enzymes our cells use to break DNA bonds before copy-ing and repair the breaks after copying. Topoisomerase inhibitors interfere with DNA repair, causing the cancer cell to die, because damaged DNA can-not be translated into proteins, such as transport and digestive proteins, that each cell needs to breathe or eat. Some topoisomerase inhibitors currently used against NHL are doxorubicin, idarubicin, mitoxantrone, daunorubicin, etoposide, and camptothecin. Camptothecin, although chemically a plant-derived alkaloid, does not behave as do the tubulin-binding vinca alkaloids vincristine, vinblastine, and vindesine. It acts instead as a topoisomerase I inhibitor. Doxorubicin, idarubicin, and daunorubicin are unique as topo-isomerase inhibitors because they are both antibiotics and cardiotoxic.

Tubulin binding agents

When a cell has made a copy of all of its chromosomes and is ready to divide, spindles made of tubulin form to pull the two copies of each chro-mosome apart into two identical clusters of 46 chromosomes apiece. Tubu-lin binding agents stop spindles from forming, thus stopping the cell from dividing. Some tubulin binding agents currently used against NHL are vinc-ristine, vinblastine, vindesine, and paclitaxel.

Alkylating agents

Alkylating agents form new bonds within the double twisted DNA strand that resemble the ladder rungs described in the earlier section, "DNA and cancer." This disrupts many normal functions of DNA, including its ability to divide. Alkylating agents are able to affect a cancer cell's DNA even when the DNA is not uncoiled and separated—in other words, they are not cell-cycle specific—which may explain their relatively high activity against many cancers. Some alkylating agents currently used against NHL are mechlore-thamine, chlorambucil, cyclophosphamide, ifosfamide, procarbazine, dacar-bazine, and CCNU.

Antimetabolites

As the word "antimetabolite" implies, these substances in some way impede the cell's metabolism—its building up and breaking down of cell parts. Each of the antimetabolites used for NHL works a bit differently from the others.

- L-asparaginase destroys asparagine, which the cell needs for DNA and RNA synthesis.

- Cytosine arabinoside (Cytarabine, ARA-C) is a close copy of deoxycyti-dine, a natural bodily substance that lengthens a DNA strand as it's being copied. ARA-C substitutes in deoxycytidine's place, and, because ARA-C differs from deoxycytidine in critical ways, the DNA is not able to be copied.

- Fludarabine, pentostatin, and 2-CDA, although their exact mechanisms of action are unknown, appear to interfere with certain enzymes that aid in copying, lengthening, or repairing DNA and perhaps RNA.

- 5-fluorouracil is incorporated into RNA and DNA in place of uracil, causing malfunction of protein synthesis.

- Hydroxyurea blocks ribonucleotide reductase, without which DNA synthesis is impaired.

- Methotrexate is a folate antagonist. Folate or folic acid, a B vitamin found in many green vegetables is needed to make the building blocks of DNA, purines and pyrimidines. If these are absent, new copies of DNA cannot be made. Methotrexate blocks the action of an enzyme called dihydrofolate reductase, which is necessary for the metabolism of folate.

- Mercaptopurine can be substituted in DNA in place of adenine, leading to a misreading of the DNA message. It also can be converted to a sub-stance called a nucleotide that inhibits manufacture of a group of build-ing blocks called purines which are needed for RNA and DNA synthesis.

- Mitoguazone disrupts polyamine manufacture (biosynthesis), thus dis-rupting formation of DNA.

- Thioguanine can be substituted into DNA in place of guanine, causing misreading of the DNA message, or it can be processed and converted to a DNA building block that inhibits an enzyme essential for RNA and DNA synthesis.

Immune suppressants

Glucocorticoids such as dexamethasone, prednisone, and methylprednisolone are manmade copies of the human corticosteroid hydrocortisone normally produced by the adrenal glands. They're used against hematologic cancers—lymphomas and leukemias, cancers of the white blood cells—to suppress the rampant growth of cancerous white blood cells.

Rescue drugs

Rescue drugs are used to offset certain dangerous effects of chemotherapy:

- **Leucovorin** is folinic acid, one of the B vitamins. It's used several days after methotrexate to offset the toxicity of this folate antagonist and allow the building of DNA to resume in healthy cells.

- **Allopurinol** is used to protect kidneys from urate nephropathy, a possible aspect of tumor lysis syndrome. Urate nephropathy can arise spontaneously in patients with a high tumor mass.

- **Mesna** protects the bladder by offsetting the negative effects of cyclophosphamide metabolites called acroleins, which are excreted in urine and can cause a severe form of hemorrhagic cystitis.

Drugs that don't fit well into other categories

These are described in Appendix E as *idiosyncratic agents*, and include:

- **Cisplatin**. Similar to the alkylating agents, platinum-based cisplatin forms rung-like cross-links on the DNA ladder that disrupts DNA function, including replication. Like the alkylating agents, cisplatin is able to affect a cancer cell's DNA even when the DNA is not uncoiled and separated.

- **Bleomycin**. Made from parts of the fungus *Streptomyces vesticillis*, bleomycin joins with one form of iron to create breaks in the DNA strands. When DNA strands are broken, many cell processes, including replication, cannot proceed.

How radiotherapy works

Radiation therapy interferes with the growth and replication of cancer cells by changing the structure of molecules that make up the cell's DNA.

A beam of radiation, which is a stream of energy, can knock the electrons from the atoms that make up the molecules of DNA. Removing electrons changes the structure of critical molecules, after which the DNA strand can no longer be copied, lengthened, paired, and twined.

Similar damage is possible in healthy cells that happen to be in the path of the radiation beam, especially if they are in the process of dividing, but cancerous cells are more likely to be disturbed by radiation because their DNA is more often uncoiled and separated.

Sometimes only local or involved-field radiation is used. This targets only the tumor and not the surrounding or extended fields. Irradiating extended fields has proven to be unhelpful against many NHLs, which do not often spread in an orderly, adjacent way.

Occasionally an area called the mantle field, involving portions of the chest, is irradiated if the tumor is in this area (the mediastinum) or is causing superior vena cava syndrome (SVCS). SVCS is a collection of symptoms including swelling of the trunk, neck, face, or arms, or their veins; difficulty breathing; cough; hoarseness; eye swelling, redness, or vision changes; chest pain; upper back pain or numbness; dizziness, headache, nosebleed; or changed cognitive abilities or mood. SVCS arises when the superior vena cava—a large vein that drains blood from the head, upper trunk, and arms—is blocked by a tumor, blood clot, or, most often, by compression owing to a nearby chest tumor or enlarged lymph node. The increased pressure in this system of veins causes fluid leakage and swelling in areas that are drained by branches of the SVC.

Total body irradiation (TBI) may be used to prepare NHL patients for a bone marrow transplant.

When radiotherapy is used for children, very undesirable side effects may occur many years after treatment. To avoid these serious effects, radiotherapy is avoided as treatment for children with NHL, except to control symptoms that are not responding to any other treatment.

How phototherapy works

Phototherapy, or light therapy, can be used for types of NHL that emerge primarily in the skin, and can be used either as single-agent treatment or as an adjunct to other treatment.

Researchers have long noted that ultraviolet A sunlight and manmade versions of it have an immunosuppressive effect on the white blood cells in our skin. Because lymphomas are cancers of the white blood cells, immunosuppressant therapies, such as prednisone and phototherapy, can slow or halt their growth. Although natural and manmade UVA light has immunosuppressive effects that are effective against benign diseases such as psoriasis and rheumatoid arthritis, when used alone they are not strong enough to combat the T-cell cutaneous lymphomas.

The immunosuppressive effects of UVA light can be boosted, however, by treating tissue first with photosensitizing compounds that make the effect of light more pronounced. Psoralen, for instance, embeds in DNA and makes it more sensitive to breakage from both natural light and from manmade UVA irradiation.

How biological therapies work

There are a number of biological therapies, and each works differently, but in general, they are manmade copies of natural body substances and enhance the action of these substances. Some biological therapies are also biological response modifiers.

Monoclonal antibodies

Monoclonal antibodies are manmade copies of proteins—antibodies—that our white blood cells secrete. Because a particular cell surface protein, or antigen, attracts a particular antibody, natural antibodies are responsible for attaching to foreign substances in the body, and for initiating an attack against invaders such as viruses and bacteria.

When mass-produced in the laboratory, antibodies can be made all of one type (monoclonal) to target only a certain kind of invader. Because cancer cells are different in some ways from healthy cells, such as in the proteins that extend from their surface, manmade monoclonal antibodies (abbreviated as moabs or mabs) can be made to aim only for cancer cells by sensing these surface proteins. A monoclonal antibody may be naked, or it may be coupled or conjugated with another substance called a payload—a toxic substance such as ricin, or a radioactive substance (radioisotope) such as iodine-131 or yttrium-90. When the conjugated monoclonal antibody attaches to the cancer cell's surface protein, the proximity of the toxic substance damages or kills the cancer cell.

Each monoclonal antibody is a bit different from the next, because each cell surface protein to which it binds plays a slightly different role in the cell's life. For instance, Rituxan, a naked antibody, couples with the surface antigen CD20 on the cancer cell and causes the cell to burst. Rituxan has also been shown to resensitize drug-resistant B-cell lymphomas to chemotherapy. Monoclonal antibodies that target the CD22 cell surface antigen, on the other hand, can take advantage of this antigen's tendency to cause whatever attaches to it to be carried inside the cell.

Cytokines

Cytokines are substances that the body uses to trigger other immunologic events.

- **Interferons.** Interferon-alfa-2B, the interferon most often used in NHL therapy, halts growth, forces cells to maturity, and interrupts cell motility. It stabilizes NHL, and in some cases, kills it.

- **Interleukins.** There are several interleukins; the one best studied for use against cancer is interleukin-2. IL-2 stimulates growth and maturation of white blood cells (lymphocytes), and can direct lymphocytes to attack tumors.

- **TNF.** Tumor necrosis factor appears to have a role in killing both healthy and cancerous cells.

Colony stimulating factors

Colony stimulating factors are substances that cause growth of new cells.

- **G-CSF.** Granulocyte colony stimulating factor is a manmade copy of a protein that causes bone marrow to grow new white blood cells called neutrophils.

- **GM-CSF.** Granulocyte-macrophage colony stimulating factor, like G-CSF, is a manmade copy of a protein that causes bone marrow to grow both new white blood cells called neutrophils and new monocytes. Macrophages, which develop from monocytes, are cells that surround and eat foreign material and microorganisms in the body.

- EPO. Erythropoietin, like the colony stimulating factors, is a manmade copy of a substance made by the kidneys (and in lesser quantities by other organs, such as the liver and adrenal glands) that causes bone marrow to produce new red blood cells.

- TPO. Thrombopoietin, like G-CSF and EPO, is a manmade copy of a body product that causes bone marrow to grow new platelets.

Tumor vaccines

For reasons still unknown, at some point the body stops attacking cancer cells, even though evidence suggests that it does mount an immune attack against cancer cells when they are still small and few in number. Tumor vaccines are an attempt to re-educate the body to attack tumor cells.

How surgery is used

Surgery is rarely used as a means to cure NHL. Rather, surgery may be used in the following ways:

- Surgery may be the best means of obtaining tissue for diagnosis.

- Surgical removal of certain organs heavily affected by NHL, such as the spleen or thyroid, may be recommended to control symptoms. Such instances of extranodal disease usually relapse elsewhere; therefore, chemotherapy usually is used in these cases, whether surgery is used or not.

- Surgery may be used to reduce tumor volume before other treatments, but it is more common to use radiation therapy for this purpose, except in specific cases such as intestinal involvement of aggressive lymphomas.

If your spleen is removed, you should discuss with your doctor the need to be revaccinated every few years with pneumococcal, *Haemophilus influenzae* type b, and meningococcal vaccines. The risk of being overwhelmed by agents capable of producing encapsulated infections is higher in those lacking a spleen.

How marrow or stem cell transplantation works

Transplantation may be recommended as first-line treatment if the patient has several bad-risk features, or if the lymphoma is particularly aggressive.

Reintroducing marrow or stem cells to the body after high-dose treatment permits very high doses of chemotherapy or radiotherapy to be used—high enough to destroy bone marrow. Moreover, if donor marrow is used, the attack of incoming alien white blood cells against your tissues, called a graft-versus-host reaction, also confers a graft-versus-lymphoma effect that may overcome any residual cancer cells.

If your doctor has recommended transplantation, ask her for help weighing the risks and benefits, particularly for an allogeneic (donor marrow) transplant. At the time of this writing, the mortality rate for an allogeneic transplant ranges from 15 to 25 percent associated with the procedure itself, that is, death associated with treatment, not from a relapse of disease. Offsetting this is preliminary evidence that allogeneic transplantation may offer the best hope for cure. Autologous (self) transplantation, while entailing a much lower treatment-related risk of about 3 percent, usually lacks the graft-versus-lymphoma effect that appears to be responsible for the higher number of relapse-free patients following allogeneic transplantation.

Marrow and stem cell transplantation procedures are discussed in detail in Chapter 20.

Treatment of special groups

Some individuals require special consideration when facing treatment owing to vulnerabilities associated with age or other health problems.

Treatment of children

The NHLs most commonly found in children are the small noncleaved cell (Burkitt's or Burkitt-like) lymphomas, large-cell lymphomas, and lymphoblastic lymphoma that melds into acute lymphoblastic leukemia, depending on a somewhat arbitrary definition that considers the amount of bone marrow involvement.

All parents of children with non-Hodgkin's lymphoma should consider enrolling their child in a clinical trial. The most current methodologies for dealing with what are usually aggressive cancers can be found in these settings. Seventy-five percent of children with cancer are treated in clinical trials, and your oncologist will almost certainly approach you about this. Call the National Cancer Institute on 1-800-4-CANCER for the pediatric oncology center closest to you.

Because NHL in children frequently is spread throughout the body by the time it is diagnosed, combined chemotherapy treatment using multiple drugs normally is recommended.

According to the National Cancer Institute's PDQ *State-of-the-Art Treatment Statement* for Childhood NHL, evidence is building that radiation therapy for children with NHL is not only of no benefit, but also poses long-term risks to healthy tissue, such as fibrosis and second cancers, that are too dangerous. Thus radiation therapy might best be avoided, except for unusual cases such as primary lymphoma of bone, a rare and distinct form of NHL that is not the same as bone marrow involvement.

Treatment of the elderly

Often, special precautions are taken for those over age sixty-five to avoid taxing healthy organs with toxic treatments. In general, older people have more difficulty metabolizing drugs than do younger people. The concern is heightened if the patient is dealing with any of the illnesses that may accompany aging, such as heart disease or diabetes.

To circumvent problems, a standard chemotherapy regimen may be adapted to the older patient by:

- Using only some fraction of the recommended dose
- Using fewer doses than are given to younger patients
- Substituting a gentler drug for a more toxic one, such as substituting pirarubicin for doxorubicin
- Using longer infusion times to spread out the delivery of some drugs, perhaps by using an implanted pump
- Using shorter infusion times for certain cycle-specific chemotherapies such as vincristine that are increasingly toxic with increased presence, as more cells entering various stages of cell division become exposed

Treatment of the immune-compromised

Immune-compromised patients who may develop NHL as a result of their suppressed immune status are:

- Those who are deliberately immune-suppressed with drugs following organ transplant
- Those with AIDS
- Those with genetic diseases that cause the immune system to fail

NHLs that appear in these patients, especially in AIDS patients, are unique in some respects. Often these NHLs appear first in the brain or other parts of the central nervous system, gastrointestinal tract, body cavity, head, neck, or nasal passages, but often they also are characterized by unusual presentations such as the pancreas, esophagus, anus, or rectum.

Frequently these tumors have not developed from a single (monoclonal) cell line as most other cancers do. In these cases, they often contain evidence of Epstein-Barr (EBV) or human herpesvirus 8 (HHV-8) infections. Usually they are high-grade, aggressive tumors that are difficult to treat.

The threat to survival often is the patient's already lowered immune status, further exacerbated by cytotoxic cancer treatment that permits infection to gain a foothold. Some studies have found that immune-compromised patients do as well following anticancer therapy as the immune-competent do, if careful measures are taken to prevent, detect, and control infection.

For transplant survivors, lowering of immunosuppressive drugs may cause the NHL to recede, especially if the tumor cell line was found to be polyclonal.

For those with AIDS, boosting of CD4+ T-cell counts can cause tumors to regress, especially if the tumor cell line was found to be polyclonal, but the presence of other AIDS-related illness also may affect outcome.

For any immune-compromised patient, excellent nursing care and social support to prevent, detect, and combat infection is needed.

Treatments that might be recommended include:

- Interferon-alfa
- Monoclonal antibodies that target CD20- or CD24-positive B-cells
- Monoclonal antibodies conjugated with toxins such as CD19-ricin

- Radiation therapy for single sites of disease

- Central nervous system treatment with methotrexate or ARA-C

- Antiviral or antiretroviral drugs such as AZT

- Combined chemotherapy as described in the sections on aggressive NHLs, later in this chapter

Classification and staging

Knowing your classification, grade, and staging information gives you a way to compare your diagnosis and recommended treatment to reports in the literature or descriptions of clinical trials. It also gives you the vocabulary you need to speak with medical professionals who might not already be familiar with your case.

Many attempts have been made to categorize the NHLs in a way that is meaningful to the treatment chosen and the best outcome. Nonetheless, owing to the variety of ways NHL can manifest, a unified system has yet to be agreed upon. See Appendix D, *Classification Systems*, for more information.

You should ask your oncologist about your classification and grading information, about which classification system was used—Kiel, Working Formulation, the REAL system, or some amalgam of these—and obtain a copy of your pathology reports.

Because there is such disparity about classifying the NHLs, you should not become alarmed if a treatment described in this chapter as appropriate for another classification is recommended for yours.

Treatment of low-grade disease

Most low-grade NHLs, also called indolent NHLs, if found in the earliest stages—many are not found until quite advanced—are small-cell and follicular, that is, occurring only within the follicles of lymph nodes. Exceptions include the low-grade MALT lymphomas that occur outside lymph nodes in other lymphoid tissue such as the stomach and salivary glands.

Low-grade disease usually progresses slowly at first. As time passes, it may convert to a more aggressive disease with larger cell appearance and diffuse involvement of the entire lymph node instead of just the follicle. This is called *diffuse* disease within the node, but please note that the term "diffuse" may also be used to describe a wider spread of disease throughout the body, or may be used to describe certain types of bone marrow involvement.

It's possible for low-grade and higher-grade disease to coexist in the same patient or even within the same node, and when this is seen, it may be assumed by some practitioners to be a transition to a higher grade and is treated as a higher-grade disease. Treatment for low-grade disease that has converted to aggressive disease is discussed in other sections for the aggressive subtypes of NHL.

It is much more common to find low-grade disease in adults than in children.

The National Cancer Institute recommends that all patients with low-grade disease should consider enrolling in a clinical trial. Many treatments in use today for low-grade disease result in remission, even in long remission, but usually these are not lasting remissions. By examining clinical trials, you may gain access to newer, better treatments years before they are made available to the general public. You and your oncologist should discuss the advantages and disadvantages of this option.

Low-grade disease may be treated with one of the monoclonal antibodies that sense particular cell surface proteins, such as Rituxan, which was approved by the FDA in November 1997, and is specific for the CD20 cell surface antigen.

A watch-and-wait approach may be suggested by your oncologist. This consists of watching for certain blood values to change, for nodes to enlarge, for other organs to become involved, or for the cell type to shift to a more aggressive grade. Visits for examination and testing, including blood tests, CT scans, and perhaps marrow biopsies, may be scheduled every three to six months, or more often, depending on your individual circumstances. This posture is adopted because studies of those treated with chemotherapy in early stages of low-grade NHL have not shown an overall increase in survival over those who wait until disease is more symptomatic to start treatment. As many people with low-grade NHL can live for twelve years or more, five-year survival statistics following treatment must be interpreted very carefully. Ten- or fifteen-year survival statistics are more meaningful.

Low-grade disease may or may not exhibit symptoms initially. If symptoms are present and serious, immediate treatment may be called for.

One survivor describes why some NHL survivors of low-grade disease call "watchful waiting" by another name, "watch and worry":

> *I can tell you it is unnerving at best not knowing when, where, or how "the beast" will strike. I wake up every day and think, "Is today the day?" When it's time for a doctor visit or a CT scan, I think, "Have the nodes grown? Is this the visit when my doctor will tell me it's time for treatment?"*

> *And just try to explain to outsiders that you have cancer, but are receiving no treatment. Outsiders are sometimes confused—sometimes they believe you're "too far gone" for treatment. You can see a look of doom come over their faces. This can be frightening or funny, depending on who's doing it, when, and so on.*

> *For those on watch-and-wait before treatment, there's an eerie aspect concerning our denial. There are moments when we can pretend not to be sick, and we do such a good job of denying our illness that when a node suddenly grows, or when the doctor says it's time for treatment, we feel foolish and betrayed.*

Many research centers are studying the effect of bone marrow or stem cell transplantation on low-grade disease.

Stage I or contiguous stage II low-grade disease

This stage, usually symptomless, can be treated, and might possibly be cured, with local radiation or surgery.

Additional treatments that might be recommended:

- Single chemotherapeutic agent such as fludarabine or chlorambucil
- Interferon
- Monoclonal antibodies

Stage II noncontiguous or stages III/IV low-grade disease

Treatment that might be recommended:

- Single-agent chemotherapeutic agents such as 2-CDA, cyclophosphamide, chlorambucil, or fludarabine

- Combination chemotherapy, such as CVP or CHOP
- Surgery to remove the spleen (splenectomy) if the spleen is affected
- Radiotherapy to selected locations
- Monoclonal antibodies
- Bone marrow transplantation

Recurrent low-grade disease

If low-grade disease relapses to a higher grade, treatment is geared to its grade, as described in the next section, "General treatment of aggressive NHLs."

For relapses that remain low-grade, one of the treatments described in the preceding sections usually is used.

General treatment of aggressive NHLs

The aggressive NHLs include a large group categorized as intermediate- or high-grade disease: low-grade disease converting to a higher grade, lymphoblastic lymphoma, angiocentric lymphoma, angioblastic lymphoma, immunoblastic lymphoma, Burkitt's or the Burkitt-like small noncleaved lymphomas, true histiocytic lymphoma, viral-associated adult T-cell lymphoma/leukemia, and others.

Not surprisingly, the most important determinant in treating the aggressive NHLs is the subtype being treated, some of which have quite specific therapies. An accurate diagnosis is mandatory for selecting the right treatment.

In addition to this general information, see separate discussions later in this chapter for lymphoblastic, small noncleaved (Burkitt's and Burkitt-like), large-cell, MALT, cutaneous T-cell, and extranodal lymphomas.

Stage I or contiguous stage II aggressive disease

According to the National Cancer Institute's PDQ *State-of-the-Art Treatment Statement* for Adult NHL, studies have shown that long-term survival or cure is achieved more often if both chemotherapy and radiation therapy are used for this stage of disease, in spite of its relatively limited spread. Usually CHOP or a related regimen is used, but important differences in treatment exist for many aggressive lymphomas such as the large-cell, lymphoblastic, and small noncleaved cell lymphomas, which are discussed separately later in this chapter.

Your doctor may determine that chemotherapy alone, or radiotherapy alone, is more appropriate for your circumstances than combined chemotherapy and radiotherapy.

Stage II noncontiguous or stages III/IV aggressive disease

Because at these stages disease usually is more widely distributed through the body, combination chemotherapy alone usually is recommended, without radiation, as radiotherapy doses to multiple sites for widespread disease would be too toxic. There may be instances, however, when local radiotherapy is needed to reduce tumor size in one location.

Usually CHOP or a related regimen is used, but important differences in treatment exist for many aggressive lymphomas such as the large-cell, lymphoblastic, and small noncleaved cell lymphomas, which are discussed separately later in this chapter.

Patients at high risk of relapse might be advised to consider autologous or allogeneic bone marrow transplantation.

Other chemotherapeutic regimens used

Some studies have shown that, for many of the aggressive NHLs that respond to anthracycline-based therapies like CHOP, other chemotherapeutic regimens have not emerged as clearly superior to CHOP, but more than forty such similar regimens in addition to CHOP are recorded in the medical literature. Often, alternate regimens containing some of the same drugs used in CHOP are used for a variety of reasons tailored to the specific patient.

Bill's story

Bill is a survivor of high-grade NHL who was treated with both chemotherapy and radiation therapy. He describes his treatment and the side effects, and offers encouragement that the discomfort is temporary:

> I was diagnosed April 1, 1996. I had a swollen neck gland and the back of my tongue had a huge hump on it. The ear, nose, and throat (ENT) doctor took a piece off the back of my tongue, sent me over for x-rays and a CT scan (both negative, by the way). I went back to the ENT doctor in two days and he gave me the news: large B-cell NHL, diffuse. I then went to an oncologist friend who I had known for twenty-five years, though not professionally. He did bone marrow studies, a spinal fluid analysis, more CT scans, all kinds of blood work, and put me to sleep for a gastroenterology look-see…all negative, so he staged it IIA, high grade.

> The tumors completely disappeared with the first CHOP (plus VP-16) treatment, which was administered three days running, every third week. I do recall several times just feeling so bad during treatment. Not nausea or digestive sickness, but just sick. Just about the sickest I've ever been. But it did pass in a few days.

> After the third of these treatments, I suffered a heart attack, but ended up with minimal to no damage. I had two stents implanted in my right coronary artery. I did nicely with that.

> After seven CHOP treatments, I had radiation to the neck area every day for four weeks. I was left with very painful yet numb feet, and tingling in my left arm, which is still there. The neurologist has not found an answer to that. He says numbness results from vincristine, but it ought not to hurt. Rest assured that I was so sick several times that death would have been a relief (not really, but it felt like it).

> One last thing: I did not taper off the prednisone dose, and I have since felt that the precipitous drop in dosage may have been responsible for the sickness. But, while taking it for those five days, I was king of the world, fit to be tied, a bundle of energy—though that got to be less and less with each session.

> Take it easy. Easier said than done, I know, but just recognize the fact that you will not feel well some of the time.

Lymphoblastic lymphoma

This form of lymphoma, usually found in children and young adults, is rapid and aggressive, and often resembles acute lymphoblastic leukemia.

Treatment is begun as soon as possible. If disease has already spread as indicated by staging at levels III or IV, the same highly successful approach that is used for acute lymphoblastic leukemia (ALL) may be used, involving two to three years of treatment, and precautionary treatment of the central nervous system. This treatment is divided into three phases: induction of remission, consolidation of remission, and maintenance. Each phase uses different drugs and timing to eradicate all disease. In adults, areas of bulky tumor involvement may be irradiated to reduce tumor mass.

It is possible for this form of NHL to lodge in the central nervous system. Treatment to kill all cells that may be lingering there might be recommended, consisting of either cranial and spinal irradiation or methotrexate injected into cerebrospinal fluid.

Postremission therapy, called maintenance, which improves the survival odds in this form of NHL, may include short-term intense chemotherapy, longer, less intense chemotherapy, or bone marrow transplantation.

Stages I/II

Several treatment regimens produce good results against early stage lymphoblastic lymphoma. Treatments that might be recommended include:

- Vincristine, doxorubicin, cyclophosphamide, prednisone, mercaptopurine, methotrexate
- CHOP alternating with infusional methotrexate
- COMP
- LMT 81 (LSA2L2 plus methotrexate)
- Sometimes for adults, CHOP plus methotrexate, 6-MP, and l-asparaginase

Stage III

The National Cancer Institute recommends that patients with a large anterior mediastinal (chest) tumor should consider clinical trials, because of the risks associated with superior vena cava syndrome and with treating such a large tumor in this location. (For a description of superior vena cava syndrome, see "How radiotherapy works," earlier in this chapter.)

If the tumor is pressing on the superior vena cava, low-dose radiation may be used to shrink the tumor.

Treatment that might be recommended:

- LSA2L2, a multiphase treatment consisting of induction, consolidation, and maintenance
- LSA2L2 plus high-dose methotrexate
- CHOP, alternating with methotrexate
- ACOP+
- BFM, a multiphase treatment consisting of induction, consolidation, and maintenance
- LMT 81 (LSA2L2 plus methotrexate)
- Addition of VM-26 (teniposide) and ARA-C (cytarabine) to multiphase therapies such as LSA2L2
- Sometimes for adults, CHOP plus methotrexate, 6-MP, and l-asparaginase

Stage IV

Although there are several FDA-approved treatment options available for this stage of disease, the National Cancer Institute recommends that all patients at this stage should consider entering a clinical trial to take advantage of the foremost improvements in treatment.

If you have disseminated lymphoblastic lymphoma, treatment for possible spread to the central nervous system should be considered.

Compression of the superior vena cava may be treated with low-dose radiation.

Treatment that might be recommended:

- LSA2L2, a multiphase treatment consisting of induction, consolidation, and maintenance
- LSA2L2 plus high-dose methotrexate
- BFM, a multiphase treatment consisting of induction, consolidation, and maintenance
- LMT 81 (LSA2L2 plus methotrexate)
- Addition of VM-26 (teniposide) and ARA-C (cytarabine) to multiphase therapies such as LSA2L2
- Sometimes for adults, CHOP plus methotrexate, 6-MP, and l-asparaginase

Recurrent disease

How relapse is treated depends on what treatments were used in the past, and where the disease has recurred. Clinical trials, intensive regimens, other regimens containing drugs not previously used, and bone marrow transplantation are possible choices you should discuss with your doctor.

Small noncleaved cell lymphomas

This category includes Burkitt's as well as the Burkitt-like lymphomas.

Treatment for adults and children is similar, and may include brief, intensive combination chemotherapy, with or without radiation.

Surgical removal of disease in the abdomen may be advantageous if the tumor can be completely removed.

Stages I/II

Treatment that might be recommended:

- COMP
- CHOP
- CHOP plus methotrexate
- BFM 86

- High-intensity, brief-duration treatment: cyclophosphamide, etoposide, vincristine, bleomycin, methotrexate, doxorubicin, allopurinol, and prednisone
- ARA-C, high-dose methotrexate, ifosfamide, and etoposide, if bone marrow or central nervous system involvement is found

Stage III / IV

Although there are several FDA-approved treatment options available for this stage of disease, the National Cancer Institute recommends that all patients at this stage should consider entering a clinical trial to take advantage of the foremost improvements in treatment.

Treatment that might be recommended:

- French LMB-89
- Total B (St. Jude's)
- BFM 86
- ARA-C, high-dose methotrexate, ifosfamide, and etoposide, if bone marrow or central nervous system involvement is found
- High-intensity, brief-duration treatment: cyclophosphamide, etoposide, vincristine, bleomycin, methotrexate, doxorubicin, allopurinol, and prednisone
- For stage IV, modified "total B": cyclophosphamide, doxorubicin, vincristine, methotrexate, cytarabine

Recurrent disease

How relapse is treated depends on what treatments were used in the past and where the disease has recurred. Clinical trials, aggressive or intensive regimens, other regimens containing drugs not previously used, and bone marrow transplantation are possible choices you should discuss with your doctor.

Large-cell lymphomas

Several types of large-cell lymphomas are found in both adults and children. These include Ki-1 anaplastic large-cell lymphoma (ALCL), and centroblastic and immunoblastic lymphomas.

Stages I/II

Treatment that might be recommended, depending on subtype:

- COMP
- CHOP
- MACOP-B, for mediastinal disease

Stages III/IV

Treatment that might be recommended, depending on subtype:

- APO
- ACOP or ACOP+
- COMP
- CHOP
- MACOP-B, for mediastinal disease
- The Milan protocol
- NHL-BFM 86/90
- POG 8106
- LSA2L2, as used for acute lymphoblastic leukemia/lymphoma

Recurrent disease

How relapse is treated depends on what treatments were used in the past, and where the disease has recurred. Clinical trials, aggressive or intensive regimens, other regimens containing drugs not previously used, treatment using regimens tested under stage III or IV small noncleaved cell lymphoma, and bone marrow transplantation are possible choices you should discuss with your doctor.

Adult T-cell lymphoma/leukemia (ATLL)

This form of NHL arises in about 3 percent of those who test positive for the virus known as HTLV-I, human T-cell lymphotropic virus. It's found among IV drug users in many parts of the world, and among those living in parts of

Japan and parts of the Caribbean. A smaller number of infected population also is found in the southeastern U.S.

Treatments that might be recommended are:

- Pentostatin (deoxycoformycin) plus interferon-beta or IFN-gamma
- Monoclonal antibodies that target CD25-positive B-cells
- Antivirals such as zidovudine plus interferon-alfa

MALT lymphomas

MALT lymphomas arise in the mucosa-associated lymphoid tissues, such as the stomach, tonsils, thyroid, or parts of the small intestine. MALT lymphomas may be low-grade or aggressive, but are usually low-grade.

The gastric MALT lymphomas, which comprise the bulk of the MALT lymphomas, usually are associated with infection by the bacteria *Helicobacter pylori* and may respond to treatment with antibiotics. If they do not, generally single-agent chemotherapeutic drugs are attempted.

A few studies have shown a possible link between *H. pylori* and MALT lymphoma in the lung.

Other sites of disease, such as the thyroid, might be treated with surgery followed by chemotherapy.

Enteropathy-associated T-cell MALT lymphoma, which is linked to inherited celiac disease, dermatitis herpetiformis, and possibly to Epstein-Barr virus, might be treated with surgery.

Monocytoid B-cell MALT lymphoma might be treated with the COP, CHOP, ABVD, or m-BACOD regimens.

Other MALT lymphomas, such as those of the lung, pharynx, salivary gland, stomach, thyroid, or immunoproliferative small intestine disease (IPSID) may be approached with combination chemotherapies such as COP, CHOP, or CVD in addition to surgeries or antibiotic treatments.

Malignancies that arise in Waldeyer's Ring, consisting of the nasopharynx, tonsils, and the base of the tongue, are considered by some researchers to be nodal NHLs, but by others to be MALT NHLs, and will be treated according to the physician's beliefs. (Note that two tonsils remain after tonsillectomy, at the base of the tongue and at the back of the roof of the mouth.)

Cutaneous T-cell lymphoma

Cutaneous T-cell lymphoma, also called mycosis fungoides, begins as low-grade disease and may entail a long survival time of twenty years or more. It may progress beyond skin involvement to a more serious and rapid disease called Sezary syndrome. Cutaneous T-cell lymphoma is treated in different ways, depending on how much of the body is affected.

This form of lymphoma should not be confused with peripheral T-cell lymphoma, adult T-cell leukemia/lymphoma, or anaplastic large-cell lymphoma, which are higher-grade lymphomas that also may present in the skin and are treated with therapies suitable for high-grade disease.

Many treatments are geared to cutaneous lymphoma still found only in the skin:

- Radiotherapy
  - Total skin electron beam therapy (TSEBT)
  - Local electron-beam irradiation
  - Orthovoltage radiation therapy
  - Carbon dioxide laser
- Light therapy
  - Psoralen/PUVA light therapy
  - Extracorporeal photochemotherapy (photopheresis): blood circulated through a pheresis machine (ECPP)
  - Phototherapy with ultraviolet B light in clinical trials
- Topical medications
  - Mechlorethamine (nitrogen mustard)
  - Carmustine (BCNU)
  - Retinoids (etretinate)
  - Phosphocholines (hexadecylphosphocholine)

Disease that has spread to other organs might be treated with multiple agents, combined with skin treatments above, perhaps including:

- Interferon alfa
- Monoclonal antibodies

- Systemic (whole-body oral or IV) chemotherapies such as fludarabine, 2-chlorodeoxyadenosine (2-CDA), pentostatin, chlorambucil and prednisone, cyclophosphamide, methotrexate, or combinations of these and other chemotherapeutic agents

Relapses might be treated with recombinations of the treatments listed above, with bone marrow transplantation, or with novel approaches available through clinical trials.

Primary extranodal sites

Disease that has not spread from elsewhere, but instead has arisen outside a lymph node or lymphatic organ, requires a specialized approach depending on the location of the disease. This appearance of an NHL is called "primary disease in an extranodal site," and characterizes several of both the low-grade and aggressive lymphomas.

Owing to the great number of extranodal sites in which an NHL can arise, a detailed outline of standard treatments for each site cannot be given here. Magrath's *The Non-Hodgkin's Lymphomas* and current research papers and NCI treatment statements are your best sources for information about the rare primary extranodal NHLs.

The tissues comprising Waldeyer's Ring—the base of the tongue, the palatine, sublingual, and pharyngeal tonsils (the latter two are not removed during tonsillectomy), the nasopharynx, and the larynx—are considered by many researchers to be either nodal or MALT lymphomas rather than extranodal sites, as these tissues are lymphatic tissue. For these sites, see the descriptions of treatment for low-grade, aggressive, or MALT diseases earlier in this chapter.

Other extranodal NHLs, such as certain intestinal NHLs, also may be determined to be MALT lymphomas if they arise in the mucosa-associated lymphoid tissues. See the section "MALT lymphomas" earlier in this chapter for more information.

Primary lymphoma of bone is distinct from lymphoma that has arisen elsewhere and traveled to bone marrow.

Each extranodal presentation is treated in a highly individualized way with chemotherapy, radiotherapy, or a combination of the two.

Summary

This chapter reflects an effort to digest and summarize the latest information regarding treatment for many of the various subtypes of NHL. New treatments evolve continuously, however, and it's in your best interest to keep abreast of these changes. Your doctor, the National Cancer Institute, and cancer research journals are your best sources of information for current treatment choices.

If you have questions about the appropriateness of the information you have found here, and in particular if you have a rare subtype of NHL that we do not address in the foregoing discussion, please rely on your doctor for clarification and updates.

Consider using the steps outlined in Chapter 24 to keep informed about changes in treatment strategies.

CHAPTER 7

What to Expect During Chemotherapy

*Surely every medicine is an innovation, and
he that will not apply new remedies, must
expect new evils.*

—Francis Bacon

The specific chemotherapy treatments patients may face to treat NHL are of consuming interest to them. For many, this may be the first chapter read. Such is the concern we feel after having heard so many stories about chemotherapy.

The non-Hodgkin's lymphomas are a collection of diseases, and the chemotherapies used to treat NHL vary widely. Consequently, the experiences and reactions that people have differ greatly.

The goal of this chapter is to acquaint you with a typical chemotherapy experience and with events that may unfold. As most chemotherapy is administered in the outpatient setting, we will walk you through an outpatient treatment, beginning with your preparations and scheduling, entering the treatment office, encountering certain medical personnel and other patients, advancing through the treatment itself, and finishing with what you can expect afterward. Keep in mind, though, that what you experience may differ.

Use of the newer and gentler treatments categorized as biological therapies and biological response modifiers—monoclonal antibodies, interferons, interleukins, colony stimulating factors, vaccines, and the like—are also discussed in this chapter. Biological response modifiers often are injected, as are other chemotherapies, and pose some of the same risks.

The theories behind NHL treatment and the side effects of treatment are discussed separately in other chapters.

The information this chapter provides is not a substitute for your doctor's knowledge. Always ask your doctor when an aspect of your treatment is unclear, and report immediately to your doctor any adverse reactions that arise during or after treatment.

The following sections will walk you through preparation, scheduling, pre-treatment testing, receiving chemotherapy, departure, and the days that follow treatment.

Preparation

People can have a wide range of responses to chemotherapy, even if they're receiving the same drug and dose. You don't know for certain how you'll respond, so it would be best to make sure you have certain supplies and assistance if you need them. Some of the drugs given for chemotherapy or to prevent side effects can cause drowsiness or affect concentration, for instance, or you might be sitting for many hours in a room that is overly warm or too cool.

For these and other reasons, during your first treatment visit it would be wise to have a friend or loved one along, not only for emotional support, but to handle issues such as safely tucking away written instructions for diet and aftercare, understanding and remembering verbal instructions, communicating insurance information and handling the co-pay, if any, and assisting with the drive home. As you adapt to treatment, you may need someone to drive if you take medication for nausea before leaving home, as many of these drugs cause drowsiness.

Comfort should be high on the list of priorities for anyone facing chemotherapy. Come prepared for a few hours' testing or treatment by wearing comfortable, easy-to-shed clothing, bringing along relaxing buddies or music cassettes, and asking in advance what to expect. Don't arrive with an empty stomach. Eat light food up to two hours before treatment.

Although the antinausea drugs in use today are excellent, store a bucket in your car against the possibility of nausea during the ride home. Call the doctor a day or two in advance to get nausea medications, and take them beforehand if instructed to do so.

Before your initial treatment, ask about wearing cosmetics, jewelry, or nail polish, because skin and nailbed color are useful ways for the medical staff to assess your well-being and response to drugs. Ask about using lotions or aftershave, as these may cause skin irritation depending on the treatment being given. If you feel strongly about wearing cosmetics and nail polish to treatment to improve your frame of mind, ask them about a compromise, such as leaving one fingernail bare for visibility or for using the thimble-like oxygen sensor that slides over your finger.

Ask if your chemotherapy will be administered into an arm vein. If so, plan to wear a short-sleeved shirt, and bring a cardigan for the parts that needn't be uncovered and might get chilled.

Tell the staff about dental appliances, contact lenses, surgical staples, pacemakers, and other manmade materials that may interfere with treatment.

Mary Butler, a survivor of a bone marrow transplant for NHL of the bone, describes how frightened she was before her first chemotherapy session, and how well the nursing staff handled her fear:

> The word "cancer" didn't cause the terror in me that "chemo" did. I had a vision of some well-meaning nurse hooking me up to a bottle of chlorine bleach. It was terrifying. I didn't even know anyone who had gone through chemotherapy.
>
> I was fortunate to find a local cancer support-group meeting the night before my first chemotherapy, and it helped calm my panic. Knowledge has always been my best defense; nevertheless, I found myself sitting in the chemotherapy room at the oncologist's office crying, with as much dignity as possible, as the nurse approached me. She was very kind and understanding. She didn't point at me and laugh, or even smirk. She explained in detail what would happen and how carefully the staff would watch me. In fact, she sat with me for at least an hour as the first bag of medication dripped into my vein.
>
> Six months later when I went in for my last chemotherapy, she commented on how far I'd come from that first day when I'd introduced myself with tears streaming down my face.

Scheduling

The schedule on which chemotherapy is administered is based on years of research that determine a drug's effectiveness at a certain dose and interval. Some chemotherapies are given daily; some are given weekly for several months; some are given once a month for many months. Those delivered via portable pumps enter the body throughout the day. Oral medications taken at home may be taken once a day, several times a day, or in a tapered dose spread over several days.

If you can't afford or don't want to miss time from work, you might prefer scheduling your treatment to occur just before a weekend break so that you'll have a couple of days to adjust and recover without the additional stress of meeting work responsibilities.

Don't be surprised if the schedule on which your chemotherapy is administered differs from the schedules you hear others discussing, because your schedule likely is tailored to your particular circumstances. You may, for instance, be receiving a drug that is known to be toxic to the heart, but on a less condensed schedule that is intended to lessen toxicity to the heart.

Depending on what drugs are being used, the timing of subsequent therapy may be influenced by the quantity of white blood cells remaining in your blood after your last treatment. Thus, for certain regimens, your blood will be tested when you arrive (or perhaps a few days in advance, if your doctor recommends or you prefer) using a standard measurement known as a complete blood count (CBC). If your white blood counts are too low, treatment may be delayed a few days or a week.

A delay of one week is not likely to affect the success of treatment, but a great many delays or a delay of long duration may. For this reason, many oncologists prescribe injections to bring your white blood counts up to safe levels, substances called colony stimulating factors, such as granulocyte colony stimulating factor (G-CSF) or granulocyte-macrophage colony stimulating factor (GM-CSF). These manmade copies of natural body products cause bone marrow to produce more new white blood cells than it otherwise would.

It's not unusual for one chemotherapy session to last for several hours. Therapies that must be administered over several days may require a hospital admission, but the trend is toward outpatient treatment for all but the most rigorous procedures or the sickest patients.

Arrival

Often, your treatment is not started until a doctor, nurse, or medical technician has weighed you, taken your blood pressure and temperature, done a brief physical, and drawn blood to check blood counts.

Although the new antinausea drugs (anti-emetics) are excellent, make a point of discussing alternative nausea medication with your doctor *before* treatment starts. Ask for suppositories in case oral medications won't stay in your stomach.

Certain specific drugs used for chemotherapy may react badly with certain foods or with sunlight. Ask your doctor if you should avoid certain supplements, vitamins, or foods such as grapefruit, smoked meats, or cheese for a week or two before or after treatment. Grapefruit interferes with metabolism of some drugs by the liver; other foods such as cheese contain tyramines that may interfere with certain drugs used, such as procarbazine. Potassium supplements may trigger a dangerous metabolic imbalance, tumor lysis syndrome, that imperils the kidneys if you have a large tumor that is killed rapidly by treatment.

You may also receive instructions about avoiding other possibly dangerous circumstances such as excessive sunlight or crowds. Some of the drugs given by IV cause skin to become overly sensitive to sunlight. Protective clothing, glasses, and sunscreen lotions may be recommended.

After you're settled in the treatment area, waiting or being treated, consider having your companion visit the pharmacy to buy ice bags, a pill organizer, to fill any prescriptions, or buy any over-the-counter drugs, including stool softeners and antidiarrheals, that you'll need later. With this arrangement, if you feel bad or fatigued after treatment, your medications and supplies will be immediately available.

Your first visit is a good chance to begin to make friends with the nursing staff. Oncology nurses are a unique breed, generally cheerful and unusually kind. Often they'll have great ideas for helping you that might not occur to your doctor to mention, such as where to buy satin pillow covers to reduce hair loss. Interaction with a good nurse may well be one of the finest and most rewarding experiences in life, exemplifying the best that humans can offer each other. Many oncology nurses say that they get much more from their patients than they give.

The setting

Chemotherapy may be administered in a doctor's office, in a hospital outpatient setting, or, if given in the form of tablets or a portable pump, by yourself in your home. If it is administered in a doctor's office or outpatient department, it may be administered by a chemotherapy nurse or by the doctor herself. It may be administered in a large room with other cancer patients who are seated in reclining chairs in partitions divided by curtains, or it may be administered on a bed or chair in a private room.

Sometimes the setting in which chemotherapy is given is dictated by what insurance companies will pay for. Injections of colony stimulating factors, for example, which may be necessary to stimulate bone marrow, may be administered safely and easily by the patient or another at home, but some insurance companies will pay for these injections only if they are administered by a doctor.

Some chemotherapies and some tumor types are known to be associated with risks that are best handled in a hospital setting. Cyclophosphamide, for example, is known to damage the bladder, and is best administered simultaneously with heavy bladder irrigation such as that provided by intravenous fluids. Large tumor masses of the chest or abdomen that die quickly when treatment is started may require IV fluids to protect the kidneys only at the start of treatment. For this reason, you may be admitted to the hospital to receive these treatments. See Chapter 10, *If You're Hospitalized*, for what to expect.

How chemotherapy is administered

There are many different forms of chemotherapy for NHL, and many different ways to administer it.

Intravenous therapy

Most often, chemotherapy for NHL is administered into a vein using a temporary or semi-permanent IV line in the forearm, or by any one of a number of venous access devices (VADs), such as a central catheter that has been implanted into a large vein in your chest.

If you have difficulty finding a usable vein, see Chapter 5, *Tests and Procedures,* for suggestions that may make this easier. If you continue to experience trouble with inaccessible veins, or if they worsen during treatment, discuss with your doctor the advantages and disadvantages of venous access devices such as central catheters.

Some of the drugs used will be in plastic bags that are hung from your IV pole. They may be mixed with a saline drip to dilute them as they enter your vein. Others, such as adriamycin (also called doxorubicin), a bright red solution, may be injected directly into your IV line from a large syringe. This method is called a bolus push.

Many of the drugs used for intravenous chemotherapy are damaging if they come in contact with skin. Notify the medical staff immediately if you experience any pain, swelling, redness, or burning near the injection site.

Certain drugs, such as vincristine (Oncovin) are damaging to the narrower veins of the arms if they are bolus-pushed, and usually will be given via IV drip diluted with saline if you don't have a catheter.

You may feel a warm flush when certain drugs are administered. Verify with the medical staff that this is normal for your drug regimen.

Monoclonal antibodies are a manmade version of a natural body product secreted by our white blood cells. They are injected into a vein via an IV. It's possible to have an allergic reaction to monoclonal antibodies, because they are formed from combined human and mouse antibodies. This is a very common reaction that is easily controlled, but it must be addressed immediately to keep it from becoming serious.

Here's one survivor's experience with the monoclonal antibody Rituxan:

> I was given Rituxan six times from November 1996 through March 1997 as part of a clinical trial testing the combination of Rituxan and CHOP on untreated people with intermediate/high-grade lymphoma. I didn't have any of the side effects others describe; in fact my breathing became slightly easier shortly after the antibody infusion. (I had a giant mediastinal mass about the size of a rugby ball which had crushed one lung completely flat at diagnosis, as well as being pretty anemic, so I felt constantly short of breath.)
>
> In general, the side effects of Rituxan are considered mild compared to most chemotherapies, and are minimized by very slow infusion rates, particularly during the first treatment. However, the nursing staff do

monitor you carefully, so they can slow down or stop the infusion if there seems to be an adverse reaction.

Oral therapy

Your chemotherapy regimen may include oral medication along with or in place of intravenous injections, or you may be given oral medication to offset nausea. You may be given tablets to take at home, perhaps several times a day, perhaps every other day, or in a dose that tapers. You may be instructed to buy over-the-counter products such as stool softeners to take with your chemotherapy. Although taking pills may seem easy, there are several potential issues to be aware of.

The chemotherapy drugs can cause some problems in swallowing pills. After several days or weeks of treatment, you may notice your mouth becoming increasingly dry as the rapidly dividing cells in your mouth die. A good habit to cultivate is wetting your mouth before attempting to swallow a tablet.

It's easy to forget what medications you've taken when you have quite a few, and when some of them are making you drowsy. Each day, keep a new list of what you must take, and check them off as you take them. Consider buying a plastic pill organizer to ensure that all doses are taken.

If oral prednisone or dexamethasone is part of your therapy, be sure to take it exactly as prescribed. If your doctor has not recommended tapering your dose, ask why. Abruptly stopping prednisone without a tapering period can cause severe physical and emotional side effects that mimic failure of the adrenal glands.

Topical therapy

Some treatments for NHL of the skin (cutaneous T-cell lymphoma, or mycosis fungoides) consist only of photochemotherapy. Photochemotherapy may consist of:

- Light-sensitive drug treatments, administered directly to the skin, followed by intense ultraviolet A (UVA) light exposure, a treatment called PUVA.

- Treatment administered to the blood as it flows through specialized machinery for this purpose, and then recirculates back into the body. This method is less common.

Phototherapy for cutaneous lymphoma usually is administered by rubbing, painting, or soaking the affected area with psoralen, a plant compound that increases skin sensitivity to light. The patient then stands or lies in a UVA generating light booth or bed. If the lymphoma is widespread, the psoralen may be administered orally. A typical schedule is twice-weekly treatment.

If you're given oral psoralen, take it within two hours after eating to reduce the chance of nausea, and limit your intake of alcohol. Most likely you will have to avoid sunlight, wear protective clothing, and wear strong sunglasses during all hours of daylight, and while under fluorescent lighting. During light treatment, you will be given protective goggles to wear.

Spinal or intrathecal therapy

For NHL that has affected the central nervous system, or is very likely to, chemotherapy is administered directly into cerebrospinal fluid, the fluid that travels in the spinal column and bathes the brain. This can be done by injecting these agents into the spine, or by installing under the scalp a rubber bulb called an Ommaya reservoir which can be used to access cerebrospinal fluid repeatedly. An Ommaya reservoir is preferred by many patients over repeated spinal taps, because spinal taps can be painful.

Subcutaneous injections

Treatments such as interferon-alfa-2B, interleukin-2, or colony stimulating factors such as granulocyte colony stimulating factor (G-CSF) or erythropoietin (EPO) frequently are injected under the skin or, less often, into muscle.

If your insurance company will pay for the drug, you may be able to give yourself these injections at home. The medical staff will teach you the quick, painless poke in the thigh, using pinching, stretching, or slapping to anesthetize the area first. Small syringes of the type used for insulin usually will do; they'll give you a "red bag" for needle disposal, which should be returned to the doctor's office when full, not put into the trash.

If your insurance company will only pay for these injections if they are administered in a doctor's office, you may have to make twice- or thrice-weekly trips to the doctor.

Portable (ambulatory) pumps

It's possible to have certain drugs administered all day long by using a portable pump. Your catheter can probably be used for this treatment. If you don't have a catheter, an IV line is established within a vein by the medical staff and taped in place. Then the small battery-powered pump is connected to the line. The pump can be implanted under the skin or carried in a satchel that you can wear around your waist or over your shoulder. Portable pumps also can deliver drugs under the skin or directly into the abdominal cavity, but an IV connection is most common. These devices can deliver multiple drugs at the same time.

Dosages

If you feel inclined to do so, you can verify your chemotherapy dosage, keeping in mind that any variation you note may be planned deliberately by your doctor.

See Appendix C for a chart of common heights and weights, and their corresponding body surface areas in square meters.

If you have a computer, you can access Glaxo-Wellcome's DoseCalc web site at *http://www.meds.com/DChome.html,* which will calculate dosages automatically given your weight, height, and a drug name. DoseCalc also lists the current chemotherapy regimens used against NHL, and the milligrams per square meter needed for each drug.

If you notice a substantial difference between the calculated and actual dose given, ask your doctor why. Often there are very good reasons for differences. For example, if oral Etoposide is used instead of intravenous Etoposide, twice the IV amount per square meter must be given, because only half survives exposure to stomach acid and digestive enzymes. Another example is Doxorubicin: if given every three to four weeks, the amount per square meter used can be up to 75 milligrams. If given weekly, however, the dose may be dropped to 25 milligrams.

Departure

Before leaving the doctor's office, be sure you have received written instructions regarding any necessary dietary or behavioral changes, information about possible side effects, prescriptions, and phone numbers for emergencies.

Do not leave feeling unwell. If you are feeling unwell, tell the medical staff.

Use the restroom before leaving if you received your treatments via IV line. Often, IV drugs are accompanied by a saline drip. The volume of fluid that your kidneys have processed from this treatment may surprise you halfway home.

Most chemotherapy regimens do not result in infection or side effects that require hospitalization. However, occasionally such problems do occur. Carefully note all symptoms and communicate immediately with your doctor if problems arise.

Patient stories

In this section, two NHL survivors describe their experiences with chemotherapy. As you'll see, each experience is unique based on diagnosis, treatment chosen, support found, personal outlook—and luck.

> My diagnosis at age 44 was stage I or II, high-grade, small, non-cleaved cell, non-Burkitts, non-Hodgkin's lymphoma. My protocol, based on a Vanderbilt University study, called for my being hit hard with high-intensity, brief-duration chemotherapy. Brief meant two one-month cycles of lethal stuff, including cyclophosphamide, etoposide, vincristine, bleomycin, methotrexate (with leucovorin as a "rescue"), doxorubicin, allopurinol, and prednisone. I lost all my hair within the first couple of weeks, and relied on scarves to get me through the rest of treatment. We had ordered a high-quality wig, which would not arrive for six weeks or so.

> I was hospitalized for the first treatment of each cycle, and once in between each cycle when my counts or condition were perilously fragile. No matter what the reason for admission, I railed against the notion of being a patient. I don't completely understand why, except it was consistent with my desire to convince myself and others that I was just passing through and I would not be back in any chronically ill capacity. My husband—a brilliant and golden presence in my life—spent the nights there with me.

> It quickly became impossible for me to drive myself anywhere. That meant my husband had to come home at noon and drive me to the doctor's office nearly every day for blood count monitoring, Neupogen or Epogen shots, changing the Groshong [catheter] dressing, more chemotherapy, or whatever was on the agenda that day.

Neupogen shots seem to have different effects on people. While I did not suffer the bone pain others do, my tolerance for the sharp sting of each shot became lower as I became weaker. I found that I preferred that they be injected in my abdomen—it seemed to be a little less sensitive there. Though it might have been more convenient to self-administer the shots, my doctor feared insurance would not cover the considerable costs under those circumstances. He did not want to take any risks there, and besides, he still wanted to see me nearly every day.

The treatments became more debilitating over time. I was often neutropenic, and there were days when I could not walk well at all. My ability to taste foods disappeared, and everything took on a metallic tinge with unpleasant odors. I tried Ensure (chocolate flavor worked best) and other things, like mild soups or small low-fat snacks, since no normal meal could be tolerated. I had prescriptions for Percocet and another strong relaxant to occasionally force me to rest during the worst of the long days of battling NHL with very little sleep.

The administration of certain treatments during my second cycle defeated my attempts to suppress the nausea, even with previously successful Zofran and Compazine. I think it was the aggregate effect of being "poisoned" once a week. I had to practically lecture my body to retain nutrients, but a couple of times it was up to an IV to get me through. Over the course of treatment, I believe I was given a couple of red blood cell transfusions as well as one platelet transfusion. The Groshong catheter had some minor blockages, but fortunately the double lumen architecture provided a secondary access. I was generally physically uncomfortable, but drew comfort from the thought that it would all soon be over, and I was going to survive all this. We just kept focusing on the countdown to the finish line.

I know I was on the edge of an abyss—close to death—more than once during my treatment. I caught myself thinking, you know, this is not so terrible. It was sort of like floating, like a feather that could be flicked into oblivion if I gave myself a self-absorbed breeze to escape on. But that feeling of floating was all more like a little mind game I played with myself. I was way too angry about being in this physical state to defeat myself that way. I honestly felt, to the core of my imperfect being, that it was not my time. I had too much left to do and I did not want to miss any more "real time" with my husband.

Another NHL survivor's story offers other insights:

> The day started with a trip to the hospital to train my family in catheter care so they could take over when I couldn't. This turned out to be very valuable because my daughter did all my catheter care for the first two weeks, partly because of the soreness that made it difficult to bend my head down to see what I was doing, and in part because I think it made her feel like she was doing something to help me recover. She was very meticulous. After the hospital visit, we took the girls (my daughter and sister) out to lunch and then dropped them off at the movies. I was glad they weren't there because the stress of the last three weeks was about to descend on me with a thud.
>
> When I arrived at the doctor's office, we had to wait about forty minutes in the waiting room. During that time, I was up to the bathroom at least six times; I could also feel the tears starting to well up. I hadn't taken the time to really accept what was happening and let my feelings out since that first night in the hospital and here it was, happening in the waiting area of the doctor's office. When I got into the exam room, the dike burst and I couldn't stop sobbing. I was so afraid. The one thing I hated more than anything else in the world was vomiting, and here I was about to get medicine that I was sure was going to make me sick. That on top of reality sinking in had me crying for what seemed like an eternity. The doctor explained that this was mostly caused by the whirlwind I had been experiencing, coupled by the prednisone I had been taking to help me breathe. She told the nurse to start me off with intravenous Ativan to help me calm down.
>
> Everyone was very nice in the office; the nurses tried to introduce me to the other patients in the room with me to ease my fears. What they couldn't understand was that I felt humiliated by my crying and the last thing I wanted to do was to talk to other people! The Ativan finally kicked in and I settled down. I tried to concentrate on the television, but couldn't. My mom had to leave in the middle to pick up the girls and take Courtney to her driver's education class. When it was finally over, the nurse gave me a sample of Kytril, a new antinausea drug, to take that night at home. I was also instructed to take the Compazine around the clock the first two days to prevent nausea.

I did fairly well the first couple of days, eating only chicken and rice soup, but by Sunday I felt miserable. I was having a tougher time breathing and I had a low-grade temperature of 100.3. By Monday morning, I was coughing so hard I started vomiting, so I called the doctor and they wanted me to come in. The doctor I saw—not my regular oncologist—decided that the problem was most likely inflammation caused by tumor breakdown. He gave me my prednisone intravenously that day, as well as some antinausea medicine and changed the schedule of my oral prednisone. I was still feeling lousy by the time of my visit with my oncologist the following Thursday and it was decided that it was most likely due to the Allopurinol. Luckily, it would end the next day.

I went to the doctor weekly for the first five weeks. After that we changed to every two weeks, and finally only every three weeks for chemotherapy. I was very fortunate that my blood counts stayed very high for a chemotherapy patient. I never needed to delay chemo, and I never needed a blood transfusion or special medicine to help my white blood cells grow. I've been told I have very strong bone marrow—hopefully a good sign and not a sign of resistance to the treatments. Looking back, I feel very lucky to have had a relatively easy go of it. I have now completed eight rounds of chemotherapy.

After four rounds of chemo, I had my CT scans repeated. While the news was generally positive, there were also some shocks to me. The good news was all the tumors had either shrunk or disappeared. The bad news was they realized I had more tumors than originally thought, discovering a shrinking tumor in my pancreas and now nonexistent nodes in my abdomen. Radiation was nixed after a consultation with my doctor and several radiation oncologists, as well as a personal visit to a radiation oncologist, because I still had tumors in my abdomen that wouldn't be adequately treated if we stopped the chemotherapy to start radiation. If I got full chemo, then the radiation could damage my heart, so it was decided to treat the greater amount of the disease with chemotherapy. Now I wait and hope the tumors don't grow back. If they do, the next plan is a bone marrow transplant.

Summary

Not surprisingly, many people have concerns about what chemotherapy will be like, and how they'll make it through treatment. This chapter, in combination with Chapter 9, *Side Effects of Treatment*, aims to make the experience a less frightening one.

Many of the topics we touch on in these chapters are well described in other books. See Appendix A, *Resources*, for several excellent books that can offer you much more information.

CHAPTER 8

What to Expect During Radiotherapy

*Poisons and medicine are oftentimes the same
substance given with different intents.*

—Peter Mere Latham

By now you have consulted with several types of oncologists and have decided that radiation therapy is a good choice for treating your NHL. Perhaps it will be used alone if you have a single tumor or perhaps one of several sites will be irradiated to alleviate unpleasant symptoms such as pressure or pain. Radiation may be used in conjunction with other therapies such as chemotherapy or surgery.

We are justifiably afraid of radiation. We know that sunlight can burn us, that x-ray technicians leave the room and wear lead aprons when they treat us. We know we should be wary of too many diagnostic x-rays, and that large amounts of radiation caused tremendous damage at Hiroshima, Nagasaki, and Chernobyl. In spite of fears about radiation, many NHL patients are pleasantly surprised to find that radiation therapy is a smooth, quick, silent, painless treatment.

As was done in the prior chapter for chemotherapy, in this chapter we will acquaint you with a typical radiotherapy experience. Most radiotherapy used for NHL is external radiotherapy and is administered in the outpatient setting, so we will walk you through an outpatient treatment, beginning with your preparation, including treatment simulation, scheduling, arriving at the treatment office, encountering certain medical personnel and other patients, advancing through the treatment itself, and finishing with what you can expect afterward.

Although there are different kinds of radiation, including x-rays and electron, proton, or neutron beams, for the sake of readability in this chapter we will not distinguish among them. We will use only the term radiation.

The theories behind radiotherapy as treatment for NHL, and the side effects of treatment, are discussed separately in other chapters.

The information this chapter provides is not a substitute for your doctor's knowledge. Always ask your doctor when an aspect of your treatment is unclear, and report immediately to your doctor any adverse reactions that arise during or after treatment.

If you would like greater detail on radiation therapy, *The Chemotherapy and Radiation Therapy Survival Guide,* by Judith McKay, Nancee Hirano, Myles Lampenfeld, *Making the Radiation Therapy Decision,* by David Brenner and Eric Hall, and *Coping with Radiation Therapy: A Ray of Hope,* by Daniel Cukier and Virginia McCullough are books that focus on radiation therapy from the patient's perspective.

The following sections will walk you through preparation and treatment simulation, scheduling, receiving therapy, departure, and the days that follow treatment.

Simulation

Your first one or two treatment visits to the radiation oncology treatment offices will be spent determining precise details of how best to treat you: positioning you on the treatment bed, marking your skin with small dots of temporary or permanent ink, and creating shields for sensitive organs. All of these preparations are called simulation, and may take several hours spread over one or more visits.

Several medical specialists are involved in this stage of your treatment. These include your radiation oncologist, the radiation therapy technician who will administer the treatment, a dosimetrist who calculates the correct dose, and the radiation physicist who calibrates the machine. Some of these staff members may work behind the scenes.

For these initial visits, which are lengthy, make yourself as comfortable as possible by wearing clothing that doesn't bind, that goes on and off easily, and has no metal zippers. Bring a cassette player if you like, and use the restroom before the simulation starts.

If parts of your head or neck are being irradiated, a mask or helmet may be made to protect the areas that are cancer-free and to help you remain still during treatment.

None of these preparations are painful, although some NHL survivors report feeling a little claustrophobic if they have a mask or helmet made, or uncomfortably stiff if they have to hold still for a long time. The substance used to make masks and helmets takes a few minutes to harden and must harden on your head in order to provide an exact fit. While you are able to breathe normally with them in place, during this time you must hold quite still.

Special shields or blocks may be made to shape the radiation beam to match exactly your tumor's shape. Beams of invisible radiation generated by the machinery are usually emitted shaped like rectangles, from two to fifteen inches in any dimension. If these beams were trained against your tumor, nearby healthy tissue within the two- to fifteen-inch rectangle would be irradiated, too, suffering damage. To avoid this effect, shields or blocks with cutaways in the silhouette of your tumor are created using your x-ray films as guides.

The masks and shields made for you are used only by you. You may see the same kinds of devices belonging to other patients hanging nearby or in other treatment areas.

The machinery used during simulation looks and moves just as the genuine radiation equipment does, but instead it generates only a plain light beam to verify positioning, ink markings, and the fit of masks and shields.

After all shields, blocks, masks, or helmets are made and your skin is marked, the entire simulation will be repeated with all pieces in place—exactly like a dress rehearsal.

As your treatment progresses and your tumor shrinks, new blocks may be made to match the new shape of your tumor, and these simulations may be repeated.

Preparation

Radiation therapy often makes many patients increasingly tired as it progresses. For this reason, once treatment starts, it would be wise to have a friend or loved one along, not only for emotional support, but to handle issues such as saving written instructions for diet and aftercare, understanding and remembering verbal instructions, communicating insurance information and handling the co-pay, if any, and assisting with the drive home.

If the area near your stomach is being irradiated, it's best to eat very lightly beforehand and to arrive with an empty stomach. This will reduce the chance of nausea.

Ask the medical staff about using cosmetics, antiperspirants, aftershaves, and lotions before treatment. They may interfere with treatment, or they may cause your skin to become hypersensitive if they are exposed to radiation.

Ask as well about clothing with metal zippers, removable dentures, pacemakers, surgical staples, and contact lenses.

Scheduling

Years of research have shown that a large amount of radiation can be delivered to a tumor safely if it's spread out over several weeks. This is called fractionating the dose, or simply, fractionation. It spares healthy tissue from unnecessary damage and gives it time to recover.

Dosage fractionation means that you will have to visit the treatment center several times a week, or perhaps every day, for two to six weeks, depending on your treatment plan. It also means that each dose of radiation lasts only two to four minutes. If your tumor is irradiated from several different angles, each angle may take two to four minutes after the machine is repositioned. After the lengthy time spent in simulation, you may feel that ten to thirty minutes of treatment time is an anticlimax.

Don't be surprised if the schedule on which your radiotherapy is administered differs from the schedules you hear others discussing, because your radiation schedule always is tailored to your particular circumstances, based on the size, number, and location of tumors, your overall health, your body size, and the subtype of NHL you have.

Depending on what treatment is being used, the timing of your radiation therapy may be influenced by the quantity of white blood cells remaining in your blood after your last treatment. Thus, for certain regimens that expose a lot of bone marrow or the spleen to radiation, your blood may be tested when you arrive, using a standard measurement known as a complete blood count (CBC). If your white blood counts are too low, treatment may be delayed a few days or a week.

For each treatment, you might want to call the treatment center before leaving home or work. Radiation therapy machines sustain heavy use, and must be taken offline periodically for recalibration or repair. You can save your valuable time by calling first to see whether appointments are running on time.

After a few treatments, you may begin to feel that all of your time is spent traveling to the office or chatting in the waiting room, because treatment itself is so brief.

Arrival

If you are receiving radiation to the head, stomach, or abdomen, make a point of discussing nausea and diarrhea medications with your doctor *before* treatment starts. Although the new antinausea drugs (anti-emetics) are excellent, ask for suppositories in case oral medications won't stay in your stomach. If you do develop nausea, subsequent treatments may be preceded by an injection of one of the new antinausea drugs, such as Zofran.

Ask your doctor if you should avoid possibly dangerous circumstances such as excessive sunlight or crowds.

Ask about skin care, too. External beam radiation, the most common radiological means of treating NHL, must pass through your skin to reach tumor sites, and irritation may result. Newer, higher voltage equipment used today causes less damage to skin because the damaging rays concentrate in deeper layers, but some skin reaction still is possible. See Chapter 9, *Side Effects of Treatment*, for a discussion of radiation therapy's effects on skin and other tissue.

The setting

The source of radiation will be a machine that either safely contains a radioactive substance, such as Cobalt 60, or generates its own radiation as needed. Like a CT scanner or a gamma camera, the radiation machine is designed to move around you and your bed as you hold still. Many models are almost silent, but some make a sound like a vacuum cleaner, and of course they may click and whir as they reposition.

The room in which treatment is given has thick walls and is lead-clad to prevent the very small amount of radiation that bounces off your shields, known as scatter, from affecting the medical staff, those in the waiting room, and random passersby. For the safety of the staff, the treatment room will contain only you when the machine is engaged. (The small dose of radiation they would sustain if they stayed with you would probably not harm them, but if they stayed with all patients, all day, every day, the dose from scatter would indeed accumulate to dangerous levels.)

The staff can see and hear you at all times, because there are microphones and cameras connecting you and them. If you feel at all bad, just let them know. Music and wall art sometimes are available in the treatment room to lower your boredom and stress levels.

How radiation therapy is administered

There are four ways to administer radiation therapy: external radiotherapy (also called external beam radiotherapy), radioimmunotherapy, internal radiotherapy, and brachytherapy. The latter two, internal radiotherapy and brachytherapy, are seldom used for NHL, so we will define them briefly and move on.

Internal radiotherapy is radiation therapy aimed directly and only at your exposed tumor while your body is open during surgery. Brachytherapy is the implantation of a source of radiation directly into or very near the tumor. If you would like more information on either of these techniques, see the books listed in Appendix A, *Resources*.

External radiotherapy

External radiotherapy, also called external beam radiation, currently is the most common means of treating NHL tumors, and is administered as described in the earlier section, "The setting," using the blocks, shields, masks, or helmets made expressly for you, along with sandbags to hold your arms and legs still, and blankets to keep you warm.

You should feel no pain, no heat, no sensation at all during treatment, although some survivors say that they feel a sensation of energizing—not quite a tingling—in the area of the tumor during treatment. It may indeed be that some of us can sense a highly active biological entity such as a tumor reacting to the disruption of its DNA.

Some find the absence of sensation eerie, but most people are grateful that the treatment is comfortable and brief.

Radioimmunotherapy

Radioimmunotherapy is a new treatment, still in advanced clinical trials, but quite promising. It combines the principle of radiation therapy with one of the newest treatments available, tumor targeting with monoclonal antibodies, which is discussed fully in Chapter 6, *How the NHLs Are Treated*.

Radioimmunotherapy involves linking one molecule of a radioactive substance, a radioisotope such as iodine-131 or yttrium-90, to a monoclonal antibody. The benefit of radioimmunotherapy over existing radiation treatments is that less healthy tissue is exposed to radiation because the antibody attaches to cancerous tissue only. Some healthy tissue is affected because the radioactive substance decays as the antibody travels to the tumor, but it is thought that this effect is less than that sustained during external beam therapy. Radioimmunotherapy is administered into a vein like chemotherapy.

The correct dose of radioimmunotherapy must first be determined. To calculate this dose, a small "tracer" amount of the substance will be injected first, and visualized using a CT scan or other imaging device. Based on what is seen, the doctors in charge will determine the total dose you should receive.

You will be kept in a lead-shielded hospital room throughout this treatment, and your body wastes will be disposed of in accordance with rules for handling hazardous waste. Face-to-face family visits will be very limited or denied entirely. The nurses who care for you may wear protective clothing.

If the radioisotope iodine-131 is to be used, your thyroid gland will be shielded first, unless it has been infiltrated with NHL. The radioactive isotope, I-131, will destroy the thyroid gland if it is absorbed.

To shield the thyroid, large doses of *nonradioactive* iodine, iodine-123, are given to you first. This substance is taken up by the thyroid in excess compared to other body tissues. After the maximum amount has been absorbed, the thyroid cannot absorb more iodine for several days. This protects the thyroid gland from absorbing subsequent doses of I-131.

This method of treatment is not likely to be used for those who have had previous allergic reactions to iodine in shrimp, other foods, or in other medications.

Dosages

For external beam radiation, a typical dosage for NHL is 180 to 200 centi-Greys (cGy) five times a week. If a higher dosage is required, more sessions are added, but the dose per exposure is not raised. This moderate dose per exposure has been determined to be the best amount for killing NHL cells while allowing healthy cells to recover.

Different subtypes of NHL require different doses of radiation. The varying doses depend primarily on the different sites involved, whether they are nodal or extranodal, and the bulkiness of the tumors. Diffuse disease, for instance, requires more radiation in order to combat growth. Other types of NHL are unaffected by all but the most extreme doses of radiotherapy, which makes this treatment useless against them owing to severe or fatal damage to other tissue.

Departure

After each of your first few treatment sessions, make sure you have received written instructions regarding any necessary dietary or behavioral changes, information about possible side effects, prescriptions, and phone numbers for emergencies, before leaving the doctor's office. Often, side effects of radiation therapy do not emerge until you've had two or more weeks of treatment. If you have prepared for these possibilities by asking questions during the treatment visits when you feel well, side effects may be easier to deal with.

You are not likely to feel unwell after your treatments, but if you do, do not leave without telling the medical staff of your problem.

Summary

Radiation therapy confuses and frightens some people. An advance glimpse at what it's like may help to alleviate this stress. This chapter, in conjunction with Chapter 6, *How the NHLs are Treated*, is intended to address your concerns and fears.

As always, you should ask your doctor about any issues that concern you, and immediately report any untoward effects to the medical staff.

CHAPTER 9

Side Effects of Treatment

The worst about medicine is that one kind
makes another necessary.

—Elbert Hubbard

Too often we recall people who have had terrible experiences while receiving cancer treatment. Yet remarkable progress has been made in alleviating this suffering. Especially impressive is the development of medications to relieve nausea and depression, and the development of low-scatter and high-voltage radiation equipment that reduces damage to healthy tissue.

This chapter will describe both common and serious side effects of NHL treatment, and what can be done about them. Because so many different chemotherapy regimens are used to treat the NHLs, it's not possible to list all side effects of treatment. Nor is it possible in most cases to state unequivocally which side effects are serious and which are not, as a side effect may be associated with more than one condition, and because patients' responses to treatments vary.

Always err on the side of caution and call your doctor if you're having side effects that are unexpected or unusual.

Please be encouraged that, although we list many side effects here, you may have very little reaction or no discernible reaction at all to treatment.

Although this text has been reviewed by medical doctors, the author of this book is not a medical doctor and is not familiar with the individual characteristics that make you and your illness unique. The information this chapter provides should never be substituted for your doctor's knowledge.

Report immediately to your doctor any adverse reactions that arise during or after treatment, and direct all questions to your doctor, regardless of other sources of information available to you.

If you don't find the information you need in this chapter, see Chapter 16, *Late Effects, Late Complications*. Some late effects occur earlier in some people, at times even before treatment ends.

Several excellent books are available that focus on treatment from the patient's perspective, including dealing with side effects. If you'd like much more detail about dealing with side effects such as nausea, hair loss, IV lines, appetite changes, or fatigue, look in Appendix A, *Resources*, for a list of titles.

Why do side effects arise?

Side effects of treatment can arise for several reasons.

First, the treatments commonly used today for NHL affect not only cancerous cells, but many healthy cells as well. Radiotherapy and many chemotherapy regimens target cells that divide rapidly, as many cancer cells do. This targeting of fast-growing cells means that many healthy cells that divide rapidly—cells in the mouth, intestinal tract, hair, fingernails, and others—will be affected, too. After treatment, these cells die all at once, instead of passing through the life cycle just a few at a time. This rapid turnover of cells causes some of the most common side effects of cancer treatment, such as mouth sores and hair loss.

Other side effects come about owing to the body's attempt heal itself. Tumor lysis syndrome, for instance, is a side effect of the body's attempt to clear itself of dying tumor cells.

Many side effects of treatment are normal and pose no danger to you. Adriamycin, for ·example, will turn urine red; this phenomenon does not mean something is amiss. Fatigue is another common side effect of treatment that does not necessarily herald a problem.

Your oncologist should give you fact sheets to provide you with information about side effects that are very serious and about which you should telephone as soon as you notice them. If your doctor doesn't offer this information, ask for it.

It's wise to keep in mind that even commonly used drugs are known to have numerous side effects. Aspirin, for instance, is known to cause any of the following in certain people: vomiting, diarrhea, confusion, drowsiness, severe stomach pain, unusual bruising, bloody or black stools, dizziness, hearing loss, ringing in the ears, swelling of hands, face, lips, eyes, throat, or tongue, difficulty swallowing or breathing, or hoarseness. Like most other drugs, chemotherapeutic agents also are known to cause a large number of both common and rare reactions.

Before we begin discussing individual side effects, it's important to note one generality: worsening side effects may be the result of synergy, increasing in number or degree as the dose or number of drugs increase. Not surprisingly, newer, more aggressive regimens that use high doses of chemotherapy and total body irradiation cause more side effects than older, standard dosages. Keep in mind as you read what follows that a drug or combination of drugs may cause more or worse side effects if given in very high doses. For instance, the standard dose of cytosine arabinoside (ARA-C) causes suppression of bone marrow; high doses may cause damage to nerves, liver, or stomach and intestines. High-dose treatment, such as that used for Burkitt's or small noncleaved lymphoma, or in preparation for a marrow transplant, may cause stronger side effects.

A word about prednisone

Prednisone, the most commonly prescribed glucocorticoid for controlling the growth of white blood cells, can be responsible for many side effects if given in high doses, and especially if long-term use is in order following allogeneic bone marrow transplantation. Side effects include a suppressed immune response, appetite increases, rapid mood changes, insomnia, stomach pain, gastric ulcer, pancreatitis, diabetes, depression, weight gain (especially in the trunk and face), changes in blood chemistry, menstrual irregularities, impotence, facial redness, thinning of skin, stretch marks, acne, bruising, changes in bodily hair, cataracts, glaucoma, protrusion of the eyeballs, weakening of muscles, osteoporosis, avascular necrosis of bone, high blood pressure, seizures, and, rarely, psychosis.

Fortunately, there is an excellent book available about prednisone and its side effects. *Coping with Prednisone*, written by patient Eugenia Zukerman and her sister, Julie Ingelfinger, who is a medical doctor, can answer just about all questions you might have about using this drug.

Neeraj, a survivor of NHL/ALL, describes the effects prednisone has on his sleep and academic performance:

> I take prednisone five days every twenty-eight days. Owing to those five days, my body has adjusted to a sleep cycle of 1:30 to 10:00 A.M. (advantages of being in graduate school: one can sleep till late), so the days when I have early meetings I have to really struggle. One day after getting vincristine and a spinal tap, I decided to risk not sleeping, and I ended up in the emergency room. However, I refuse to take any medication. I think I have had more than my entire family's share of medicines.

If you are taking prednisone for about fourteen days in a row as part of CHOP or a similar chemotherapy regimen, you may notice elevated mood or euphoria while taking this drug, followed by moodiness, depression, fatigue, and pain if the dosage is ended abruptly. Ask your doctor if you can taper the last two or three days of your dosage. Some physicians recommend a taper after as little as fourteen days' use. Other doctors feel that fourteen days is not long enough to disturb the interaction of the adrenal, the pituitary, and the hypothalamus, but many patients report these side effects when their prednisone dose is finished.

> If it hadn't been for the energy I got from the prednisone given as part of chemotherapy, I can't imagine how I could have continued to work. There were times during that period when I felt more energetic than I had in months. I was always quite hot, though, and wearing a wig didn't help. I gained about forty pounds, and my "moon face" was so round I was unrecognizable. At Thanksgiving that year, my nieces and nephews asked their mother, "Who is that woman with Uncle Steve?" Learning that I am not my body was a big part of the cancer experience for me. I felt like me, but I didn't look anything like me.

Side effects of treatment

Listed alphabetically are the most common and most serious side effects of treatment, with the most common being nausea, hair loss, and fatigue, although great variability exists in patients' reactions to treatment. Included within the various sections are tips from NHL survivors for dealing with side effects.

Abdominal pain

Abdominal pain might occur following treatment regimens utilizing vincristine or prednisone, but it also may signal a serious condition known as typhlitis, an inflammation of the cecum, which is the first part of the large intestine near the appendix.

Typhlitis is emerging as a side effect of newer, aggressive chemotherapeutic regimens used against lymphomas and leukemias. Phone your doctor immediately if you experience these in combination: nausea, vomiting, swollen abdomen, diarrhea, fever, and soreness in the lower right side.

Typhlitis results from unusual bacteria thriving in vulnerable parts of your intestine when your white blood cell counts are abnormally low. Your doctor can confirm this diagnosis with an ultrasound. Typhlitis also is known as neutropenic enterocolitis, necrotizing enterocolitis, or ileocecal syndrome. It's more likely to follow aggressive, high-dose treatments, and can be fatal in a high percentage of patients if not caught early.

See "Constipation," "Metabolic imbalances," and "Radiation enteritis" for other causes of abdominal pain.

Appetite or taste changes

Chemotherapy and radiotherapy can affect your taste buds to such an extent that you can't taste food, or it tastes metallic or disgusting.

Adequate nutrition in spite of food aversion is a very important part of your recovery. Eat what you like, but eat as much nutritional food as you can. Ask your doctor about vitamin supplements and liquid supplements such as Nutrical or Ensure.

One survivor describes experiences with taste and appetite changes:

> This is more annoying than anything else. I have become extremely sensitive to smells. I can smell every medication I take on my skin, in my pillows, in my excretions, etc. This causes you to look for good smelling items! Also, my sense of taste eventually changed so much that toothpaste left a bad aftertaste. I also need more salt on my foods than usual. The only thing to do is to experiment. Luckily the problem crescendos about day seven after chemotherapy and slowly gets better after that. For me, the magic taste was cinnamon. I got cinnamon mouthwash and lots of Tic-Tacs to suck on.

One of the oddest things about all of this is a craving for red meat. I began to crave/need red meat like a diabetic craves sugar when his blood glucose is too low. I have checked with others and this is a pretty common phenomenon among lymphoma patients. I would have days when I felt nauseous and dizzy and eating a hamburger cured me. Strangely, non-meat forms of protein didn't work for this. I believe the body craves what it needs. Maybe all the meat I ate is what kept my red blood count from becoming too low?

Others note that, rather than craving particular foods, they are repelled by them, particularly by meat. Foods that once were favorites now have a repugnant or metallic taste and scent.

Blood clots, pulmonary embolism

Large tumors of the abdomen or chest are implicated in the formation or dislodging of blood clots in certain cases. At the beginning of treatment, a large abdominal tumor may shrink rapidly and dislodge a pre-existing blood clot. Chest (mediastinal) tumors may contribute to the formation of blood clots around a central catheter, as may certain imbalances in blood levels of mineral and electrolytes (see "Metabolic imbalances").

If you have a large abdominal or chest tumor, and have either just started treatment or have a central catheter, be especially aware of deep pain or difficulty breathing that may signal a dangerous blood clot dislodging or capable of dislodging and traveling to the lung.

Bone pain

Steroid drugs such as the glucocorticoid prednisone or the colony stimulating factor G-CSF can cause aching bones and joints. Ice packs may relieve this pain; if not, ask your doctor if the dose can be lowered.

Bone pain associated with G-CSF is temporary. That associated with steroid treatment is usually transient, but may become permanent if it causes avascular necrosis of bone.

Severe back pain may be associated with degenerative changes to the spine following radiation therapy. The spine is not able to sustain as high a dose of radiation as some other organs can. Surgery to fuse spinal discs may alleviate this pain. See also "Metabolic imbalances."

Breathing problems

Many treatments for NHL, such as monoclonal antibodies, radiation, or certain chemotherapy drugs that affect the heart can cause difficulty breathing.

Rapid breathing (tachypnea) can be the body's effort to lower levels of excessive acid, called acidosis. Acidosis is a very early sign of certain conditions such as serious infection, kidney damage, or diabetic complications that should be treated immediately.

Rarely, circulatory or respiratory distress can be linked to untreated, intractable constipation. Constipation in its most serious form, fecal impaction, can be fatal.

Call your doctor immediately if you have trouble breathing.

Cognitive changes

Many NHL patients report that treatment makes them feel fuzzy-minded or forgetful. These symptoms should improve over time, although they may improve very slowly.

More serious changes such as delirium or dementia may occur as well, often dependent on the drugs being used. Methotrexate, ifosfamide, fluorouracil, vincristine, vinblastine, bleomycin, carmustine, cisplatin, asparaginase, and procarbazine are known to cause delirium or dementia.

Steroid drugs such as the glucocorticoid prednisone are particularly notorious for causing a wide array of aberrant mental processes, ranging from minor and rapid mood swings to severe mania or depression. These changes usually develop within the first two weeks of steroid use, but this is just a general guideline, as these changes may occur at any time, including during subsequent use following an uneventful first use.

Often the actions of these drugs or the cancer itself interfere with normal levels of minerals and metabolites. This is clearly the case with prednisone, which alters levels of cortisol and adrenaline. See "Metabolic imbalances."

Treatment consists of modifying drug dose, controlling symptoms with sedatives or neuroleptic drugs, or waiting for the effects of the drug to wear off. Call your doctor if these symptoms are very disturbing, or if you or a loved one feel that these side effects represent a danger to the patient or the family.

Constipation

Constipation can be a very serious problem during NHL treatment, because inactivity, other illnesses, and certain drugs such as painkillers, vincristine, vinblastine, antidepressants, or antihistamines may slow or paralyze the intestine or mask the urge to move one's bowels.

Constipation in its most serious form, a total blockage of the intestine called fecal impaction, can present as circulatory or respiratory distress, and can be fatal. Call your doctor immediately if you feel constipated for more than three days, or if you have difficulty breathing or symptoms of heart failure.

> *Constipation was a real problem because I already suffer from hemorrhoids since the birth of my daughter. The vincristine in the chemotherapy seems to just shut down your bowels. The big danger here is if you take too many laxatives you end up treating yourself for diarrhea. Then you take antidiarrheals and end up constipated again.*

> *I finally discussed with my doctor that I had no urge, and was unable to even push to have a bowel movement for the first five days of chemotherapy. We tried a medicine called Reglan which stimulated the small bowel to contract. This took care of the problem and I never went five days again between bowel movements.*

> *This is an embarrassing problem that people don't like to talk about, but [you should]—there is help. Before discussing this with my doctor, I tried Metamucil, Senakot, docusate sodium (a stool softener), and Biscodyl. The Reglan, even though it was a prescription, was cheaper and more effective than all of those. It even had no rebound effects that the others had. Later I would learn that my seasonal favorite, hazelnuts, provided me the helpful fiber I needed [and enabled me to] even stop the Reglan.*

If your doctor agrees, experiment with small amounts of different foods until you have a sense for what will maintain a balance between constipation and diarrhea. Increased fluid intake, regular exercise, increased dietary fiber, warm or hot drinks, privacy and quiet time in the bathroom, easy access to a toilet or bedside commode, and stool softeners may be tried to ease constipation. Do not make dietary changes or greatly increase your fluid intake without first verifying these choices with your doctor.

Dehydration

Dehydration is a very serious side effect of vomiting or diarrhea, as cancer patients must have adequate fluid to remove toxins from the body as well as proteins released from dying cells. Moreover, the quantities of electrolytes and minerals such as phosphorus, calcium, potassium, magnesium, and sodium already are disrupted in the NHL patient, both by disease and by treatment. Dehydration exacerbates this imbalance.

If you suspect you are dehydrated, call your doctor immediately.

The most reliable symptom of dehydration is thirst. Other signs include the inability to urinate about once an hour, the production of very little urine, or the production of urine that is both dark and low in volume. Other symptoms, such as faintness, dry lips, thick saliva, or loss of appetite too closely resemble the side effects of chemotherapy to be reliable indicators of dehydration.

Take in as much fluid as possible, but do not drink products containing electrolytes (such as the products marketed to sports enthusiasts) unless your doctor says that your kidneys are in good condition and that these drinks will do you no harm.

See "Metabolic imbalances" for hypercalcemia.

Diarrhea

Diarrhea frequently is caused by radiotherapy to the abdomen as dying cells are shed from the intestine, and by chemotherapeutic drugs that disturb the balance of electrolytes such as potassium and sodium.

Phone your doctor immediately if diarrhea is combined with a fever more than 1.5 degrees higher than your normal temperature, general malaise, severe chills, night sweats, burning or pain while urinating, headache, neck stiffness, coughing, or trouble breathing.

Your doctor can recommend anti-diarrheal drugs, which you will have to balance carefully with drugs such as stool softeners to control constipation. Experiment with small amounts of different foods until you have a sense for what will maintain a balance between constipation and diarrhea.

Dry mouth, difficulty swallowing

Normal saliva contains an antibiotic. If saliva is not present, dry mouth can lead to serious dental problems that result in whole-body (systemic) infection and tooth loss.

Gentle but scrupulous dental care is a must. Avoid spicy, sour, or acidic foods. Examine your mouth daily for fuzzy white patches that might be a fungal infection. Ask your doctor for drugs to increase saliva flow, or for a homemade mouth rinse that can be used several times a day.

Problems with swallowing that develop after radiotherapy can be corrected with surgical devices that stretch the esophagus.

Extravasation

Sometimes, chemotherapy that is administered by IV can leak out of the vein into surrounding skin, an adverse event called extravasation. The reaction of the body to a high concentration of chemotherapy in the skin can be serious and painful. The vein may be unusable for chemotherapy thereafter; the skin may die, slough off, and fail to regrow. A response resembling an allergic response, known as recall sensitivity, may happen later—sometimes even years later—if the same drug is used again, even if the drug is injected elsewhere.

Symptoms of extravasation include pain, redness, swelling, or burning at the IV site during or after the administration of chemotherapy.

Notify the medical staff immediately if you have these symptoms during or just after IV treatment.

Eye problems

Cranial irradiation, PUVA treatments for cutaneous lymphoma, or long-term, high-dose use of the corticosteroid drugs such as prednisone are known to cause cataracts, or the redness and soreness of the cornea known as keratitis, in some NHL survivors. While keratitis may resolve on its own, surgery to remove cataracts is the only known cure.

> Unfortunately I developed two problems as a result of my chemotherapy. Due to insurance company politics, I went several months without treatment. The easiest one to treat was dry eye syndrome. All I

needed to do was simply get lubricating drops and use them generously. The second problem was cataracts. Apparently all the prednisone has caused me to develop cataracts prematurely. The only treatment will be surgery in the future.

Fatigue and sleep disorders

Those being treated for cancer list fatigue as the most debilitating symptom they experience. 95 percent of those being treated for cancer report fatigue.

> *I have felt increasingly weak with each chemotherapy treatment. I've been told it's simply the build-up of toxins in my body compounded by not drinking enough. I just can't seem to drink adequately. I also give myself permission to let the house go unkempt and to sleep in when I feel like it.*

While being treated, you may be able to offset some of the effects of fatigue on well-being and performance by getting as much rest as possible, eating well, and exercising moderately. Nonetheless, you may do best to adjust your demands on yourself to these new circumstances: let the less critical things go and attend only to what matters the most.

Symptoms of fatigue should improve after treatment ends; however, many cancer survivors report fatigue years after treatment.

Sleep disorders also are common, and in some cases persist years after treatment. Insomnia, "night horrors," and corresponding daytime sleepiness plague many NHL survivors.

Because fatigue can have so many causes—nutritional deficit, drug interactions, tumor activity, tumor death, inability to exercise, depression, changed sleep patterns—it is difficult to treat fatigue with other than trial-and-error methods. Ask your doctor for suggestions for dealing with this problem, and see Chapter 11, *Stress and the Immune System*, for additional ideas.

Neeraj, NHL/ALL survivor, describes his attempts to overcome fatigue:

> *My doctor said I got so much chemotherapy it was the equivalent of a bone marrow transplant. I have been totally off school and am going back full time next semester. I do not know what to expect with a hematocrit of 36 to 38, and hemoglobin of 11; I tend to get tired. Maybe naps in the noon would be something I should do, or maybe I will have to do. I guess I am going to start a totally new chapter in my recovery, and worst of all*

my mom, who has been with me for a year, won't be here (on my insis-
tence). I would like to know what the future is going to be like in terms of
energy level.

Fever, chills, sweats

Although fever is common following some NHL chemotherapies such as G-CSF or bleomycin, fever should always be reported to your doctor, especially if other signs of illness accompany fever. Fever can be the first symptom of life-threatening infection when white blood cells have been destroyed by therapy.

Unattended fever in the absence of sufficient white blood cell numbers can be fatal and is a medical emergency requiring immediate attention.

Hair loss and growth

Radiotherapy and many chemotherapeutic agents cause hair loss—alopecia—although there is a wide range of individual responses to treatment in this regard. Some people lose just a little hair; others lose all hair, including body hair, eyebrows, and eyelashes. Others report losing gray hair earlier than hair that contains pigment. Those receiving radiation therapy may lose hair only on the spots irradiated.

New hair should regrow in the weeks or months after treatment. In some instances, it may not regrow, although this is more common after radiotherapy, busulfan therapy, or following the high-dose treatment associated with bone marrow transplantation.

Methods to spare the scalp from exposure to chemotherapeutic agents, such as ice-packing or tourniquets, are not recommended, because small amounts of NHL may be sequestered in the skin or blood vessels of the scalp. Denying chemotherapy the opportunity to kill all NHL cells may result in failed treatment or relapse.

> *Two weeks to the day after the first chemotherapy, my hair started*
> *falling out. That was on a Thursday. By Saturday, I sat in my aunt's liv-*
> *ing room pulling my hair out. My daughter Courtney helped. We kind of*
> *made a joke out of it. "Hey, it's a party game," I proclaimed. All I had to*
> *do was run my fingers through my hair and it would fall out.*

My aunt was a little dismayed by it all. She didn't want to take a picture of the event, saying, "I don't think this is something I want to remember." I let Courtney "buzz" the last of it the next day. She loved doing that!

I never got a wig: they all looked so fake. I got a lot of hats, but after about two weeks I got my nerve and just went bald unless I was cold. I got a "wiglet," little bangs you put in a hat, but that gave me a rash. I figured if people couldn't accept me the way I was then phooey on them.

My eyelashes, brows, pubic hair, and underarm hair followed in the next two months. I sunburned my head a couple of times, but other than being cold occasionally at night, it's been kind of nice being able to shower and be dressed and ready to go in less than ten minutes.

Conversely, two drugs used for NHL, interferon and cyclosporine, may cause excessive growth of hair, called hirsutism. Some women taking interferon-alfa-2B report growing long eyelashes for the first time in their lives.

Heart damage

Radiation therapy to the chest and certain drugs used for NHL, such as doxorubicin (adriamycin), are known to be cardiotoxic. Although it is more common for damage from the anthracycline drugs to emerge slowly months or years after treatment ends, immediate and rapidly serious or fatal damage is also possible.

Call your doctor immediately if you experience any symptoms that resemble a heart attack, such as chest tightness or pain, difficulty breathing, or numbness in the left arm or shoulder.

Hypercalcemia

See "Metabolic imbalances."

Infection

Infection can result when neutropenia, a lowering of white blood cell counts, occurs after treatment. The danger period for most patients is five to ten days after treatment. In general, chemotherapy is more likely to cause neutropenia than radiotherapy, but whole-body irradiation can suppress blood counts.

Preventive measures include hand washing, avoiding scratches and cuts via gentle handling of the skin, such as using an electric razor and patting skin dry, rather than rubbing, thorough cooking of food, reducing human contact, and avoiding gardening and handling pet waste.

If you have a fever more than 1.5 degrees higher than your normal temperature, general malaise, severe chills, night sweats, burning or pain while urinating, headache, neck stiffness, coughing, or trouble breathing, phone your doctor without delay.

If an infection develops, your doctor will examine you, and you may be admitted to the hospital, placed in an isolation room, and given a combination of immunoglobulin therapy, antibiotics, antiviral agents, or antifungal agents.

> *Even though I had "high WBC counts for a chemo patient," they were still low enough for infection to creep through. I have experienced one exit site infection around my catheter. It came on very fast, with pain in my breast, redness and drainage from the exit site. I called the doctor on call first thing in the morning since it was a Saturday. I knew I was infected and since it was eight days after chemotherapy I wasn't going to mess around. He had me report to the oncology ward at the hospital as an outpatient. There, the nurses drew blood for a CBC (complete blood count) and collected a culture of the exudate. The doctor then came by and took a look, wrote me a prescription for Keflex and sent me on my way. By Monday, it was as if it had never happened.*

Kidney damage

Temporary or permanent damage to the kidneys may occur with certain drugs such as ifosfamide, CCNU, methotrexate, or cisplatin. Notify your doctor immediately if you have symptoms of kidney failure such as unusually high or low levels of urination, swollen limbs, yellowing skin, decreased sweat, or heart or circulatory symptoms.

Liver or gallbladder dysfunction

Mild liver or gallbladder problems sometimes develop when you are fed only by IV line (TPN, total parenteral nutrition), and the problems go away when you resume eating normally.

An NHL survivor describes the careful monitoring of his liver function during consolidation therapy he received for NHL/ALL:

> My induction and consolidation therapies were quite intense, and the consolidation had to be curtailed a bit due to rising liver enzymes, ALT, and bilirubin. We started the maintenance therapy once the enzymes came down, but the drugs 6-MP and methotrexate (which I took both orally and via spinal taps) caused them to go up again. We tried experimenting with taking 6-MP in small doses and stopped the methotrexate to see the effect on the liver; however, mild doses of the 6-MP elevated the bilirubin and ALT enzymes. So, after a lot of deliberation, we decided to stop the 6-MP and replace methotrexate for the spinal taps with cytosine arabinoside (ARA-C). There doesn't seem to be much literature on such problems during maintenance and what one should do in a situation like this.
>
> I am currently in the experimental phase with the oral methotrexate wherein I am gradually increasing its dose. The liver seems to be doing okay at ten milligrams of methotrexate with the ALT a little elevated to 45, and the bilirubin at 1.5. I have also noticed that the bilirubin remains around 1.0 to 1.3 generally when I go for the blood test after lunch, but goes up if I don't eat, or if I have an empty stomach before the test.

Later, during the year-long maintenance therapy he received, liver values continued to be monitored:

> Blood counts go down during maintenance for NHL/ALL, but believe me, it is the easy phase. After being off school for one and a half years owing to my induction and consolidation therapies, I am doing almost everything as before while on maintenance chemotherapy. The consolidation therapy which lasted ten months has made my liver sensitive, so the doctors have had to be very careful with my maintenance dosage. I am glad that they are also giving a lot of consideration to my quality of life in this phase.

Lung damage

Cyclophosphamide and bleomycin may cause pulmonary fibrosis; methotrexate may cause pneumonitis. Notify your doctor if you have any symptoms of lung impairment such as chest pain or difficulty breathing.

Metabolic imbalances

The drugs used to treat NHL, sometimes in combination with the action of the tumor itself, may disrupt natural levels of electrolytes, minerals, insulin, or antidiuretic hormone. Hypercalcemia, an excess of calcium in the body, is associated with certain NHLs such as T-cell lymphoma/leukemia, some tumors of the head or neck, or myeloma. Disorders known as diabetes insipidus and syndrome of inappropriate antidiuretic hormone (SIADH) also may develop, or symptoms of delirium or adrenal disease may emerge.

Tumor lysis syndrome, arising from the death of large tumors and more common among lymphoblastic and small noncleaved B-cell lymphomas, may arise shortly after chemotherapy is started. Symptoms of kidney failure owing to excessive amounts of calcium, phosphate, and potassium being released by dying tumors are noteworthy, and can be offset with oral or IV hydration, alkalinization of the urine prior to chemotherapy, careful monitoring of electrolytes, use of diuretics, and low initial doses of chemotherapeutic agents, such as those outlined in the French LMB81 protocol.

If you or your loved ones notice any unusual symptoms, especially excessive thirst, unusually high or low levels of urination, swollen limbs, yellowing skin, decreased sweat, abdominal pain, bone pain, seizures, heart or circulatory symptoms, severe mood changes, dementia, delirium, cognitive changes or psychotic behavior, call the doctor.

Mouth or rectal pain (mucositis)

Most people remember stories about vomiting when they think of chemotherapy, but treatments for NHL and other cancers actually may affect the entire gastrointestinal tract, from mouth to anus.

If you experience severe mouth sores, rectal pain that feels like hemorrhoids, or painful or bloody bowel movements, don't suffer in silence. Painkillers and perhaps IV feeding for about a week will help immensely. Some oncologists may prescribe a rinse called Magic Mouthwash that contains a painkiller, an antibiotic, and an antifungal.

Muscle cramps

Many NHL survivors report muscle cramping, especially in the legs and at night, during and after chemotherapy. Often the chemotherapy regimen in use contains vincristine or doxorubicin.

Various remedies exist, such as quinine, calcium, potassium, or magnesium. As calcium, potassium, or magnesium can damage the kidneys, none should be used until you have discussed this issue with your doctor.

Some NHL survivors report that heat treatment, or alternating heat and cold treatment, temporarily reduces pain. Others report that vibrators, massage, or acupuncture help.

Nausea and vomiting

Nausea and vomiting are the result of some, but not all, of the drugs and radiation treatments used for NHL treatment. Nausea associated with radiation therapy usually occurs only if the area just above the navel is irradiated; nausea associated with PUVA treatment for cutaneous lymphoma occurs in 25 percent of patients.

It's important that nausea and vomiting are controlled, not just to reduce suffering, but to allow your body to absorb nutrients to heal, to keep you well hydrated and thus able to flush chemotherapy drugs from body, to support your kidney function, and to allow you uninterrupted sleep during which the immune system is rebuilt. You should not suffer nobly through nausea and vomiting as a mark of strength: you may harm yourself if you do.

Fortunately, excellent drugs are available today to control nausea and vomiting. Zofran (ondansetron) and Kytril (granisetron) are two such anti-emetics, and anti-anxiety drugs such as Xanax, a drug similar to Valium, may work for brief episodes of nausea. Some steroids such as Decadron also work, for reasons that are unclear. Older, less effective drugs, such as Compazine, are also still in use, sometimes in combination with newer drugs.

Phone your doctor immediately if nausea and vomiting are combined with any of the symptoms described under "Infection."

Take your antinausea medications on time, even if you feel well. They work by priming your body before nausea sets in. Moreover, if you wait to take them until you feel bad, you may lose them as you vomit.

Keep your doctor informed about the success of these drugs, because they can be recombined and substituted by others until a good solution is found.

Some oncologists start by prescribing older, less expensive nausea drugs because their use is more acceptable to insurance companies—even though many patients report that drugs such as Zofran are more effective than other drugs. If your pharmaceutical insurance option is liberal, tell your doctor so that he will feel free to prescribe his best choice first.

> Make sure you eat before chemotherapy. It helps—trust me. Also, take your nausea medications with food because they can cause nausea too. Invest in a bland food that you like: for me, it was chicken and rice soup with soda crackers. Sometimes just having food on your stomach helps alleviate the nausea.

Conversely, you may have less nausea after abdominal irradiation if you have an empty stomach when undergoing treatment.

Sometimes just the aroma of food can bring on nausea. If so, you might try eating foods that have been chilled.

If you are unable to keep food down in spite of nausea medication, feeding by IV line for a period of time will give your stomach a chance to recover.

See also "Metabolic imbalances" for hypercalcemia.

Anticipatory nausea also is normal for many cancer patients. If you had treatment in the past that made you ill, during subsequent visits your central nervous system may react with nausea to visual cues or odors in the doctor's office before treatment is begun. You're not crazy: many people report this reaction, even years after treatment. Chapter 11 describes this subconscious and unbidden learning process more fully.

This survivor of NHL/ALL describes with humor how he dealt with nausea:

> A tip for nausea is distraction. My nausea was so bad that during chemotherapy I could throw up on demand. However, one strategy that really worked for me was telling myself that I had no time for nausea and vomiting, and it helped.

Neutropenia

See "Infection."

Numbness, tingling

See "Seizures, paralysis, numbness, tingling."

Pain

Pain can be caused by several of the drugs used for NHL or by radiation therapy.

The vinca alkaloid vincristine clearly is associated with the development of peripheral neuropathy, which may include temporary or permanent pain in hands and feet. Vincristine's negative effects are made worse when G-CSF also is used.

Severe back pain may be associated with degenerative changes to the spine following radiation therapy. Surgery to fuse spinal discs may alleviate this pain.

Painful radiation fibrosis, a reaction of the immune system after exposure to radiation, can develop in any tissue that has been irradiated.

Many other examples could be listed, as pain is a symptom of many aberrant physical processes. The best treatment depends on a correct diagnosis. Consult your doctor or a pain management specialist to find the best treatment for your pain.

Pancytopenia

Pancytopenia is a lowering of all blood cells counts. It's treated with transfusions of red cells and platelets, or irradiated whole blood. See "Infection" for additional information.

Peripheral neuropathy

See "Seizures, paralysis, numbness, tingling" and "Pain."

Pulmonary thrombosis

See "Blood clots."

Radiation enteritis

Radiotherapy can cause abdominal or rectal pain, diarrhea, bloody stools, or mucus in stools when the abdomen is targeted. It may be a short-term effect that fades in four to eight weeks after treatment ends, or, in 5 to 15 percent of patients, it may become a long-term chronic problem.

Interference with the absorption of nutrients is the chief concern. Enteritis is treated by controlling diarrhea with Kaopectate, Lomotil, Paregoric, Cholestyramine, Donnatal, Immodium, or narcotics. Steroid foam may be prescribed if the rectum is quite sore.

Radiation pneumonitis

When the lungs are in the path of radiation targeting NHL in the chest, pneumonitis may develop. The symptoms of pneumonitis resemble pneumonia, and it must be distinguished from pneumonia. Pneumonitis is treated with steroids.

Recall sensitivities

Certain chemotherapies and radiation therapy may damage tissue in a way that leaves it reactive to further treatment for months or years afterward. Drugs that accidentally leak from a vein, for instance, can cause recall sensitivity in that part of the body, even if the drug is injected elsewhere during a subsequent administration. Radiation to an area can cause tissue in that area to react with pain and dysfunction when chemotherapy is administered afterward.

Seizures, paralysis, numbness, tingling

Side effects related to the central nervous system are sometimes seen after certain chemotherapeutic agents are used for NHL.

Seizures may follow use of drugs such as methotrexate, cytosine arabinoside (ARA-C), cisplatin, or ifosfamide. Only about 3 percent of patients receiving these agents experience seizures, and it is more likely to occur in patients who have had cranial irradiation, but it is also possible that seizures will occur in a patient whose metabolic balance has been affected by NHL or its treatment. Seizures can be controlled with antiseizure medication and are usually transient.

If you are receiving methotrexate or ARA-C administered under the scalp or into the spine, you may be at risk for ascending myelopathy, which is numbness in the legs and back, and the loss of bowel and bladder control. It usually develops rapidly, and may progress to paralysis. Seizures also may follow. Usually the symptoms abate on their own, but there are instances of permanent damage and even death. Some doctors will administer these drugs only at intervals of forty-eight to seventy-two hours in order to reduce the chance of this side effect.

The vinca alkaloid vincristine clearly is associated with the development of peripheral neuropathy, which may include numbness, tingling, or pain in hands and feet, and, more rarely, twitches or palsies. Vincristine's negative effects are made worse when G-CSF also is used. Peripheral neuropathy usually is temporary, but may become permanent.

Some NHL survivors who receive radiation report odd head, neck, or arm symptoms when they tilt their head or twist their neck. Called Lhermitte sign, some report this as dizziness, and others as an odd sensation that spans the gap between noise and movement. This is most likely caused by demyelination, a temporary form of radiation damage to the material that insulates our nerves. As electric wires are insulated by rubber, so our neurons are insulated by myelin, which serves to protect our neurons from crossover of electric current and loss of signal. Lhermitte sign is an indication that two nerves are crossing over in a demyelinated area and are confusing their signals. This symptom should abate in several months.

See also "Metabolic imbalances."

Skin problems

A wide variety of skin problems—pain, itching, burning, discoloration, scaling, wrinkling, dryness, rash, redness—are associated with just about all of the treatments used for treating NHL. Many chemotherapies, radiation therapy, and photochemotherapy for cutaneous lymphomas can cause these problems.

Ask your doctor for help before tackling this on your own, because dermatology problems can be complex and hard to diagnose. Common remedies, such as lotions that contain alcohol, may make the problem worse, especially if itching is your chief complaint.

One survivor discusses this common reaction:

> One of the most troubling things happened almost immediately. I always have had somewhat sensitive skin, but now it really got out of hand. I couldn't wear any tape or adhesives at all, they all gave me a rash. This made securing my catheter difficult. I finally had to start wearing a bra twenty-four hours a day, seven days a week, to hold the catheter in place. I couldn't wear a dressing over my catheter so I just scrubbed it daily with antibacterial soap. I couldn't use my normal moisturizer for sensitive skin and the chemotherapy was drying me out even more. I finally stumbled on oatmeal soap and cream. This did wonders, and didn't burn. I would later learn that the skin problems were caused by the action of chemotherapy on quickly replicating cells, into which category epidermal (skin) cells fall.

The change in skin color that may accompany treatment is often a tanned effect. This is not a true suntan that will protect you from the sun's rays. In fact, your skin will be overly sensitive to sunlight, and prone to wrinkling, freckling, or premature aging, and should be protected accordingly.

If you notice any unusual lesions in the treated areas, such as moles, tell your doctor.

Sore, red, stiff veins

If administered into the arms, the vinca alkaloid vincristine (Oncovin) may cause pain and swelling of veins, even if no leakage has occurred.

If you notice lengths of rigid, painful, swollen, or red veins in the days or weeks following receipt of vincristine, tell your doctor, because these symptoms are the same as those associated with blood clots.

Ice packs or warm (not hot) compresses may relieve the pain associated with veins that have reacted to chemotherapy.

To spare your veins from additional damage, your doctor may recommend that you have a venous access device such as a PICC line or central catheter installed.

Tumor lysis syndrome

See "Metabolic imbalances."

Urinary bladder pain, hemorrhagic cystitis

Drugs such as cyclophosphamide (Cytoxin), ifosfamide, CCNU, and platinum-containing drugs such as cisplatin can damage the bladder. Simultaneous administration of a drug called Mesna (mercaptoethane sulfonate), along with hydration by mouth and IV, are critical to protect the bladder from this painful and sometimes chronic condition. Sometimes this combination is administered during a brief hospital stay to allow close monitoring to guard against bladder or kidney damage:

> It was a difficult process (for me) to receive these high doses of chemotherapy followed by loads of saline to flush and hydrate my system. It meant feeling bloated for about a day, and dragging all the tubes and IV rack back and forth to the bathroom every hour or so. When I was too weak to do that, it meant pushing a call button all day and night to summon a nurse with a bedpan. And of course, it meant monitoring the output of urine, which gradually transitioned from burning to normal, until the doctor was convinced we had compensated for the toxicity of treatment. Some of this protocol must have been surprising to the nurses. I recall hearing my doctor's voice telling hospital staff at the nursing station that this would be bringing me to the point of death in order to save my life.

Radiation therapy that cannot avoid the bladder also may cause temporary or permanent changes in bladder function. The bladder may become less elastic, and the urge to urinate may become more frequent.

Weight gain or loss

One of the myths about cancer treatment is that it always causes weight loss. For any cancer treated with steroids, however, the reverse may be true.

The corticosteroid drugs used against NHL, such as prednisone, may increase appetite and cause weight gain. When treatment has ended, the weight may drop away on its own, or changes in diet and exercise patterns may be necessary to lose weight. Attempting to lose weight while being treated is not recommended. Maintaining excellent nutritional intake to help your body slough off damaged tissue and rebuild new tissue is difficult enough during treatment without limiting the intake of calories.

It's quite common to develop chubby cheeks, known as moon face, if you're taking prednisone for NHL. This accumulation of fat in the cheeks will abate after prednisone therapy ends.

If you are losing weight during treatment in spite of, or in the absence of, steroid therapy, notify your doctor, and see the suggestions included in the sections, "Appetite and taste changes" and "Nausea and vomiting."

Summary

Many cancer survivors expect that treatment will make them feel bad, but they're not sure exactly what to expect. Some are delighted to find that they experience very few side effects of treatment, or none at all.

This chapter may serve as a reference for you as treatment unfolds. Knowing which effects of treatment are temporary, which are harmless, and what to do about those that are not is a useful beginning to dealing with treatment.

Some side effects linger and can be classified as late effects. Some effects that usually do not emerge until months after treatment may emerge sooner in some patients. Chapter 16 describes these more fully.

See Appendix A for excellent books that describe side effects, and how to deal with them, in greater depth.

CHAPTER 10

If You're Hospitalized

*Such patients as are able shall assist in
nursing others, washing and ironing linen and
cleaning the rooms and such other services as
the matron may require.*

—Regulations of the Philadelphia
General Hospital, 1790

Treatment of the non-Hodgkin's lymphomas has evolved in sophistication and accuracy to the point that most treatments are no longer given in an inpatient setting. There are a few circumstances surrounding NHL, however, that might result in your being admitted to the hospital. Treatment for infections that arise during chemotherapy, delivery of drugs that require offsetting with other, protective drugs, the care surrounding bone marrow transplantation, and certain surgeries are most successfully addressed in an inpatient setting.

Some people are frightened by the idea of being admitted to the hospital, even while realizing that the best care for a particular problem can be delivered only with the round-the-clock medical scrutiny available in a good hospital.

This chapter will help you view the experience in a positive light, and will highlight the precautions you can follow to make your stay brief and fruitful. We will examine the experience chronologically, beginning with preparation and admitting procedures, and finishing with discharge and home care.

In the United States, generally you are limited to using hospitals at which your doctors have admitting privileges. It's best to consider this in advance, as discussed in Chapter 2, *Finding the Right Oncologist*. Ideally, the hospital should be an NCI-designated comprehensive cancer center or affiliated with a medical school. At the very least, it should be accredited by the Joint Commission on Accreditation of Healthcare Organizations (JCAHO). Call JCAHO at (708) 916-5800, and ask the hospital's administrators about the outcome of their latest evaluation by JCAHO. For more detailed information on selecting a hospital, see *A Cancer Survivor's Almanac*, published by the National Coalition for Cancer Survivorship.

If you have a child who is facing hospitalization, you're probably aware that children have unique fears and misunderstandings about hospital care. You can address your child's concerns using the collective advice of more than forty parents presented in the book *Your Child in the Hospital: A Practical Guide for Parents*, by Nancy Keene and Rachel Prentice.

Preparation

If you know in advance that you'll be admitted to the hospital, you can plan to make your stay brief and successful. If your admission is a planned one for a transplant or for surgery, copious helpful information, including what to bring, will be given to you in advance by the staff.

On the other hand, you may be admitted to the hospital hastily if an infection or unusual side effects develop after chemotherapy is administered. If you have symptoms of an infection, your doctor may insist, for example, that you proceed directly to an isolation room in the oncology wing while your loved ones deal with the admitting paperwork in the germ-filled front lobby.

You may be admitted via the emergency room if symptoms are unusual, have a rapid onset, or are associated with immediate danger, such as difficulty breathing. It's best to avoid the emergency room, though, by careful tracking of symptoms and timely communication with your doctor. Emergency-room care may be greatly delayed, or may vary in quality, based on several factors beyond your control, such as the seriousness of the illnesses of others waiting or the experience of the medical staff on duty. If you must use an emergency room, be sure to call your oncologist and let her know what's happened.

Arrangements

Here are some general tips for preparing in advance for a hospital stay:

- You can smooth the path of abrupt admissions by having an overnight bag ready that contains much of what you'll need. See the next section, "What to bring."

- If you're being admitted for surgery or any other procedure, call your insurance company to see if the procedure must be precertified. Keep a written log of whom you spoke with and when.

- If you're being admitted for surgery, verify that the surgeon and the anesthesiologist are board certified in their areas of expertise. The *Official ABMS Directory of Board Certified Medical Specialists* is a publication that can be found in a local library, and the American Medical Association also can verify board certification. (See Appendix A, *Resources*.) Your state licensing board or state medical society can verify how many years of experience your surgeon has. If you're having a tumor-affected ovary or uterus removed, consider consulting a gynecologic oncologist, a surgeon who specializes in removing cancers of the female reproductive organs.

- If you're being admitted for surgery, obtain and review all consent documents. Strike any clauses that connote that staff other than your surgeon may be participating in your procedure, unless you and your doctor have already discussed who else might be participating and you're comfortable with these additional personnel.

- Hospitals that receive federal funding or are governed by certain local laws must adhere to federal or local laws regarding informed consent prior to use of human subjects for research. Government-funded hospitals include most university, state, and nonprofit hospitals. Verify whether your hospital receives any federal funding, and phone your state health department to determine if your state has its own laws regarding consent issues. If your hospital is a private for-profit hospital that receives no federal funding and is not governed by similar local laws, question closely any treatment suggested for you. Ask your doctor if your proposed treatment represents state-of-the-art treatment as defined by the NCI, or if you'll be treated in an investigational study.

- Ask if you can donate your own blood (autologous donation) in advance of surgery.

- Read as much as you can on the procedure you'll be having.

- Make notes about all health problems you have, related to NHL and otherwise. Make several photocopies of these notes, because each group of medical caretakers you meet will ask the same questions again.

- Arrange for child care, if appropriate. Most likely this care will be provided by a well-informed friend or relative, but if not, prepare abundant information well in advance, in writing, including phone numbers of relatives and pediatricians.

- Contact a pet-sitter, if needed. Provide clear written instructions regarding feeding and any health problems. Provide your veterinarian's address and phone number, and those of an emergency all-night veterinary service. Leave all supplies, including carrier and medications, in a prominent place.

- Have the mail and newspapers held if nobody will remain at home. Make arrangements for a plant-waterer, if needed.

- Pay any upcoming bills in advance.

- Plan transportation to and from the hospital, allowing plenty of time in everyone's schedules for check-in and check-out procedures. Hospitals are not very good at checking patients out quickly, especially if you need special instructions about home aftercare.

- Call the hospital and ask about parking arrangements, such as less expensive long-term passes for those who will be visiting you during an extended stay, special parking for outpatient units, or discounted or waived fees for those accompanying you during a surgery.

- Arrange to use your laptop computer during your stay if you enjoy Internet email support from friends or other people with NHL. Ask first if the hospital has digital phone lines. If so, borrow or buy an adapter so your modem won't be ruined. Tell email friends if you'd love to receive email during your stay, but point out that you might not be able to respond. Ask them not to be offended, but to keep on writing.

- Contact your employer, not only to arrange for use of sick time or disability pay, but to ensure his emotional and professional support when you return to work. Ask for a copy of company leave policies and the federal Family and Medical Leave Act in order to become acquainted with all employment-related options.

- Check your calendar and cancel any commitments that conflict with your hospital schedule.

- Arrange for a visiting or live-in home nurse if you think you or your caretaker will need extra help after your hospital stay. Many insurance companies will pay toward this service if your doctor says you meet certain conditions, such as being temporarily unable to bathe.

What to bring

Some people pack too little, assuming that the hospital will provide everything. Here are some suggestions:

- Prepare several copies of lists of your medications, both prescription and over-the-counter. Never assume the hospital has spoken with all of your doctors.

- Bring your health insurance card and your certificate showing you donated your own blood, if applicable.

- Bring your own over-the-counter medications if you suffer from hemorrhoids, athlete's foot, tooth sensitivity, or other conditions not related to NHL. You must remember to inform the staff first, though, if you need to use these supplies: they are medications, and they may interact unfavorably with the medications your doctor has ordered.

- You may feel better in your own clothing if you have someone who can launder it for you. Don't bring any clothing with metal zippers or snaps, which may interfere with diagnostic tests such as x-rays or MRI. If you're having surgery, choose clothing that won't press on your incision or cause you undue strain as you dress. Choose shirts with easy sleeves that can accommodate IV lines. Add something dashing or seductive to the overnight bag if you think an ego boost will help. If you're being hospitalized for a transplant, pack loose cotton garments that can withstand sanitizing procedures involving high heat.

- If you pack a razor, avoid the plug-in electric variety, as the local fire code or the proximity of hospital oxygen supplies may regulate against these. Battery-operated razors generally are most acceptable; however, a disposable razor may do, provided you're able to manipulate it while feeling less than your usual self, and provided you're not told to avoid cuts and scrapes while your blood counts are low.

- Bring eye and ear coverings for sleep. Hospitals can be noisy places at odd hours.

- If music will help you relax and sleep, bring a personal player with a headset to avoid disturbing your roommate.

- If you anticipate a long stay, bring pictures of home, family, pets, and loving experiences.

- Remember warm socks. (The nursing staff love wild socks.)

- If this is a return trip, bring the phone the hospital may have sold you during your prior stay.

- An old sock full of quarters will help you and your family make postsurgical phone calls, pay for parking, buy newspapers, or buy those dreadful but sometimes unavoidable vending-machine meals. Unlike a purse or a wallet, a ratty old sock doesn't look worth stealing.

- If you bring a laptop computer, bring a bike lock to anchor it to the bed if the hospital has experienced theft.

- Pack a list of phone numbers of friends and family.

- Most hospitals provide some toiletries, such as soap, washcloths, and a toothbrush, but you may prefer your own. Avoid heavily scented products, though, as these may make you or your roommate ill.

- Prepare several copies of your advance directives to inform the staff of your wishes for or against extreme life-support measures.

- Bring books that are lightweight, both tangibly and intellectually. You may be groggy and achy for a spell. Don't plan to read and analyze the Hardy-Weinberg equilibrium or to hold open a seven-pound tax code manual during your hospital stay.

- For females, pack a long, loose shirt or tunic top for the times when you're told to "take everything off, and put on this gown with the opening in the front." Sooner or later you will indeed have to open these in the front, but you'll feel less the victim of someone else's poor sartorial taste.

- For both males and females, pack a pair of baggy boxer shorts for the times when you're told to "take everything off, and put on this gown with the opening in the back."

What not to bring

Some people bring too many things or inappropriate things to the hospital.

- Leave all jewelry at home. If you want to wear your wedding band, ask the staff about this first. They may secure it with tape during a surgery, for example.

- Scented toiletries. You may feel nausea after certain procedures and scents may tip you (or your poor, captive roommate) over the edge of gastric comfort. Moreover, you may come to associate your once-favorite scent with a hospital stay.

- Leave your purse, wallet, credit cards, and money—beyond incidental change for newspapers and the like—at home or in a safe-deposit box.

- Leave your worries and your work behind. Let your family and the hospital staff coddle you with backrubs. Channel-surf and watch sleazy TV shows for the utter decadence of it. Order everything on the hospital menu and share it with your pals.

Admission

Admission will start with paperwork, phone calls, questions about next of kin, phone and TV service preferences, attachment of a plastic ID bracelet, and directions to the correct room and floor. Have copies of all insurance paperwork and medical records ready

After admission, a volunteer may be assigned to stay with you briefly until you've arrived in your room and become oriented, especially if you're having surgery.

Once you have arrived in your room, the nursing staff will take control and prepare you for whatever care you will need. They'll check vital signs such as pulse and temperature, and may start an intravenous line (IV) for administering drugs. You'll probably find that nurses will return a hundredfold any small effort you make to be friendly and kind.

Ask now about the meal menus, as there is usually a delay in getting meal preferences to newly admitted patients.

The staff

The nursing staff are the first group you're likely to encounter in your hospital stay, but they're just one group of a confusing array of medical personnel you'll meet.

Note that you may refuse care administered by any staff member with whom you don't feel comfortable, and may ask for a more experienced person to attend to you.

Nurses

Hospital nurses will provide most of your care:

- Nurses' aides and licensed practical nurses (LPNs) will help wash you, help you in and out of bed, make your bed, and perform simple nursing tasks such as checking your pulse and temperature. LPNs, but not nurses' aides, have completed vocational training and may provide medication.

- Registered nurses (RNs) have earned a college degree in nursing and passed a licensing examination. RNs are able to provide more complex and critical medical care than LPNs, such as changing wound dressings, starting IVs, and administering IV medications.

- Nurse practitioners or clinical nurse specialists are RNs who have undertaken extensive additional training and are licensed to provide many of the same services that doctors provide. In some states they are able to prescribe drugs under the auspices of a physician. In some hospitals or clinical settings they may perform simple surgeries and procedures, such as lancing abscesses.

- Head nurses and nurse managers are in charge of other nurses, entire floors, or patient centers. Although all nurses now face the additional burden of administrative work that deprives them of time they prefer to spend with their patients, head nurses and nurse managers usually handle administrative issues exclusively, and seldom provide patient care unless staffing is inadequate.

Doctors

In teaching hospitals, you'll encounter the full spectrum of doctors in various stages of training. In some community hospitals, you'll encounter just residents and attending physicians. In other community hospitals that have agreements with nearby medical schools, you may find an amalgam of the two systems. Doctors in various stages of training include:

- Medical students have completed four years of college and are undertaking four additional years of medical school. Medical students do not treat patients, although they may accompany an attending physician on rounds, and the physician may elicit their opinions.

- Interns, also called first-year residents, or postgraduate year-one students, have completed four years of medical school and are in the first year of three to six years of primary specialty training. They will not give you care unless supervised by much more experienced personnel, such as the attending physician or a more experienced resident, but that supervision may be distant. If you prefer not to be treated by an intern, say so.

- House officers (once called residents) may be postgraduate year-two students, postgraduate year-three students, and so on. These physicians are still receiving primary training that can last from three to six years, depending on the field.

- Fellows, or teaching fellows, have completed their six years' primary training, and have undertaken three years of additional training in a subspecialty.

- The attending physician is in charge of all fellows, residents, and interns. In university hospitals, she is likely to be a faculty member. In community hospitals, she is hired to oversee patient care in her area of specialty based upon her reputation in the medical community.

Treatment

Although reasons for hospitalization among cancer survivors vary greatly, certain treatments for NHL fall into a pattern. Occasionally, complex exploratory or diagnostic procedures, such as biopsy of a chest tumor, may require hospitalization. In general, however, abdominal surgery, isolation against and treatment of infection, and supportive care during certain chemotherapy regimens are the three most common hospitalization experiences among NHL survivors.

Surgery

Surgeries for NHL that require hospitalization include removal of the spleen, an ovary, a portion of the intestine, or biopsy of lymph nodes in the abdomen or pelvis. Occasionally, neurosurgery may be performed to treat NHL found in the brain.

You'll receive extensive instructions, will meet with the anesthesiologist, and will be monitored to ensure that no food is taken about 12 hours before surgery. Certain tests such as CT scans or MRI may be repeated to precisely target tumors that need to be removed.

If you do not have a central catheter, an IV will be placed in your arm or hand before surgery—perhaps one day before or directly before.

The site of the incision will be cleaned, shaved, and possibly marked just before the surgery. If you're an especially hairy male, ask that a large area be shaved, including the IV site on your arm. Sticky bandaging can hurt terribly when it's removed if it pulls against hairs that have not been shaved.

If you're feeling nervous, ask for a sedative. The hour or two directly before surgery are likely to be the most tense.

If you're having general anesthesia and have had nausea associated with this procedure in the past, tell the anesthesiologist.

You may be asked to walk into the surgical suite, or you may be taken in on a rolling bed and shifted to the table. If you're having general anesthesia, a rubber oxygen mask may be placed over your face to check for fit. If you're having epidural (spinal) anesthesia, most likely you'll also be given a sedative by IV to help you relax. Your arms may be positioned on armrests that facilitate giving medications by IV.

For general anesthesia, most likely a breathing tube will be inserted from your mouth to your upper lungs, but this intubation will be done after you're asleep, as may the insertion of a urinary catheter or a nasogastric tube to keep your bladder and stomach empty. Coating your eyelids with a lubricant while you're asleep to keep them from drying may also be done, as presurgical medication may include drugs to dry body fluids and reduce bleeding.

And now, the good part: you'll fall asleep, and you won't care what they do.

When you reawaken slowly, you'll be in the recovery room. You may notice that you've acquired rubber support stockings or a series of tubes attached to various body parts—but you won't care too much, because you'll be groggy for several more hours. You may also notice that your hearing returns first, well before sight does, and that you can remember odd or humorous things the staff said as the surgery was ending.

You may feel some pain, too, upon waking. The nursing staff will not administer painkiller, though, until you're clearly awake, in order to avoid overdosing a patient possibly still affected by anesthesia. This means that, if you're feeling pain, you must tell them distinctly as soon as you are able. Groaning, for example, is not considered a clear indicator that you're awake.

Eventually you'll be returned to your room, but the first twenty-four hours may be a hazy memory if you've received general anesthesia. If you received a sedative instead of general anesthesia, you'll be groggy, too, but it will resolve more quickly than the aftereffects of general anesthesia.

If you received spinal anesthesia, you may be required to lay flat for twenty-four hours to avoid getting headaches. If you develop a headache following a "spinal," do tell the nursing staff, because small leaks at the puncture site in epidural tissue that cause headaches are easily repaired.

If you feel any nausea at all, even transient nausea, tell the nursing staff immediately. Vomiting, especially with a fresh abdominal incision, is a very unpleasant experience.

A PCA (patient-controlled analgesia) pump may be attached to your IV line so that you can administer micro-doses of painkiller as needed. (Don't worry about overdose. The pump won't allow it.) Alternately, you may be given oral painkilling medication on a fixed schedule or as needed.

Use of anesthesia and painkillers slow the activity of various organs, including the kidneys, urinary bladder, and intestinal tract. Your liquid and solid waste may be monitored after surgery until the staff note that your body systems are once again functioning as they should.

Infection

About seven to ten days after certain chemotherapies are given, it's common for one's white blood cell counts to drop to dangerously low levels. Without adequate numbers of white blood cells, the body cannot fight infection.

If you're hospitalized for infection, most likely you'll be placed alone in a hospital room, a procedure called isolation. The air may be scrubbed with a high-energy particulate air (HEPA) filter or controlled via laminar airflow.

Although some studies have shown that infection during neutropenia most often arises from pathogens already within the patient's body, restriction of visitors, gifts, and certain foods will be enforced:

- All who enter will be expected to adhere to safety measures such as vigorous handwashing and covering the mouth with a mask.

- Gift plants with pollen-bearing stamens, potting soil, or silk plants with mossy, fungus-bearing camouflage at their base may be returned or held outside your room.

- Certain foods, such as fresh fruit or yeast breads, may be denied you.

Isolation procedures may seem odd—after all, you're already infected—but the goal is to prevent your coming in contact with additional and potentially very serious infectious agents.

You'll be given oral or IV antibiotics, antivirals, or antifungals, depending on your symptoms and the results of various cultures. You may also be given drugs to help you grow new white or red blood cells.

You'll stay in isolation until your white blood cell counts rise and the infection is bested, either by the antibiotics you're given or by the infection-fighting ability of your own increasing white blood cells.

Chemotherapy

Some chemotherapies are given as inpatient treatment in order to simultaneously administer additional agents that offset the damage to healthy organs or to monitor the state of affected organs. A frequently noted example is the use of Mesna to prevent damage to the bladder and kidneys when the anticancer agent cyclophosphamide is used.

The procedures used will vary, of course, depending on the agents being given, but most likely you can expect an IV line to be inserted if you don't have a permanent venous catheter, and you'll receive frequent and perhaps somewhat embarrassing attention from nurses regarding normally routine and personal phenomena such as blood pressure, how much urine or feces you've passed, whether bowel movements are painful, and so on.

If copious oral or IV hydration accompanies your treatment, unless a urinary catheter is in place, you'll be compelled to rise frequently to urinate, and you may become quite tired owing to lack of a full night's sleep.

Thriving versus surviving

Almost nobody wants to be hospitalized. The goal is to make the stay short and successful by remembering that ultimately it's your life, and, in spite of perhaps temporarily diminished capacities, you're still very much in charge.

Here are three key points:

- **Read your medical chart.** Ask questions if anything is unclear. Ask for definitions of terms the staff may use, such as NPO (*noli para os*, nothing by mouth). If you're not well enough to do this, have a friend or relative do so.

- **Verify all drugs given to you.** Ask about oral medications before swallowing, and read the contents of the IV bags on your pole. If you're not well enough to do this, have a friend or relative do so.

- **Tell the nursing staff right away if something seems wrong.** Don't let seemingly simple things, like feeling constipated, become major problems.

Additional ideas for dealing with your hospitalization:

- Move about your room and the corridors as much as possible. You'll heal faster and diminish the likelihood of serious complications if you move about. If you feel too bad to get out of bed, flex your arms and legs a good deal. If you're neutropenic, ask if you and your IV pole can cruise the corridors wearing a mask and surgical slippers. (If you feel conspicuous wearing a mask, you might try making a prank of it by adding a toothy grin with waterproof ink.)

- If you've had surgery, do the physical therapy, coughing, or breathing exercises you're given as soon and as often as possible. Like overall body movement, these exercises will help you heal more quickly, and will reduce the chance of developing complications such as the form of pneumonia that's associated with lying flat for long periods. If you have an abdominal incision, hold a pillow against it for comfort while you cough.

- If you brought your laptop, use it to read email from friends. Don't feel obligated to respond if you're feeling bad. Ask a loved one to reply for you if a reply seems much needed.

- If you have trouble getting in and out of bed after abdominal surgery, ask the nursing staff to tie something rope-like to the footboard so you can experiment with using arm muscles instead of abdominal muscles to pull yourself up and, especially, to lay yourself back down.

- If you're not on a restricted diet, coerce friends and loved ones into bringing you your favorite foods. This will make you feel better, and will help those friends who would otherwise not know what to do feel useful and loving. Most hospitals now permit outside food to be brought into the patient's room, a change more in keeping with the European model of families caring for patients.

- At first, take pain medication on schedule, even if you think you won't need it, because you'll heal better and can be more mobile if pain is adequately controlled. As time passes, you'll be a better judge of how much painkiller you really need.

- Befriend the staff. They'll repay you tenfold for your kindness. It's surprising how much can be asked of others if it's done in a nice way.

- If you're a caretaker, pitch in and do what you can to help the nurses help your loved one. Stay overnight if at all possible; if the staff decline, insist.

When my husband was hospitalized after his abdominal surgery, he was on morphine which slowed his ability to urinate. Often during the night he needed to use the john, and he and his IV pole would stand there in front of the toilet doing not much of anything for ten or fifteen minutes. Because I stayed with him overnight, I was able to help him in and out of bed repeatedly without his calling a nurse.

Discharge and departure

Discharge may be an anticlimax after your hospital stay, but you should use this time to have the staff answer all of your questions about aftercare. Make sure you understand:

- First, whether you're really going to be able to handle being at home. If you're not reasonably mobile or pain-free, ask for additional time in the hospital.

- If your spleen is removed, you should discuss with your doctor the need to be revaccinated every few years with pneumococcal, *Haemophilus influenzae* type b, and meningococcal vaccines. The risk of being overwhelmed by agents capable of producing encapsulated infections is higher in those lacking a spleen.

- The medications you may be taking.

- Whether the hospital pharmacy can fill your prescriptions before you leave. If not, get the doctor to phone your pharmacy or get a family member to fill prescriptions beforehand.

- How to care for your incision if you've had surgery.

- What side effects or aftereffects you should watch for that might signal a problem.

- What follow-up appointments should be scheduled, and any diet restrictions.

- Your bill. Always ask for an itemized bill.

The person helping you with your trip home should bring the car to the exit in advance, and should make as many preliminary trips as necessary to remove your personal effects and gifts from your room, perhaps warming or cooling the car in advance as well. Most important, though, is that by leaving you for last your escort can devote attention to you alone as you're exiting. This is a useful arrangement because you may need help getting into the car, for example, but the hospital's assistance and liability end at the door.

Use the restroom before you leave, even if you think you don't need to. Even a small amount of stress on the trip home, or cold temperatures, for example, can cause the brain to signal the bladder or bowel to empty.

Most hospitals have a regulation stating that you must be escorted to the door in a wheelchair. This reduces the chance that patients possibly weakened by extended bed rest will pass out or suffer a misstep while exiting. While many people leaving the hospital find using a wheelchair embarrassing, it safeguards both you and the hospital. Fortunately or unfortunately, you'll have plenty of chances to prove you're mobile again once you're out the door.

Note that all of the circumstances addressed in this chapter—surgery, treatment of infection, and receipt of chemotherapy—may cause feelings of fatigue that may last for weeks after your hospital stay has ended.

Summary

Current treatment for NHL has evolved away from inpatient hospital treatment, but there are a few circumstances that may require hospitalization. This chapter offers insights and checklists to help make your stay successful.

For several good books that deal exclusively and in depth with being hospitalized, see Appendix A, *Resources*. For many excellent ideas on dealing with surgery and recovering afterward, see *Surgery and Recovery*, by Kaye Olson, RN.

CHAPTER 11

Stress and the Immune System

A good laugh and a long sleep are the best
cures in the doctor's book.

—Irish proverb

Some people believe that their non-Hodgkin's lymphoma was caused by stress, or that it will be made worse by stress, or that perhaps they have a cancer-prone personality. Many research studies have attempted to discover links between cancer, stress, depression, personality, and coping skills. The connections are complex:

- First, there is no consistent evidence that stress causes or worsens cancer. Studies done using animals and humans do not consistently show a positive association between stress and cancer, not even when underlying disease already exists. In fact, in some animals, some forms of stress cause tumors to shrink. More details are provided in the section "Stress and cancer."

- Second, the few studies that hint at a link between personality and cancer are not conclusive for various reasons, such as the design of the study. Details are discussed in the section "Is there a cancer personality?"

This chapter will describe the known associations—or the lack of them—between stress, the immune system, illness, and cancer. A definition of stress is offered, then physical and emotional responses to stress are described, followed by a discussion of the evidence, or the lack of it, regarding stress and cancer. This chapter concludes with ways you can minimize stress or make stress a useful experience.

What is stress?

Experts in various fields of medicine and psychology recognize many different circumstances and events as stressful. Depending on the circumstances or point of view, stress could be viewed as a threatening object or the event itself, the physical reaction within our bodies to the threat, or the state of mind that precedes our taking some action in response to threat.

To the psychiatrist studying brain chemistry, our awakening in the morning and the corresponding rise or fall in levels of several hormones may be viewed as a stressful event for the constantly adapting brain. For the psychologist, overcrowding of humans in urban areas can be viewed as a stressful event. For an orthopedic surgeon, the impact sustained by cartilage within the knee when one runs on concrete is viewed as stress.

The psychoneuroimmunologist, however, views the interaction of the immune system with the central nervous system as an adaptation to stress. This interpretation, which can accommodate both physical and emotional stress, will be the chief focus of this chapter.

For the sake of readability, we won't differentiate between responses and reactions, nor between anxiety and worry. We will assume that the stress of a cancer diagnosis causes distress, although some authorities maintain that not all stressors cause distress.

Responses to stress

Our bodies and minds respond to stress in many ways. These adaptations may change with the type and intensity of the stressor, the amount of time we have been exposed to it, our previous experiences trying to adapt to similar stressful events, the person experiencing stress, and his or her physical and emotional state at the time.

Although many emotional responses to stress are possible, such as anger and withdrawal, the responses most often reported by cancer survivors are fear, anxiety, and depression. The National Cancer Institute reports that during and after diagnosis and treatment, almost half of all cancer patients report anxiety and about a quarter report significant anxiety. Twenty percent experience transient or long-term depression, and 15 percent are diagnosed with post-traumatic stress disorder. Estimates by other researchers are sometimes much higher.

Fear is sometimes useful

Several bodily changes occur as a reaction to a fearful event. During fear, hormones that prepare us to adapt to stress are released in a chain reaction, first from the brain, which trigger in turn the release of antistress hormones from the adrenal glands. Our heart rate increases, blood is redirected to body parts associated with fight or flight, and extra sugar is made available in the bloodstream via the liver.

Fear can be a useful, goal-oriented reaction to a stressor. Each of these physical changes is aimed either at our fleeing from danger or conquering it bodily.

Fascinating research into brain structure and function has shown that the amygdala, part of the "old brain" conserved in most creatures from reptiles up through the primates, including humans, is the brain organ responsible for finding safety quickly when fear arises. Direct connections between the amygdala and our sensory organs bypass the higher brain centers of decision-making, allowing us to react very quickly to threats, sometimes without our being aware that we have perceived them. For instance, if you hike in the woods, have you ever stopped abruptly after sensing just a muted change of color or pattern, and upon closer inspection realize that subtle difference is a snake? This brain connection is probably responsible for the immediate, calm, highly effective, goal-oriented behavior that some people exhibit in unbelievably horrifying situations.

Although fear doesn't feel good, it can be a useful, goal-oriented reaction to a stressor. It galvanizes us and prepares us for action. The extreme and immediate physical reaction to fear, however, does little or nothing to prepare us to deal intellectually with a fearful situation that requires extensive analysis, planning, and decision-making, such as absorbing the technical medical information about our cancer diagnosis. On the contrary, research has shown that both very low and very high levels of the antistress hormones from the adrenal gland interfere with learning new tasks. Short of our ability to jump up and flee the doctor's office or our sudden acquisition of strength to throttle the bearer of bad news, we have been poorly prepared by evolution for dealing with cancer as a stressful event. As a result, an out-of-phase mismatch of events is what many of us experience when being told of the cancer diagnosis—with a strong likelihood that we will remember forever and with great acuity the perceptual cues that were present, instead of the key points that the doctor attempted to relay.

Anxiety is unhealthy

Most adults have experienced the difference between fear and anxiety. Fear is an acute, strong, visceral response to stress. Anxiety is a nagging, chronic, or generalized fear response. Although some would choose the chronic physical distress of anxiety over the pronounced physical distress of fear, anxiety may be the more physically harmful of the two experiences.

Unresolved fear may convert to anxiety as we begin to grow accustomed to a threat. When we're anxious, the same physical changes that accompany fear occur at lower levels, with deleterious effects on our body. Sustained increased heart output and constriction of blood vessels to rechannel blood to certain organs can contribute to the development of high blood pressure and cardiovascular disease. Altered sugar metabolism can worsen diabetes. The tendency for digestive activity to increase in times of stress can exacerbate underlying gastrointestinal disease.

Worry and anxiety involve recycling the same fear, repeatedly examining the outcomes and evaluating interventions. We sometimes use this activity to justify worry, assuming that repeated scrutiny will result in knowing what to do if worse comes to worst, but this continual rehearsal of negative events in search of solutions may not benefit us should danger actually arise. The two thought processes, worry and planning, center in different parts of the brain. On magnetic resonance imaging, those who worry show activity in the emotional part of the brain, whereas those who plan show activity in the opposite hemisphere, the so-called logical half of the brain. This may mean that, from the standpoint of providing a good solution in the face of danger, worry is not the best strategy. Worry does not determine the best solution and move on to the next problem. It prevents us from detecting and dealing with new problems in a timely and effective way.

Physical symptoms of anxiety may include any of these: shortness of breath, sigh breathing, dry mouth, inability to swallow, trembling, weakness, incessant crying, circular or obsessive thoughts, inability to concentrate, paralytic or manic movements, insomnia, headache, recurrent nightmares, or extreme fatigue.

What feels like anxiety is not always caused by worry. Sometimes it can have physical causes. In some cases, symptoms that are indistinguishable from anxiety can be caused by the tumor itself:

- NHL tumors in the lung can cause shortness of breath

- Tumors in parts of the kidney can stimulate the adrenal gland to over-produce cortisol, a hormone released during fearful episodes

- Tumors of the brain near or in the pituitary can stimulate hormones that in turn stimulate the adrenals to overproduce cortisol

These medications taken as anticancer therapy also can cause anxiety:

- Corticosteriods such as prednisone

- Bronchodilators and certain other drugs used for asthma

- Newer antidepressant drugs to control nausea and pain, such as Prozac

- Cessation of the use of the quick-acting antianxiety drugs, such as Valium or Ativan

Certain physical changes that accompany incipient medical conditions are heralded by feelings of anxiety:

- Pneumonia

- Heart attack

- Electrolyte imbalance

- Angina

But the chief cause of anxiety among cancer survivors is worry and sustained, unresolved fear. Fear of pain, of abandonment, of dependency, of financial ruin, of professional ruin, of relapse, of death.

When we worry for a long time about one problem, new electrical circuitry is laid in our brains. Sometimes conditions resembling or related to our problem will trigger anxiety symptoms or symptoms of physical distress. Many cancer survivors report anticipatory nausea just smelling the rubbing alcohol used to clean the skin over a vein before chemotherapy is administered. Studies have shown that this response can cause their blood counts to drop—even if they are not given chemotherapy in that session.

Obviously this reaction, called a conditioned response, can have a direct impact on the immune system, as has been demonstrated many times in animals. For example, when rats in one experiment were fed a combination of immune suppressant and saccharine dissolved in water, their white blood cell counts dropped afterward, as expected. When the experiment was repeated using only saccharine in water, white blood cell counts still dropped. This demonstrates that the association of event and outcome does not require knowing, for example, what chemotherapy is intended to do. Physiological cause and effect can occur in the absence of the cognitive processes as we know them today.

This does not imply, of course, that you can skip chemotherapy because just thinking about it may have some of the same effects. There's no evidence that a conditioned drop in blood counts coincides with an attack by the immune system on tumor cells.

Beth, the daughter of a man with NHL, describes how long-term anxiety has taken its toll on her and her family:

> I need to try something to reduce stress. I don't think I really deal with things head-on, and I end up transferring the stress to my body. I've just had horrible chest pains and insomnia lately, and my stress level is becoming horrendous. I've never been that great at dealing with it. I'm not even the one who has lymphoma, but it seems all I can do is worry, worry. I've tried meditation, but I can't keep up with it. I even work out at least weekly, and I have a pet. I don't know what to do next.

Depression

Research has shown that those who are depressed often have suboptimal immune system function.

Most cases of depression that coincide with cancer are called situational depressive episodes, directly related to the stress of adjusting to cancer. These depressive episodes differ from organic disturbances such as manic depression or unipolar depression, unless the person has had episodes of these diseases in the past, well before the cancer diagnosis.

Depression may be diagnosed if one or more of the following symptoms persist for more than two weeks:

- Despair
- Excessive sleepiness
- Insomnia
- Appetite disturbance
- Irritability

- Inability to function

- Loss of interest in sex and other pleasurable activities

- Thoughts of suicide

Cancer-related problems that seem to have no solution can cause depression. When we experience repeatedly that our efforts to solve problems don't work or are punished, we cease trying. This is called learned helplessness by experts, but we know it as despair, and it is linked to depression. Subsequently, when new problems arise that we could indeed solve, or when new methods of dealing with old problems emerge, those exhibiting learned helplessness fail to act. A therapist trained to deal with depression can help overcome learned helplessness and despair.

In addition to the psychological factors surrounding cancer that can cause depression, so might the following:

- Chemical treatments for cancer that are neurotoxic or toxic to the thyroid, such as Taxol, prednisone, interferon alfa, or interleukin-2 can cause chemically induced depression.

- Hemorrhagic stroke that may result from untreated symptoms of some NHLs can cause depression after blood products that cannot be cleared settle in the brain.

- High doses of cranial irradiation for NHL therapy that are not accompanied by steroid therapy may cause depression. Depression is but one of a constellation of symptoms following cranial irradiation.

Please note that the preceding three points are possible side effects that do not necessarily occur in every person.

The effect of stress on the immune system

The stress hormones released by the adrenals during episodes of fear and anxiety also affect white blood cells, the infection-fighting army within our blood. Initially, the surge of brain and adrenal hormones that accompanies stress causes an increase in circulating white blood cells. When cortisol remains high, however, white blood cell numbers are reduced. As stress, anxiety, or depression continue unabated over weeks or months, output of the adrenal hormone cortisol is consistently high and white blood cell numbers remain reduced.

Stress and cancer

If prolonged stress and resulting anxiety affect the number of white blood cells in our body, does this mean that cancer can be caused by or made worse by stress? The answer, based on animal and human research, is unclear.

Animal studies support what many recognize intuitively: if stress had an unequivocal link to the development of cancer, just about every one of us would develop cancer. If stressful life events within the last three years were responsible for the emergence of cancer, then everyone who survived imprisonment in Auschwitz and other Nazi annihilation camps ought to have been diagnosed with cancer soon after being freed by the Allies. Continuing with the same analogy, all people who are diagnosed with cancer should either develop a second cancer triggered by the stress of the first diagnosis or should never be able to recover from the first cancer. Likewise, all loved ones of those diagnosed with cancer should then develop a cancer from dealing with the stress of their loved ones' suffering.

In fact, animal studies show a very wide range of tumor response to stress, depending on the type of stressor used, the ability of the animal to modify or escape the stressor, the species being tested, the gender, the animal's previous experience with this stress, whether the tumor was chemically induced or transplanted, whether the tumor is primary or a metastasis, and so on. In some cases, stress causes animal tumors to shrink.

Human studies have been to date somewhat less direct in measuring stress and tumor response, because few humans would tolerate having tumors chemically induced or transplanted, or being deliberately subjected to stress. The best study design would follow cancer-free people for years, recording stressful events and subsequent cancer diagnoses.

Most human studies so far have relied on retrospective self-reports of stress levels prior to the cancer diagnosis. This method of collecting information is often criticized as of dubious reliability. For instance, a person who has just been diagnosed with cancer and who has agreed to fill out a questionnaire on life factors may report that other recent stressful life events were not very stressful. Compared to this newest problem, cancer, these events indeed may, in retrospect, seem not to be that stressful. Yet at the time the previous stressful events occurred, they may have been perceived and reacted to as very stressful events.

In short, while stress has been undeniably linked, over and over, to increased rates of some illness such as upper respiratory infection and certain autoimmune disease, there is no clear causative link between stress and cancer. Several excellent texts on the topic of stress, the immune system, and cancer are listed in Appendix A, *Resources*.

Is there a cancer personality?

If stress causes both emotional and physical changes, but does not consistently have a part in the development of cancer, what other factors might be responsible? Can the ways a person adapts to stress affect his or her health? Do habitual ways of adapting hint at a "cancer personality"? The evidence, based on animal and human research, is conflicting.

Obviously, animal studies on this topic are difficult to perform because we can't know with certainty what animals are feeling, so most studies are done on humans. Often the design of these studies has been criticized.

For instance, melancholia, or what we would call depression today, received attention in the past as a personality trait possibly linked to cancer, but we know today that depression is less a personality trait or coping mechanism than an imbalance in brain chemistry with many different causes including genetics, situational adjustment, influenza, and stroke.

One study of breast cancer survivors assessed personality and coping styles, using a questionnaire and interview the day before breast biopsy. They concluded that women who were stoical and "psychologically morbid" rather than expressive and emotional were more likely to have malignant findings in biopsied tissue. Here are some reasons why the design of studies of this kind are criticized:

- Those of us who have had biopsies know that this is often a stressful experience, likely to derail our responses, if we are able at all to take such an interview seriously in this very emotionally charged setting.

- Suppose those found to have a malignancy already had a good idea what their diagnosis might be? Suppose this idea had time to develop for a week or two while they waited for the surgery? Would the women questioned be likely to display more evolved, thought-out, stoical coping styles, perhaps not consistent with their usual more spontaneous reactions? In fact, some of the women in this study indeed had been informed by their radiologists that the lesions appearing on mammography were most likely malignant.

- How can we know that the answers on a questionnaire, even when the anxiety surrounding a biopsy is not an issue, reflect how someone really behaves?

- Suppose coping styles early in life predispose us to breast cancer, but our coping styles at maturity are what is measured by these questionnaires?

- What kind of person volunteers to fill out a questionnaire? (Questionnaire studies always face this criticism.) Would emotional women be more likely to decline, and stoical women more likely to comply? Or if a small honorarium is offered, say about thirty dollars, as is common for many psychological studies, will less affluent women be over-represented because for affluent women the invasion of privacy and the time lost isn't worth thirty dollars? If so, do less affluent women have other life conditions that would predispose them to breast cancer, such as living in an air-polluted neighborhood?

- Suppose the behavior described as stoical is an artifact of some other circumstance, such as working long, exhausting hours under artificial light for several years? Other, equally plausible theories suggest that the increasing rate of breast cancer is linked to increasing lifetime estrogen exposure. Studies have demonstrated that estrogen exposure begins earlier now, for the age of first menstruation has steadily decreased in industrialized countries since the use of electric light became widespread in the twentieth century.

- And finally, if this study had been designed in an era when being stoical was admired and being expressive was considered "psychologically morbid," would the researchers have attempted to prove that expressive women were more likely to develop breast cancer?

In my family, we have had five cancers: one male denier who has survived eight years, a female outspoken fighter who has died, an emotional, expressive man who has died, an introverted female who has died, and an outspoken, complaining female who has survived twenty years. In each case, type of cancer—lymphoma, prostate, breast, and colon cancers—and stage of disease at diagnosis were far more meaningful to survival than personality type.

No doubt each of us can think of similar cases within our own experience, in spite of the findings of studies published on this topic. Indeed, some studies have found no association between personality, coping style, and breast cancer.[1]

As you can see, the supposed link between personality and the development of cancer is a tenuous one.

What can we do?

If fear is not very useful in dealing with cancer, and anxiety and depression pose risks for long-term health problems, what reactions and responses deal effectively with cancer-related stress? And if stress is not linked conclusively to the inception or growth of tumors, and may in fact shrink tumors in some cases, why attempt to reduce the stress that is associated with the cancer experience?

First, most people prefer feeling good to feeling bad. Stress reduction techniques can help you feel better.

Second, increased levels of stress clearly are tied to the worsening of certain illnesses, such as upper respiratory infections. If you've decided on a course of chemotherapy or radiation therapy, your immune system may be compromised for a few days or a week during each cycle. It's best to avoid infections and to minimize those that may arise during these troughs. Stress reduction techniques may help you keep secondary health problems at a minimum while undergoing anticancer therapy.

Third, high levels of stress for long periods of time can contribute to the development of high blood pressure, gastric disease, migraine headaches, certain autoimmune diseases, and other stress-related illnesses.

Behavioral and medical ways to interrupt the worry cycle are discussed next.

Stress reduction techniques

A chapter of this length cannot do justice to the history of theories of stress and stress reduction, and the ways of life that arose to accomplish this. Nonetheless, stress reduction has always been of interest to humans, albeit under different names, and has received close scrutiny in the twentieth century after the chemical link between stress and hormones was delineated. Thus, various ways to reduce stress have been discovered or rediscovered.

Following is an alphabetic list of techniques that many have found useful for reducing stress. Not all of these will work for any one person; in fact, it's possible that none of these will work for you during particularly stressful times such as during periodic checkups, or if you have a symptom that causes fear of relapse. We hope, though, that the following ideas will help you discover your own ways to unwind.

Acupuncture

Acupuncture is a versatile way to reduce stress and pain, and is particularly good at relieving certain kinds of pain.

The ancient Chinese mapped the flow of energy in our bodies through pathways called meridians. These pathways are thought by Western medicine to be neuroelectric, although there continues to be discussion about the exact nature of these meridians. Eastern medicine believes that the misdirected flow of energy through these meridians accounts for most of the imbalances that occur within our bodies, and that these imbalances cause illness, and can be detected in twelve pulses.

The central nervous system produces hormones for which receptors exist on the surfaces of white blood cells. Recent gains in knowledge regarding this interaction of the central nervous system and the immune system may explain more fully some of acupuncture's mode of action.

An experienced acupuncturist will spend at least an hour taking a comprehensive medical and emotional history; will use few needles, perhaps no more than six; may prefer Japanese to Chinese needles because they're thinner; and will be skilled at using the needles in a way that is not perceptible or barely perceptible.

The needles come in packets for single use only. You'll be able to see your practitioner opening these packets, which is reassuring if you have well-justified doubts about the reuse of needles. All body surfaces on which needles are used are cleaned first with rubbing alcohol.

If you have asthma or hyper-reactive airway, tell the practitioner. Certain acupuncture treatments call for the burning of an herb called moxa, which may irritate your breathing. When moxa is used, only a sensation of warmth is felt on the skin.

Shoes should come off last and go on first. The easiest and most regrettable way to find a tiny, thin, lost acupuncture needle on the floor is with your bare foot.

It's becoming increasingly common for health insurance companies to pay for part or most of acupuncture treatment, although they generally pay less for psychological diagnoses such as stress than they do for medical diagnoses such as migraine or endometriosis.

In some states, an acupuncture practice must be supervised by a medical doctor. Verify the licensing and credentials of your practitioner with your state health department. You can contact the following organizations for more information about acupuncture:

American Association of Oriental Medicine
433 Front Street
Catasauqua, PA 18032-2506
Phone: (610) 266-1433
Fax: (610) 264-2768
Email: *AAOM1@aol.com*

National Acupuncture and Oriental Medicine Alliance
P.O. Box 77511
Seattle, WA 98177-0531
Phone: (206) 524-3511
Email: *76143.2061@compuserve.com*

National Acupuncture Foundation
1718 M Street, Suite 195
Washington, D.C. 20036
Phone: (202) 332-5794

The following two web sites have useful information about acupuncture:

* *http://www.acupuncture.com/Referrals/ref2.htm*
* *http://www.acupuncture.com/StateLaws/StateLaws.htm*

Biofeedback

Biofeedback is a way to relearn how to relax, usually monitored by a psychiatrist or psychologist.

During initial biofeedback sessions, sticky sensors are attached to various muscle groups on the part of your body that seems tense or is in pain, and a graph of muscle tension is displayed on a screen that is similar to a home computer screen. Relaxation tapes or the guiding voice of a therapist are used to establish a calm atmosphere.

When you have relaxed these muscle groups, you can tell you've succeeded because the indicators on the screen have changed.

After a few sessions with the sensors and the screen, you no longer need them to echo success, and you switch to doing relaxation exercises on your own. It is important to rehearse this stage of independence over and over with a therapist so that soon you can do the exercises independently in any setting.

As with acupuncture, it's becoming increasingly common for health insurance companies to pay for part or most of biofeedback treatment, although they generally pay less for psychological diagnoses such as stress headache than they do for medical diagnoses such as migraine.

Counseling

Counseling sessions with a mediator or therapist who is experienced in cancer survivorship issues have proven very helpful to many people. Three randomized studies, including Dr. David Spiegel's work with breast cancer survivors, have shown increased survival among melanoma, lymphoma, and breast cancer survivors who received counseling.

Group counseling or support with other cancer survivors is a wonderful way to reduce stress. The group generates camaraderie, reduces feelings of isolation, offers practical as well as sympathetic support, and can become the source of many new friendships. See the section "Support groups" for more information.

Counselors might be a psychiatrist, a psychologist with a Ph.D. or a master's degree, or a licensed social worker. Some insurance companies pay a larger percentage of the cost for sessions with a psychiatrist or psychologist, but often social workers charge less to begin with.

Exercise

Moderate, regular exercise is a wonderful, well-documented way to reduce stress as well as improve overall health. Exercise also generates endorphins, the body's natural opiates, which reduce pain and ease depression.

Be careful, though, not to be too strenuous, for very strenuous exercise, such as training for a marathon, can lower white blood cell counts for about twenty-four hours. Do only what feels good, stopping before the point of exhaustion. Check first with your oncologist before starting a new exercise regimen, especially if you have had doxorubicin chemotherapy or radiation therapy in the chest area. Both of these treatments, if given in high doses, entail a risk of cardiac damage.

Family

Of all social support factors that appear to contribute to the positive outcome of an illness, including cancer, the support of family or very close friends appears to be highest. This effect has been shown most clearly in studies of white males recovering from heart conditions, though. The beneficial effect is less clear when other illnesses, females, and members of non-white ethnic groups are studied.

Most people are both blessed and cursed with family. Cancer survivors report family members who range from saintly, indispensable soulmates to those seemingly hatched by fate as an example of how not to behave. Nonetheless, at times, there's something uniquely comforting about being surrounded by those who resemble you, share your body language and your mother tongue, regardless of their inclination, or lack of inclination, to offer support. If nothing else, the less helpful ones can unintentionally provide wry entertainment.

Occasionally people have family members who need more support than the cancer survivor does, or who are tooth-grindingly insensitive to what they're going through. And once in a while, stories surface about family members who actually blame the cancer survivor or family "rivals" such as a daughter-in-law for the cancer.

Don't berate yourself if you find you frequently need a vacation from family members who put themselves first at all costs. Often these unhealthy imbalances in family dynamics were present all along, but remained subtle and bearable until the cancer experience highlighted them.

Friends

Few other stress reducers are as good as having sympathetic, listening friends.

When friends offer to help, don't be too noble to say yes. Keep in mind that often they don't know quite what to say when they learn of your cancer, especially at first, so they may prefer to act instead.

If they're good listeners, let them know if you do or do not feel like talking about cancer today—and that tomorrow might be different. Undoubtedly there will be days when reducing stress means talking about cancer, and other days when one more word about cancer will make you want to run for cover. Try to sense or ask if *they* feel like listening, too.

Far too many cancer survivors report that friends, even very good friends, disappear when cancer appears. These friends are speechless, sad, frightened, or guilty that they're healthy—never mind that perhaps we're much more sad and frightened than they are.

Each of us has to decide on a way to handle this abandonment that meshes with our system of ethics. Many cancer survivors say that they just don't need additional sources of sadness and stress in their life, and they move on to find new friends, often in cancer support groups. Other cancer survivors try to keep their old friends by never talking about cancer. Bear in mind, though, that for those who are very fearful about cancer, just being around someone with cancer might be frightening.

If you have healthy friends who have remained a presence in spite of cancer—lawn-mowing, grocery-buying, baby-sitting friends, friends who have listened to you when you're scared, or friends who have just spent time with you if talking about cancer is not your style, you're very lucky. Show them that you're glad they're around. The harmony that results is a guaranteed stress-reducer, as Mary, a transplant survivor, has found:

> *I get to see sunsets, laugh with my friends, and even get a massage. How many friends from my cancer support group would have given anything to enjoy the quality of life I have—or any life at all? I live a little of each day for them. I'm grateful to be here, and to be in the presence of those I love. I love life, even diminished life. It's a gift.*

Take solace, too, in the goodwill of those you may never meet. The daffodils that appear in hospitals during the American Cancer Society's Daffodil Days in March, for instance, are from someone who wants you to feel better.

Gaining knowledge

Not surprisingly, a book such as this supports the belief that gaining knowledge about your cancer, and thus gaining some control over your cancer experience, is an excellent coping mechanism. Learning about your illness and your options has been proven to reduce anxiety and stress, and may be the crucial factor in your illness and its outcome. Not only can obtaining a correct diagnosis and learning about new, more effective treatments result in sound choices, but animal studies have shown that those who perceive that they have a means to escape stressful situations maintain higher white blood cell counts than those who perceive otherwise. Bear in mind as well that, while our doctors often must master information about a broad variety of cancers, or are immersed deeply in their own research projects, we have the luxury of going narrow and deep, learning a great deal about our own illness.

If your doctor seems unreceptive about things you've learned, seek a second opinion or consider changing doctors. An excellent book on this topic is *Working with Your Doctor*, by Nancy Keene.

Worthy of mention is the observation that some doctors react badly to the idea that their patients find information on the Internet, because the information available on the Net ranges from abysmal to superb. If you use the Internet to research your illness (see Chapter 24, *Researching Your Lymphoma*), avoid using the word "Internet" when discussing your findings with your oncologist. Instead, use terminology that credits the sources on which your findings are based: Medline, the PDQ database of the National Cancer Institute, Cancerlit, certain reputable medical journals, and so on.

Hobbies, volunteer work

As a form of healthy denial and, in some cases, a form of exercise, hobbies are an excellent stress reducer. Immersed in an activity you enjoy, you're likely to forget cancer, breathe and laugh more easily, and feel capable.

Hobbies are especially important for reducing the stress that may be linked to the lowered self-esteem of those who are temporarily or permanently unable to return to work.

Charlie describes how satisfying he finds it to immerse himself in his volunteer work at the zoo, for him a microcosm of life in general:

Probably the best thing that has happened to me in the realm of stress relief has been my signing on and participating in training as a docent at the Roger Williams Park Zoo in Providence, Rhode Island. I have been meditating for a number of years, but the stress of NHL was taking me deeper into depression.

To watch the constant cycle of birth, growth, and occasionally the death of animals at the zoo inspires awe. To see the pleasure and wonderment on the faces of children and adults as they gaze on the panoply of nature around them is relaxing, comforting, and at the same time energizing and expanding to my psyche. Perhaps nature in the wild is more awe-inspiring, but the training this opportunity offers in biology and animal facts, as well as the teaching of nature to another generation, is very fulfilling. To be involved in the many varied tasks of a docent with a crew of great people, all lovers of life and of God's creatures, is also a source of pleasure that takes my mind away from my problems.

It is not for everyone, I suppose, but for me it has been great. Like many other NHL survivors, I, too, have screamed into space from the confines of my car while driving in traffic. Sometimes just the enormity of my situation—knowing that I am dying with or from NHL, with the attendant financial and emotional strains that are placed on my family—make me want to scream. When I am with my friends at the zoo, however, I would rather purr.

Laughter

In his book *Anatomy of an Illness as Perceived by the Patient*, Norman Cousins says we should take humor seriously. Cousins was diagnosed in 1964 with ankylosing spondylitis, a degenerative disease of the connective tissue that causes disability and pain. He undertook to improve or cure his condition by focusing on positive, happy thinking, and he believes he succeeded.

Funny friends, books, and movies are good ways to forget about cancer for a while, and can invoke some of the healthy bodily changes that come about when we laugh and relax. Two studies have found that mirthful laughter reduces blood levels of the hormones associated with stress.

The following story illustrates one patient's need to escape from cancer's darkness:

About halfway through his chemotherapy, my husband decided he'd had enough of it. He dressed me up as him—bow tie, glasses, and mustache—and we waited for the oncologist in the treatment room, with me on the table.

On another occasion, his doctor asked him to stop by and bring his latest CAT scans. We borrowed our cat's x-rays from the veterinarian for the occasion. The oncologist was very puzzled when he put the films on the viewer.

I think the doctor now enjoys seeing us twice a year for checkups, in spite of the pranks we pulled. And I know it gave my husband a sense of control over his situation, a sly, gentle sense of "getting back" at his oncologist—the expert brandishing a syringe about a foot long filled with doxorubicin—and an opportunity to briefly break loose of cancer's hold.

Massage therapy

The backrubs and neck-rubs given to you by loved ones will release endorphins that reduce pain and depression.

The lymphatic strokes practiced by massage therapists, on the other hand, are location-specific and utilize a lot of pressure. Always check with your doctor before having massage therapy, because massage may hasten the spread of lymphoma, although the exact mechanism by which NHL spreads is unknown. There is a possibility that it may be spread through lymphatic vessels, but this may be more likely for the Hodgkin's lymphomas, which tend to progress from one node to the next, than for the non-Hodgkin's lymphomas.

Your doctor may determine that professional therapeutic massage of certain parts of the body, those that appear unaffected by lymphoma, is acceptable.

Massage therapy is licensed by some states, and recognized by a national organization, the American Massage Therapy Association (AMTA). In some states, massage therapy can be performed only under the supervision of a doctor, nurse, physical therapist, or chiropractor. Your local phone book will list the nearest chapter of the AMTA for verifying your practitioner's credentials, or you can contact the national office:

American Massage Therapy Association
820 Davis Street, Suite 100
Evanston, IL 60201-4444
Phone: (847) 864-0123
Fax: (847) 864-1178
http://www.amtamassage.org/

Meditation

Meditation is a way to interrupt negative, cyclic thinking by focusing on one soothing word or peaceful scene. Those who practice meditation regularly eventually are able to lower their blood pressure and levels of stress hormones. These reductions persist beyond the end of the meditation session, sometimes well beyond.

Lowering of blood pressure is beneficial for those who have cardiac or vascular damage following doxorubicin or radiation therapies.

One study has shown that those who meditate have higher levels of melatonin in their urine, and another study has shown that higher levels of melatonin are found naturally in those with certain cancers. The significance of higher levels of naturally produced melatonin, or melatonin supplements, in NHL survivors is not fully understood, but a few studies have shown that melatonin can increase the growth of myeloma cells in the test tube. (Myeloma is a cancer of the blood and bone marrow related to NHL and leukemia.)

Owing to this unquantified risk, the FDA requires a warning on melatonin dietary supplements made or distributed in the U.S. about possible health risks for those with white blood cell disorders.

It is likely that naturally elevated levels of melatonin associated with meditation do not have an undesirable effect on tumor growth, and that only the higher doses associated with dietary supplements do. It is also possible that all relaxation efforts, not just meditation, increase urinary levels of melatonin, and that future studies will demonstrate this—or that blood levels, not urinary levels, are significant for an effect on cancer. Clearly, more research on melatonin's effects on the lymphomas is needed, but it's not likely that meditation will harm you.

A five-year survivor of a transplant for NHL describes how meditation has helped her:

I used meditation and visualization throughout my treatment. It was something I could do, and helped me feel like I was contributing to healing. I had three noncancer friends that came over once a week for a support group meeting at my house. It was a way to feel connected to others and to Spirit, working and playing on all levels to promote healing.

Mini-vacations, healthy denial, and escapism

Denial is a healthy coping mechanism as long as it doesn't cause us to neglect the care we need for cancer. Some healthy ways to take a mini-vacation from cancer are:

- Drive to work along a prettier route.

- Schedule day trips away from daily stress.

- Buy your favorite author's latest hardcover edition instead of waiting for the paperback or library version.

- Grant yourself permission not to worry for one hour, one day, one week, and so on.

- Take a nap on your lunch hour.

- Buy a pair of wild golf pants or lipstick that "isn't your color" and wear it anyway.

- Spend all day Saturday in your bathrobe reading old *New Yorker* cartoons.

- Write a limerick and mail it anonymously to a friend.

- Odd though it may sound, you might enjoy celebrating the parts of your body that still work. Most of them still do work, of course, and rejoicing in this and using our bodies may have healing effects as yet unknown to medicine.

Music, song, and dance

Dr. Albert Schweitzer once said that he couldn't imagine life without music or cats. Schweitzer was an extremely productive, altruistic, humorous man who lived and worked in a difficult setting well into old age. He was a strong believer in the doctor within each of us, and thought himself but the facilitator of his patients' own healing processes.

Music can lower stress and enhance emotions. You can experiment with music to see which type suits your needs at different times. Some people find the relaxing or soul-thrilling effects of classical music best. Others find that loud pop or rock music numbs pain, and that its relatively simple, repetitive rhythms and singable melodies interrupt incessant worries. Still others enjoy ethnic music. Listening to a type of music you've never heard before, such as the Australian didgeridoo or Tibetan chord-singing, might distract you from the worries of cancer.

Singing can release cares from your soul, and may realign anxious breathing. Singing out loud in the car when you're alone, like screaming, can lower tension levels.

Classes in dance for people of all ages and both genders are available in many community centers. If you feel that you need greater control in your life, ballet's discipline, controlled breathing, and classic beauty may make you feel better. If, on the other hand, you feel there's too much control in your life, jazz or aerobics may allow you to set free some inhibitions. Flamenco might help you rediscover the sexuality that may have gone to sleep when you heard the word cancer. Yoga, t'ai chi, and Feldenkreis movement, all of which span the disciplines of exercise and dance, are fine ways to stretch and relax.

Nutrition

In general, the diet that is recommended for those without cancer—a diet high in vegetables, fruit, and grains—remains the best diet for those with cancer, although those who are losing weight and suffering from loss of appetite should consult their oncologists before substituting vegetables for meat.

A few nutritional factors seem to have some effect on mood:

- A diet high in animal protein has been linked to anxiety and panic attacks. Other studies have found that certain flavonoids, compounds found in plant but not animal tissue, are similar to Valium in their relaxing action. This might mean that it's not reducing meat intake, but increasing vegetable intake, that lowers anxious episodes in some people. If you're suffering from severe anxiety symptoms related to your cancer diagnosis, you might try modifying your diet to contain more vegetables and grains—but check first with your oncologist.

- Drinking milk at bedtime or eating turkey for dinner are known to help with relaxation. These foods are high in tryptophan, an amino acid that aids sleep. Tryptophan is used by the body to make serotonin, a neurotransmitter that affects mood and is the target of many of the newer antidepressants.

- Low blood levels of zinc have been correlated to treatment-resistant depression and to an increase in the undesirable immune system inflammatory response sometimes seen in depressive patients.

- Cachexia, the weight loss experienced by some cancer patients, has been linked to depression, which is thought to be triggered by nutritional deficits, or by the tumor's commandeering of dietary substances otherwise needed for the manufacture of brain neurotransmitters.

Note that chemotherapy regimens that contain procarbazine may require that you avoid certain foods high in tyramines, including bananas and some cheeses. Always verify a change in diet first with your oncologist.

Pets

You may find that your pets, considered family members by some, are a unique solace to you through the cancer experience. Animals seem to have a knack for knowing when we need help, and they don't care if we smell funny or if our hair is missing. They don't become instantly bashful because of our diagnosis, and they aren't afraid they'll catch cancer from us. How many humans will sit by us for an hour in the bathroom while we're sick, as our cats will? And who's funnier than the puppy who barks at the wig on the dresser?

Mary, who has survived a bone marrow transplant for NHL, describes how her cat and Mother Nature have helped her become rebalanced:

> There were quiet 3 A.M. mornings with the cat purring on my lap and the back door open while I listened to the dark and the night sounds. It would hit me all of a sudden that I didn't know how much longer I would have those times to sit and listen. I made a pact with my cat: while I was so busy surviving, was I living? It's all borrowed time anyway.
>
> Now we often pause to appreciate the moment, whatever may be happening. There is more depth to the colors, richer notes to the music. Did I have to survive cancer to find this kind of abundant life? I don't

know, but I do know that it was only through cancer and all its related events that I grew into the kind of person who wanted to find the abundance of life.

Positive thinking and visualization

Positive thinking and visualization have been shown to increase immune system function in some studies. Oddly, one study has shown that when cancer survivors visualize an immune system attack of the tumor, using attack images that are incorrect according to what is known today about immune system function, immune system parameters still improve. This may reflect the "taking charge" phenomenon: the belief that you can escape stress tends to lessen the effect of stress on the immune system.

Visualization can be used to attempt to direct inner forces against the cancer or to relax by calling to mind pleasant experiences, places, or dreams. Initially it might be useful to practice visualization in a quiet, relaxed atmosphere, but eventually you can do it anywhere.

Reading

As a form of escapism, reading is a good way to reduce stress. As a means of learning more about your illness, reading may make you feel more stressed temporarily, but this may be offset by long stretches of peace of mind after you're able to make better medical decisions based on what you've learned by reading.

If you have a computer, reading from and writing to the various cancer discussion groups on the Internet can provide a cathartic outlet for you. See the section "Support groups."

Relaxation training

This technique is similar to biofeedback, discussed earlier, and incorporates visualization techniques, described in the section, "Positive thinking and visualization."

Sleep

Research shows that even one night of missed sleep lowers levels of natural killer (NK) white blood cells. Although NK counts recover quickly once sleep is restored, persistent lack of sleep is an opportunity for illness.

Animal research on the artificial shifting of the phases of lightness and darkness shows that the immune system is depressed by the shifting. Fishes that occupy parts of the ocean that receive low light in winter experience an additional breeding cycle if artificial light is increased, and simultaneously their white blood cell counts decrease.

Snuggles and smooches

Being kissed, hugged, and patted by people who love you causes endorphins to be released within the central nervous system. Endorphins are natural opiates produced by our bodies, capable of reducing pain and depression, and producing feelings of well-being.

Hugging, kissing, snuggling, and giggling with a child who has cancer has been shown in several nursing studies to lower the child's pain and anxiety levels.

Hugging and kissing your partner can be enjoyable and healthy, even if you're feeling too tired at the moment to enjoy all of the sexual activities you enjoyed before diagnosis.

Spirituality, religious beliefs

Your religious beliefs may provide comfort when little else is making sense. Some people find that their spiritual beliefs sustain them in spite of a seemingly arbitrary infliction of suffering, either because their religion provides answers for the question of human suffering or because of theological beliefs they have developed independently.

Other cancer survivors, however, experience a crisis of faith after their cancer diagnosis. They find it difficult, for instance, to reconcile the emergence of a seemingly undeserved, life-threatening illness with their belief in a kind, nonpunitive deity.

On a more human level, the support that fellow church or temple members furnish to those who need help is clearly an asset in stress reduction. Support might take the form of emotional support (cards, calls, hugs, visits), prayer, practical support (drives to and from the doctor or casseroles for supper), or financial support for someone who is underinsured.

The May 1995 issue of the *Journal of the American Medical Association* contains an article showing a correlation between religious practice and prayer and increased good health. At least one other study has shown that a person who is prayed for improves when ill, even if he or she is not aware that prayers are being said.

An NHL survivor describes how her faith helped her cope with a marrow transplant:

> When I was first diagnosed with NHL at the age of twenty-nine, I was in a state of terror and fear that I had never known. I knew at that point that I alone would not be able to deal with the diagnosis or the treatment. My worst fears had come true. At that point I turned it over to God. I knew that He was the only one that could handle such a horrifying diagnosis.

Support groups

For some of us, support groups can be the difference, literally, between life and death. The opportunity to exchange information with those who have already weathered NHL can provide you with everything from emotional support to the knowledge to question your treatment and seek medical help elsewhere. Support groups are an immeasurably useful way to do this, bringing together a variety of skills, sometimes including medical and legal knowledge.

Moreover, Dr. David Spiegel's work with breast cancer survivors shows longer survival among those who were part of support groups, a serendipitous finding from a study intending to highlight other aspects of survival.

Support groups are offered locally in many areas by organizations such as the American Cancer Society, the Wellness Community, or local hospitals. If you have Internet access, support groups are also available on the Internet. See Chapter 13, *Getting Support*, for instructions about subscribing.

Water

In the 1930s, marine biologist Sir Alister Hardy noted that humans have features in common with water mammals, features not found in any other primates, such as a subcutaneous layer of body fat, hair that grows in one direction to reduce water resistance, a protective dive reflex within the respiratory system, a nose that blocks water during a dive, residual webbed toes, and fully webbed toes in 7 percent of humans. He argues that we humans may have spent a period of our evolution in water.

Anthropologists may settle this point eventually, but for our immediate use, it means that, for some of us, water is a wonderful way to relax. A good swim or a warm tub with salts and a good book can make you briefly more than just human.

Writing

If you have an urge to write, you'll be encouraged to know that those who write very honestly and emotionally about their frightening, negative experiences increase the function of their white blood cells. Writing can be in a range of formats. You can write for yourself in a journal, write letters to friends, write letters for your children to be read when they're older, or write email to cancer discussion groups on the Internet.

Stress medications

Stress associated with cancer responds well to anti-anxiety and antidepressant medication. Research has shown, though, that these medications are most effective when used in combination with counseling and behavior modification training.

There are many drugs to choose from to ease anxiety or depression or to aid sleep. The newer drugs available today have fewer side effects and are less likely to be addictive than drugs used just a few years ago.

Anti-anxiety medication

Anti-anxiety drugs (anxiolytics) fall broadly into two groups, the fast-acting drugs and the slower-acting drugs. The fast-acting benzodiazepine drugs such as Valium, Ativan, or Xanax are potentially addictive, and can cause rebound anxiety when they're stopped. The newer anti-anxiety drugs such as Buspar (buspirone) cross the boundary between anti-anxiety and antidepressive drugs, are not addictive, can be stopped abruptly with no ill effect. They take two to three weeks to work.

The mood change following use of the older anti-anxiety drugs in the Valium family is pronounced and rapid, similar to the effect of alcohol. It's unwise to drive or operate heavy machinery when using drugs in the benzodiazepine family.

The mood change following use of newer anti-anxiety drugs such as Buspar is more subtle and gradual, and sleepiness, if present, is less pronounced than with the benzodiazepines.

The anti-anxiety drug Ativan, a benzodiazepine, is often used just prior to chemotherapy to control nausea.

Antidepressant medication

The availability of today's more effective, safer antidepressants is a blessing for those coping with cancer. Unlike the antidepressants of a few years ago, which caused sleepiness, weight gain, or other undesirable side effects, today's antidepressant medications are far safer and less disruptive of weight and sleep patterns.

Some of the newer antidepressants can cause restlessness and insomnia for the first two or three weeks they are used. You might discuss with your doctor the temporary use of a sleeping pill until your body has adjusted to the antidepressant.

Antidepressants are also good pain relievers, although their mechanism as such is not entirely clear.

Improvement in mood is gradual with most of the antidepressants used today, changing slowly over a few weeks or months. The fullest effect is gained if the drugs are used continuously for months. Always check with your doctor before stopping an antidepressant lest gains in improved mood be lost.

The best source for antidepressant medication is a psychiatrist. This specialist is the one most likely to be familiar with all antidepressants and their side effects, and can rotate you through several until the best one for you is apparent.

Sleep medications

Sleep medications range from the very mildest, including over-the-counter antihistamines and Tylenol, to the stronger medications necessary for those using prednisone, or those coping with moderate to severe anxiety.

The anti-anxiety drugs in the benzodiazepine family, such as Ativan, are also used as sleep aids. The section "Anti-anxiety medications" contains cautions about these drugs.

One of the newest sleeping pills available is Ambien, a drug that aids those who have trouble falling asleep. It's cleared very rapidly from the body, so it's less useful for those having trouble staying asleep. When Ambien first was approved by the FDA, it was marketed as a nonaddictive sleeping pill, but postmarket experience has shown that, for at least some people, it may be addictive.

Drugs prescribed for severe pain, such as codeine and morphine, also induce sleep.

Some people use melatonin, a substance marketed as a food supplement, to aid sleep. Melatonin has been shown to increase the quantity of white blood cells. This is a risky phenomenon for a person with lymphoma, a cancer of the white blood cells, because the white blood cells increased could be the cancerous cells. Accordingly, the FDA requires a warning on melatonin dietary supplements made or distributed in the U.S. about possible health risks for those with white blood cell disorders.

Always consult your oncologist before using any drug, whether prescription, nonprescription, or a "natural remedy" marketed as a food supplement.

Summary

The effects of stress and personality on the inception and growth of cancer are unclear and are still being studied. Animal models indicate that a wide range of tumor responses to physical and emotional stress is possible, depending in some instances on species, gender, stressor, season, previous exposure to stress, and biological state.

Regardless of the effect of stress on cancer, there are good reasons to reduce stress. Your sense of well-being will improve, and you can lessen or prevent the chance of secondary illnesses.

CHAPTER 12

Interacting with Medical Personnel

How was it possible that he, a doctor, with his countless acquaintances, had never until this day come across anything so definite as this man's personality?

> —Boris Pasternak
> *Doctor Zhivago*

Your doctor's staff has phoned late on Friday to say that the doctor would like to meet with you to discuss your latest scan results. By the time you hear this cryptic message, it's too late to contact them for an appointment. On Monday, you're told that no appointments are available for two more days.

During your appointment on Wednesday, the doctor explains that the scan showed unusual shadows in new spots that may or may not be problematic, but additional tests are needed to clarify these results. He describes the purpose of the tests, but you don't hear much, because you're in shock. Your mind is tumbling with questions and doubts, and you find yourself losing track of what he's saying.

When you arrive home, you realize you forgot to set up the test appointments. You realize that you didn't write down the names of the tests—one of them sounded sort of like "pet"—nor did you ask what they'll entail or how to prepare for them.

Parts of this scenario unfold every day for NHL survivors, or we may have other experiences that are equally hapless and frustrating. In contrast to receiving caring, intelligent, concerned, and respectful treatment from our doctor, instead we may experience condescension, paternalism, coldness, impatience, or black humor. We may experience indifference at the hands of certain medical personnel—in each case a grotesque imbalance between some of society's most vulnerable and most privileged members.

The relationship you experience with your oncologist will play a critical part—indeed perhaps the most critical part—in your recovery from NHL. It's imperative that you communicate well with each other, and that you, the patient, feel free to ask questions. You should be well-informed in order to make decisions. There should be enough mutual respect to disagree with each other amicably while adhering to a productive plan of treatment and care. This chapter will help you learn how to communicate with medical personnel, improve communication, handle problems that arise, and move on to new and better patient/doctor relationships if improvements are not forthcoming.

What issues arise?

Oncology personnel are human. Because they are human, they will at times be tired. They may be less successful listeners on busy days or thoughts of problems at home may interrupt their concentration. They have likes and dislikes that may be irrational, and they'll experience treatment failures that make them sad and depressed. They are busy people who need to keep abreast of advances in care for many different types of cancer, not just the NHLs. Often these demands emerge in their dealings with us. Doctors and nurses may develop techniques for dealing with patients that are in some measure a defense against their own pain.

Unfortunately, outright rudeness, ineptitude, or blatant lack of concern may also manifest, and must be dealt with promptly before your health is placed in jeopardy.

Only you can define what matters in your relationship with your doctor. You may prefer to have your doctor make all decisions for you, shielding you from uncomfortable details, or you may prefer to be privy to both the worst and most minute details concerning your care. You may find that you occupy a somewhat passive patient role initially, but at some point you may evolve into a more proactive patient. You may enjoy a joking, casual relationship, or it may make you feel belittled.

Keep in mind that, in the absence of your forthright requests for a certain quality of interaction, a doctor's assumptions about your needs are likely to shape how she interacts with you. The NHL experience, like most cancer experiences, can be a volatile one, and thus your needs may change from day to day. You're entitled to say, for instance, that, for today only, you want your doctor to do your thinking for you, or that jocularity is not on the agenda today.

Keep in mind, too, that the medical staff deserve the same respect you do. If your oncologist was the first person to give you the bad news about your having cancer, for example, you may unknowingly harbor resentment and anger toward him, just because he was the bearer of bad news.

Connie's story

The following passage describes Connie's interaction with her oncologist during a visit when she wasn't feeling well and he wouldn't listen to her:

> "You have wonderful looking sinuses and your urine specimen was normal, thank you very much. Gee, you look so healthy. But wait…oh, yeah. Those pesky fevers you're getting? Just don't know. Keep a journal for a week, write down your temperature morning, noon, and night, and we'll see you next Friday. Who told you to take .88 milligrams of aspirin for your arm? No, no, no. You're anemic, and we need to keep track of your temperature. So, let's forget the arm pain. Chest pain, too.

> "You still look good, too. What was that look on your face? Surprised the lowest blood pressure we can get on you is 150/98? Ha, ha. On your last visit the lowest of three tries was 144/100. Don't worry about this, because we're not going to worry about this. We'll keep an eye on it.

> "What could be causing it? I don't know, but don't worry. Stress? Could be. That's funny, after all you've been through, your blood pressure has remained in the pretty normal range. Hmmm. And guess what? The bonus for your being sick is three pretty cream-cheese size containers for you to have your diarrhea in. Don't forget these gloves: it may get messy. Quit mentioning your arm and chest pain. I thought I was doing a good job of ignoring it, but you keep annoying me telling me about it. I would just prefer that you have your out-of-town specialist keep track of your problems. What's that you say? You can't afford all those long distance calls, nor afford to ride back and forth from Green Bay, Wisconsin, to Omaha, Nebraska? Then call them and I want all your records faxed to me so I don't repeat tests.

"Yes, I remember that you don't like the long distance calling. I choose to ignore that. You know who you've been dealing with. Now give these to the receptionist and I'll see you next week. Did I forget something now? Did she mention fatigue, shoulder and chest pain? Nah, must have been someone else. Dum de dum de dum…"

And that was my day. I'm going to cry now. There should be joy in the remission. I'm a good person. Why am I going through this? Life is a mystery. If I'm not berserk yet, I'm earning a one-way ticket there soon. I'm gonna chop off my arm soon, and hand it to the doctor and tell him that it's the one that hurt me so. I have scarring from the double Hickman catheter, and narrowing of the blood vessel because of it. Could that be the source of my pain? Why don't they know or check into it? Asking them does no good. AAAAAHHHHHHHH! I'm going to go chase after my sanity now.

When should we raise our concerns?

It's ideal if you have developed the habit of clarifying your expectations at the start of a medical relationship. Few people, however, do so—or need to—until serious illness entails complex long-term communication with the medical community.

If you're feeling disappointed with your care and haven't communicated your concerns to your oncologist, don't postpone doing so. Having an angry discussion regarding a long string of past disappointments is much less likely to succeed than realigning the relationship soon after you feel uncomfortable with it.

If you're the victim of blatant mistreatment or you sense an unacceptable lack of concern for your well-being, it's best to address the problem immediately. It may be an honest mistake, and if so, the doctor and staff will be grateful to you for bringing it to their attention. Conversely, rudeness or indifference may be a bad habit that other patients have been too intimidated to challenge. Delay won't make these problems go away.

Who are the players?

This chapter assumes that the most common failure of good communication arises between you and your oncologist. Nonetheless, most of the strategies and tactics that may work in improving patient/doctor communication also might prove useful if problems arise with an oncology nurse, a radiotherapy technician, a member of the clerical staff, or your HMO gatekeeper.

Doctors have different styles of interacting with patients. The best among them may vary this style based on the perceived needs of the patient or a patient's changing circumstances over time. A certain core style generally will emerge, though, and you may or may not be comfortable with it. The following sections discuss a few common styles found among doctors.

Paternalistic doctors

The paternalistic doctor is likely to be a fine, skilled practitioner who will provide you with excellent care. He views his responsibility to you as all-encompassing, and is likely to err on the side of total, but accurate, control. If you're in need of a doctor who will make all decisions for you—and this is not at all a criticism, if this is what you want and need at any point—you'll be very happy with this doctor.

Your first clash with the paternalistic doctor may arise if you want to understand everything about your illness, to ask many questions, and to receive patient, detailed answers. Sooner or later, he's likely to ask you if you'd like to have your very own medical degree. He may even suggest that you ought not to read articles from medical journals, perhaps saying, "They'll just frighten you."

These replies hint that the accrual of medical knowledge is the province only of the doctor, never of the patient, and is the hallmark of the paternalistic style.

Given that you may not be able to change doctors owing to certain constraints such as geography or insurance requirements, here are a few ideas for dealing with the paternalistic doctor.

- Do your homework carefully. Find information from the National Cancer Institute or from reputable medical journals. He may never respect your efforts as much as you would like, but it will be harder (not impossible) for him to argue with substantiated medical facts in print.

- Be matter-of-fact and forthright; don't slouch; use appropriate eye contact. Note that if you use humor with this kind of person, unless it's terribly urbane it's likely he'll decide you're someone he doesn't need to take seriously.

- Be kind, but direct. Subtleties may waft right past this ego.

- If you're really annoyed by a particular exchange, you might try saying in a level tone, "Please don't say that. It sounds condescending, although I realize you didn't intend to sound that way."

The impatient, insensitive doctor

Any doctor can have a bad day, perhaps seeming impatient or even cruelly insensitive, but if it happens consistently, you should consider finding another doctor.

If you are unable to change doctors, you should discuss with her as soon as possible your unhappiness about being offended or hurt. You may have some success in being very forthright and firm with this sort of doctor. When humane factors cease being honored, what remains is a business relationship, and you're the paying customer.

Ironically, this doctor may be a very good and knowledgeable technician, but you're not likely to benefit fully from her expertise if she upsets you each time you see her. Moreover, the stress of having to deal continually with a vexatious person might reduce the ability of your immune system to fight off infection, might disincline you from adhering to a chemotherapy regimen, or might discourage you from phoning her if you notice unusual symptoms.

Mary, a survivor of a transplant for NHL, describes how the human factors were mishandled by a doctor during her diagnosis:

> A week after my surgery, my husband accompanied me to the doctor's office. We sat waiting and joking in one of the examination rooms. The doctor came flying into the room, hovered above a chair as if he couldn't bring himself to sit down, and announced that "the really bad thing about this is that it's lymphoma." The room started to swim. When I appeared upset, he said, "I don't know what you're upset about. After all, it's not like it's cancer. That man across the hall—he has cancer."

> I have never been rushed out of an office so quickly in my life. The doctor told me to see an oncologist and flatly refused to offer another ounce of information. I told him I'd find my own oncologist, thanks, and that was the last time I saw him.

The aloof, guarded doctor

Some doctors seem to want to distance themselves from patients. It's difficult to know if this person is cool by nature, or is suffering the pain and burnout of being overexposed to the bittersweet results of practicing oncology. More often he is genuinely concerned about you, as a patient and as a person, but momentarily lacks the emotional wherewithal to express it.

You may find that this kind of doctor opens to you gradually, in response to certain aspects of your own attitude, your sense of humor, or to things you have in common, such as children. Many patients report finding a meeting ground with an aloof doctor gradually, as experiences are shared. To the extent that you warm to each other over time, you probably can expect expressions of compassion, support, and understanding from your doctor regarding your circumstances and the decisions you make.

The equitable doctor

This is the doctor most people probably prefer. She's able to sense whether you'd like a little information or a lot, and when. She seems to know when you need help making a decision or just more time to think. She doesn't react personally if you decide to learn as much as you can, or if you decide to get a second opinion. If you're having an especially bad day, she seems to understand and doesn't hold a grudge.

You can tell clearly that she hurts when you hurt, and she's happy to be able to help you. She rejoices when she sees you evolve through the cancer experience into an informed patient, capable of making sound choices, and when she sees you succeed in finding a perspective that will give you some respite from worry.

The oncology nurse

The oncology nurse is the third most important person involved in your treatment, following only you and your doctor as key players.

Oncology nurses are a uniquely loving breed. Not surprisingly, in some hospitals this specialty of nursing sees a high turnover of personnel owing to feelings of vulnerability and burnout. They care deeply for their patients, often thinking of their charges long after returning to their own homes and lives.

If you take the time to befriend the nurse, you'll have an intelligent, well-informed, soothing ally to help you deal with treatment and its side effects.

The HMO case manager

Cancer survivors report disparate degrees of satisfaction with their health maintenance organizations (HMOs). Often the case manager is the pivotal factor.

The case manager's role is to streamline your treatment approval process, to keep costs down by eliminating redundant tests and treatments, to review your proposed care plan to ensure it meets certain standards, and to intercede for you to bend rules when your care must deviate from the standards of the HMO.

Some, but by no means all, HMOs use registered nurses or physician's assistants to oversee the approval of your care. When this is not the case, it means that decisions about your care might be made by someone with no medical training at all, one who simply is basing decisions on rules provided by his superiors.

It's to your advantage to get to know your case manager well and to communicate as thoroughly as possible. If you feel you are not being fairly treated, however, do not hesitate to ask to speak with a superior or to have the case reviewed by the HMO's medical doctor. HMOs often keep doctors on retainer for this purpose. At times, just the suggestion of a review by an M.D. is enough to cause the HMO to bend rules in your favor.

Family members and medical personnel

Family members and others intimately involved in the patient's care may find that they are in an awkward position when dealing with a loved one's doctor. Some oncologists cleave to the concept that their relationship is with the patient alone, and, without instructions to the contrary, all communication is considered the patient's privilege. If you sense this, clarify your wishes to your doctor regarding sharing information with your loved ones.

General suggestions for interacting successfully

Now that the players and the circumstances have been defined, specific ideas for improving communication can be discussed.

In general, the more you communicate, the better your chances of getting good care, even if the exchanges are not always smooth. Many patients make the mistake of not telling their doctors enough, perhaps because they feel intimidated or feel they'll be perceived as whining, or because they suspect they're wasting the doctor's time. Here are a few tips to facilitate communication:

- Keep a journal between appointments of things you notice and questions that arise.

- Before each visit, make a list of all your concerns, side effects, unusual happenings, and so on, and number them in order of priority—but be sure to relay all of them. What seems insignificant to you may be quite meaningful to your doctor.

- Allow the doctor to distract you only briefly. If she interrupts, be sure to get back to your list after answering her question. If she interrupts often, say calmly that you want to finish this thought before moving to another topic.

- Between appointments, do not hesitate to call your doctor about anything unusual that arises. At your next meeting, remind the doctor of these calls and reiterate your understanding of the content of her replies.

- Use a tape recorder to capture the doctor's wisdom. If he seems uncomfortable with this, you might offer a nonthreatening explanation, such as the well-documented fact that one's memory doesn't work well when under stress. After the meeting, review the recording with a friend or caregiver.

- If you don't have a recorder, ask your friend or caregiver to accompany you as an advocate. Lowell S. Levin, a professor at the Yale School of Public Health and Chairman of the People's Medical Society, says you should take along a family member or friend who is assertive but diplomatic. You're likely to feel more relaxed and focused, and you'll be perceived as wanting to be on top of your own issues. Your friend may remember issues you'd discussed but forgotten, or may think of things that neither you nor your doctor had considered. Make it clear that you want the medical staff to communicate as fully with your advocate as they do with you.

- As mentioned in Chapter 14, *Insurance, Finances, Employment, Record-Keeping*, get copies of all of your medical records and acquaint yourself with them.

- If you have many questions, offer to make an appointment just for this purpose. It's unfair to the doctor and to other patients if your fifteen-minute follow-up exam turns into a ninety-minute discussion.

- If your doctor is willing to have a phone consultation to answer many questions, offer to pay for her time.

- Tell your doctor's staff whether it's okay to phone you at the office. Clarify whether they may leave detailed messages on your answering machine without concern for violating your privacy. If waiting over a weekend for clarification of disturbing news is unacceptable to you, tell your doctor, and find out her policy about being paged on weekends and holidays.

- Ask how you can reach the doctor or his staff during off hours.

- If you have a complaint, voice it first in a calm, objective way, and suggest possible solutions. Explain that you understand the stress many oncologists face, but that this problem has caused you considerable distress. This leaves you with the option of being increasingly strident later if necessary, and reassures the medical staff that they're dealing with a reasonable, tactful person who understands compromise and human error.

- Keep written details of complaints you've expressed: when and how often.

- Above all, strive to have good relations with all of the medical staff by remembering to say thanks, telling them if you're feeling especially stressed, giving them an idea how much information you're comfortable hearing, and by treating all people you come in contact with kindness, as if they're facing the same problems you're facing—because in fact, they may be.

Here's a story told by the wife of a man who has been hospitalized many times, and who has developed excellent skills for interacting with hospital personnel—among them, humor:

When Ron was hospitalized for a brain abscess that developed while he was immune-suppressed, he insisted on writing a joke a day for the nursing staff—even though he had been paralyzed, couldn't speak, and had little control of his body and his eyesight. He labored to write the joke, and his handwriting was barely legible, but he did it, and it was appreciated by the staff.

Second and subsequent opinions

A second opinion is always in order if you have any concerns at all about the decisions made for your care. While you may have to justify getting a second opinion to your insurance company, and while you should tell your doctor you want a second opinion, you do not have to apologize to your doctor for doing so. In fact, the Hippocratic Oath requires your doctor to seek outside advice when your well-being is in question.

The National Cancer Institute or the nearest medical school can supply you with the names of hematologic oncologists available for consultation. See Chapter 2, *Finding the Right Oncologist*, for more information.

Conflict resolution

Occasionally, problems arise between the patient and medical personnel that require more than tact and compromise.

Mary Butler, who is a five-year NHL survivor following an allogeneic bone marrow transplant, describes an experience from her past when her husband was ill with heart disease. She notes her difficulty in putting aside the high regard she had for the medical profession, a level of respect that was silencing her, and discusses her success in dealing with the problem in a very assertive way:

> *I know how exasperating it is to deal with medical professionals who suddenly decide that they don't need to communicate what is going on with the life of the person you love desperately. I remember the fury I felt about having to be demanding, and then, how utterly shocked and numb I felt at the lack of compassion of these people I was trusting with saving my husband's life. I, too, learned that the only way to get things done was to bulldoze my way through, to suddenly unlearn everything I had valued about respectful relations with physicians who seemed far more*

interested in the purchase of new hospital equipment than with the care of my husband who was quite possibly dying...all this in a state far from family or any support system of my own.

It wasn't until I broke through that block that kept assuring me this couldn't possibly be happening, and realized with horror that these "professionals" were not communicating—not with me, not with one another—and they really were going to push my husband off into a corner and let him sink or swim, alone...without the courtesy of even informing me of their lack of interest.

I didn't want to have to be strong, demanding, and rude, but I learned I was the only one who cared enough to get to the bottom of things. I was falling apart, my world was crumbling, I didn't think I could exhibit the kind of behavior it took to get results, but I did. I learned quickly that I could not depend on these people to give freely.

Negotiation

If your concerns evolve around occasional mishaps and miscommunication rather than grossly inadequate care, trying to work through the problem with your doctor may be worthwhile. Schedule an appointment just for discussion, write down your main points and examples, and, unless you have had a great deal of experience negotiating, rehearse what you'll say first:

- Use "I" phrases or neutral phrases instead of accusations. "I felt belittled when you joked about my question on infertility," or "I'm afraid that kind of answer about my questions seems condescending," rather than "You like making your patients feel stupid, don't you?"

- Use a level, calm tone and appropriate eye contact. Getting angry will be a less useful tool in achieving good care than an honest attempt to communicate. Either staring down the other party or avoiding eye contact entirely are often interpreted as hostile, obstructive body language.

- Make it clear that your purpose is a permanent, workable solution, not revenge.

- Be specific. For example, don't say, "Whenever I..., you always..." Say instead, "When I needed your help last week with understanding side effects, you looked at your watch and told me to just stop worrying."

- Don't repeat gossip heard from other patients, no matter the volume or apparent accuracy of such third-hand information.

- Recognize that anything perceived by the doctor as an insult is not likely to advance your chief goal of receiving good care. If, in order to satisfy your pain, you corner the doctor into admitting that she learned virtually no social skills in medical school or in life, plan to find a new doctor, because you'll almost certainly be punished for this victory later if you continue in her care.

- Demonstrate calmly that you understand occasional mistakes or miscommunications may occur, but that you expect them to be fixed promptly and tactfully, and ask how you can help make this easier.

- Don't threaten to change doctors unless you mean it. If your doctor feels defensive, your care may suffer instead of improve.

Third-party intervention

The medical community is a rigid hierarchy: use this to your advantage. If the doctor's staff continually disappoints you in spite of your tactful efforts to get satisfaction, tell the doctor. If a specialist to whom you were referred was unkind, tell the doctor. If the doctor repeatedly mishandles your concerns, say so. Unlike many relationships in life that require a great deal of subtlety and finesse, in this instance you can be quite overt as long as you're not cruel, incorrect, or unfair. Altruism and humanity aside, you are a paying customer. While tact is usually fruitful, superhuman efforts to be tactful, far exceeding those of the medical staff, for example, are not called for. It's your life at stake, not your reputation.

If you feel you have a problem with your current or previous doctor that you cannot resolve, you might contact your state health commission, the administrators or social workers at the hospital where the doctor treats you, or the local chapter of the Medical and Chirurgical (MEDCHI) Society, a group that acts as arbiters in disputes between doctors and patients.

Changing doctors

The decision to change oncologists is a wrenching one for many NHL survivors, but it need not be. If you believe you've done everything you can to resolve difficulties with your doctor or his staff, and if your medical insurance allows, a clean break and a new start may be the best option.

It isn't absolutely necessary to tell your doctor you're leaving—the fact will become obvious soon enough when your new doctor requests information from your former doctor—but you might feel better if you handle this transition courteously, and certainly it will facilitate the pragmatic aspects of changing doctors, such as getting timely copies of medical records and doctor-to-doctor communication.

All states have laws providing for transfer of records, accomplished by sending the records directly to the new doctor or to you. Expect to pay photocopy and shipment fees for this service.

Summary

Successful communication with medical personnel, especially with doctors, may require a variety of tactics. A combination of skills—language skills, listening skills, body language, assertiveness, diligent checking of facts, tenacity, compassion, and tact—are required.

If a doctor is not inclined by nature or training to accord you kindness and respect, it will be up to you to attempt to level the playing field. If your needs for care, information, or emotional support from your doctor are continually unmet, however, or are met with hostility, do your best to discuss this with your doctor or consider finding a new oncologist.

CHAPTER 13

Getting Support

Falling down you can do alone, but it takes
helping hands to get back up.

　　—Yiddish proverb

Cancer can be a terrible burden in its physical aspects alone, but to face NHL without support is far worse. Cancer can be an isolating experience for the patient, because for others, it calls to mind issues that many people dread, such as chronic pain and the surrender of physical independence. Many people, especially younger people, have never experienced any form of long-term illness in their families, much less the chronic and very serious aspects of cancer or cancer treatment.

This entire book is, of course, about getting you the support you need. Support can take many forms. Detailed legal and financial support are dealt with in Chapter 14, *Insurance, Finances, Employment, Record-Keeping.* Various organizations offer an almost staggering variety of services to NHL survivors, most of them free, and Appendix A, *Resources,* contains a full list of such services, including emotional, informational, medical, financial, travel, research, and legal services. Still other forms of institutional support are discussed in chapters such as Chapter 21, *Traveling for Care,* and Chapter 24, *Researching Your Lymphoma.*

The goal of this chapter is to get you the help you need by priming you to anticipate difficulties in communication, offering tips on articulating needs in a reasonable way, and helping you re-evaluate your expectations of others. How can you ask for what you need, and how can you reconcile yourself to being disappointed or to seeking help elsewhere, if support is lacking? How do you keep the physical problem of facing NHL from growing into additional emotional and social problems if you have a misunderstanding with someone who tries to help you? The support you ultimately receive is, in some measure, a result of how good you are at asking for help and expressing appreciation.

This chapter first details specific issues that may require the help of others: the emotional and practical support needed to deal with everyday issues such as transportation, child care, housecleaning, medical care within the home, workplace issues, keeping a positive attitude, and so on. Next, a few general aspects of communication and support are addressed, such as some typical reactions that the "healthy unaware" have to serious illness.

We'll examine in detail the groups of people you might ask for support. We'll work outward from the circle of intimacy, first discussing your strongest, most abiding relationships with family members and loved ones, then friends, support groups, coworkers, and social contacts. Please note that emotional issues specific to the end of treatment and the beginning of remission are discussed in Chapter 15, *After Treatment Ends*.

Cancer counselor and NHL survivor Nan Suhadolc points out that those we must deal with tend to fall into three categories—nurturing, supportive, and toxic—whether they're family, friends, or acquaintances. In other words, your closest family members, upon whom you may hope to rely, might be negative and unsupportive, emotionally toxic to you. Those who are less close actually may be more nurturing than family members. In the discussions that follow, the term "loved ones" implies those who are nurturing, even if they are not related to you by blood or marriage.

The chapter ends with some examples of challenging moments in communication, and how you might handle them.

Specific needs

The word "support" means different things to different people, or different things on different days, depending on what you're dealing with at the moment.

First, there are very tangible, instrumental ways that others can support you, such as:

- Offering to locate and interpret medical information about your illness (see Chapter 24)
- Offering their points of view for your decision-making process

- Organizing blood donor or marrow donor drives

- Helping you move around at home after surgery

- Offering to do some of your cooking, cleaning, laundry, or shopping

- Driving you to and from treatment visits

- Acting as an advocate for you when you're not well enough to express your needs or demand better care

- Keeping track of medications you must take if you're too groggy to do so on your own

- Monitoring your reactions to specific medications and your health in general

- Organizing fundraisers

- Calling insurance companies, medical offices, or employers to iron out misunderstandings

- Being a surrogate parent to your children

- Offering to stay overnight with you if you need nursing care

- Offering to temporarily assume some or all of your workplace responsibilities

- Understanding that fatigue is the most common long-term effect faced by cancer survivors, often lasting for years, and remaining constant in their efforts to help and understand as time unfolds

Next, there are ways that others can provide emotional support:

- Empathizing, at least in principle, with the terror of facing a life-threatening illness

- Attempting to understand how you feel, however alien it may seem to them

- Just being around when you want company

- Sending gifts and cards if you're housebound or hospitalized

- Attending to your children's emotional needs

- Not assuming they know how you feel

- Avoiding asking nosy or inappropriate questions, offering instead to listen when you're ready to talk

- Saying, "I'm sorry this happened to you. Please let me know what I can do for you"

These issues are faced by almost all cancer survivors. There also are several issues NHL survivors face, especially those with low-grade disease, that other cancer survivors may not face:

- Lengthy but uncertain survival for low-grade disease in the absence of an absolute cure

- Inaccurate, frightening, and frustrating comparisons of NHL to other cancers, especially to Hodgkin's lymphoma or to cancers that metastasize to lymph nodes and bone

- The financial devastation that may accompany the lengthy course of some NHLs, which may require retreatment or transplantation, entailing fatigue and side effects that impede your ability to work

- Looking and seeming healthy while harboring a malignancy, and the misunderstandings about this that develop among the healthy unaware

- The loss of support over time; frequently, others get tired of hearing about illness from those who have low-grade disease

Communicate these details

Those who have no experience with NHL seldom can understand intuitively what you're facing. You should consider communicating very clearly about the following issues.

For low-grade disease, they need to be told that:

- Your illness may recur after several years; that is, long remission does not currently equate to cure.

- The path is an uncertain one regarding recurrence of disease and the success of subsequent treatment.

- You may look and seem healthy even while harboring stable disease or a progression of disease.

- Your disease may progress to a more active or aggressive state.

For all subtypes of NHL, the healthy unaware need to be told that:

- It's often characteristic for lymphoma to arise or lodge in bone marrow or lymph nodes, and that this is not necessarily a spreading of disease (metastasis) that signals no hope for treatment or cure. (For detailed information about this issue, see Chapter 4, *Prognoses*.)

- Repeated treatment, and the fatigue that may follow, may leave you unable to work for long periods of time. Following transplantation, for instance, you might be unable to work for a year or more, yet the bill for transplantation still must be paid. Insurers often will cover only 80 or 90 percent of the cost, which can range from $150,000 to $500,000 depending on the follow-up care required and the type of transplant performed.

- The path and long-term side effects of this illness may be lengthy, perhaps requiring their patience and understanding for many years.

- There are differences between the few subtypes of Hodgkin's lymphoma, which generally enjoy a good chance of cure, and the many subtypes of non-Hodgkin's lymphoma, which vary considerably in behavior, treatment, and prospects for survival.

Typical reactions

In an ideal world, we would be surrounded by people who come forward as soon as we need help. They would know what we need before we need it, would give lovingly and unselfishly, and would never become exhausted. Money would flow without a second thought, and those who help us would expect nothing from us in return. In reality, it's not often that way.

Often others are only partially aware of what we're going through. Nausea? Fatigue? While they may have had nausea and fatigue in the past, it's likely that they were quickly remedied. They may not realize what it's like to experience nausea for days each week, even before the chemotherapy treatment has begun. They don't truly understand what it's like to be tired all day, every day, as soon as they wake in the morning. Most people may have considered their own mortality, but seldom have they done so with the sense of immediacy that a cancer diagnosis entails.

At times, others would like to offer support, but don't know what to do or say. They may say the wrong thing. In some instances, others find it easier just to avoid discussing the issue of your illness. They hope—it is presumed—that if they dwell on other topics you (and they) will feel normal again.

In very rare cases, the motives of others are not at all honorable, and they may say or do things that are despicable.

Frequently there are good explanations for what you may perceive as the failure of others to provide adequate support. Other people, being mortal, have finite logistic, emotional, and financial resources. They still have their own responsibilities and needs to address.

If they are loved ones, they may have assumed some of your responsibilities as well. They might be attempting to manage this on a reduced income if the NHL survivor is unable to contribute financially. They may be concerned that the time they're missing from work to provide care will jeopardize the family's only remaining source of income. The thought of losing a loved one is probably highly threatening to them, perhaps causing anger, terror, sadness, and a host of other debilitating feelings. None of these issues justifies unkind behavior, of course, but hidden concerns might cause loved ones to seem distracted, inattentive, overly controlling, or insensitive.

Fortunately, it appears that many NHL survivors receive most of the support they need when they need it, with just an occasional bump along the way—if they make their needs known. A nurse with NHL discusses the wonderful support she received from family and friends:

> One of the most amazing things that happened to me during this disease was learning how much people cared. I had friends call and visit me in the hospital that I thought were mere acquaintances. When I was finally diagnosed, I learned that I wouldn't be allowed to return to work during treatment. This meant that I would need to go on disability but there was a thirty-day waiting period.
>
> A coworker who I thought of as a friendly acquaintance I shared my commute with took up a collection for me at work. Within three days she had collected almost $300. I was just flabbergasted. I work at a state prison that has around 600 workers in various units. In my unit, we don't see a lot of the other workers because we are so isolated. A bake sale was held in my honor, and the employees' association run by the same management I had been so outspoken about gave me $200. The union gave me another $300. I received checks from people I didn't even know. Those who couldn't give money donated their sick leave to me.
>
> It was the most overwhelming and generous support I'd ever received. I feel like I owe them all so much for their support and kindness that I can't even think about leaving now. I never made a secret about

what was going on. I shared my disease openly, even sending a lymphoma education booklet to work with my particulars highlighted.

My coworkers in my immediate unit have also gone grocery shopping for us three times now. I protest, but they seem to receive joy in doing it. It really has helped too. They call occasionally for a status update, and sometimes I fax a letter to them. I am now anxious to return to work. I need the companionship and to get my life back to normal.

My family also became a haven of support. The cancer strengthened ties that were slipping by the wayside. I spent more time with my mother; the days I had chemotherapy treatments, my mother took off work so she could take me. My father moved back to the northwest from Missouri. He says he was planning to anyway, but I think the disease hastened his plans. He wanted to arrive in time for my first chemotherapy, but couldn't make it. He took me to most of my doctor's appointments after that, though, and I found out later that he went to see my doctor privately to discuss my prognosis. My mother also helped me out financially, even though it embarrassed me to have to ask for money. She is now paying my propane bill so that I can have heat during the winter; she even called them and had them bill her directly, so now they just come automatically and I never even see a bill. Again, it embarrasses me that I need this help, but I'm so grateful.

I have also heard from extended family members who live out of state. My cousin has called his mom with information he got from the Internet. I started writing to family members that I hadn't talked with in years.

Some of the most interesting friendships I've developed because of this illness have come via the Internet. I joined a support group for lymphoma patients and have been overwhelmed by the caring and support that "strangers" can offer each other. I've had advice, private email with words of support, offers of financial help when things were bleak—it has been truly amazing. I have cried quietly when others were in pain or at the support and caring shown members.

Most of all, I feel this has made me closer with my daughter. She has been such a help, even scolding me for not taking my medication or "overdoing it." The most important thing I want, though, is for her to have a normal life. I don't want her to skip things because she's worried we can't afford it or worried about my health. I want her to challenge my authority and to have the normal teenage angst. I haven't learned how to convey that yet, but I think things are slowly getting back to normal for her, too.

How to communicate about needs

There's no one way to communicate successfully with others about your needs. Even among people who believe they know each other well, misunderstandings and hurt feelings arise because of daily variations in mood or circumstances of which they're unaware. Your own skills in dealing with NHL come into play, too, when what was not upsetting yesterday may be upsetting today, if you're sick, tired, and discouraged.

Despite these ups and downs, many NHL survivors have learned by experience about communicating with others. Details regarding how to discuss your illness will be touched on in each section below, but some very general guidelines are:

- With your closest loved ones, be as honest as possible, as gently as possible.

- With those to whom you're not very close, use your judgment about what, and how much, to say in order to protect yourself and them from undesirable consequences until you can assess the quality of their responses. You may choose, for example, to tell some family members, social acquaintances, and coworkers a few things about your treatment while avoiding lengthy, painful discussions or topics they're likely to misunderstand.

- For that group in the middle comprising good friends and perhaps some other family members, try to sense the boundary. Just as you have limits to what you can bear, few friends are able to absorb all of your pain all of the time. Asking, "Are you in the mood to listen to this today?" or "Do you have the time and energy to be my sounding board?" are two possible approaches. And the reverse is true: you need to be clear but tactful if you don't feel like discussing your circumstances, for instance, or if you aren't feeling sturdy enough to have visitors.

Exceptions to the rule

The general suggestions above are probably no surprise to you. Nor will be the fact that there are exceptions to every rule.

The general guidelines of telling your closest loved ones the most, with greatest honesty, may not hold. For example, you may have a close relative who handles bad news better if you joke about it a little, but who will never be able to react appropriately to the rawer emotions. He or she may turn tail and run if you cry, for instance. Conversely, you may have a casual friend with a medical background who is a skilled listener, and who can at times provide you with more objective support than your family can. From such an interaction a very deep friendship may grow.

At times, you just can't predict how someone else will react. This experience is retold by a survivor puzzled over the reaction of her husband:

> When I was in the hospital with pneumonia six months after my stem cell transplant, my legs began to swell because of the fluid I was receiving by IV. My blood pressure rose from its normal 120/80 to near 200. I was getting scared. I rang for the nurse and insisted that someone consult with the doctors for a diuretic. My husband stood up and said, "I'll be back in an hour." Who knows what was going through his mind?

Although most loved ones will support you, it's not unheard of for some family members and friends to disappear when they discover you have cancer. There's no one solution to this very painful problem. Often, NHL survivors just move on to find new friends, but some justifiably neither forgive nor forget. Sometimes the absentee friend will reappear and apologize, perhaps not until years later.

Cultural and gender differences

Gender and cultural differences in communicating about illness can affect the outcome of asking for help, especially in the U.S., as our population is composed of so many cultural groups.

Insight into possible cultural and gender differences can help us understand how we're being perceived, how we react to others' responses, and can help us make corrections if needed. For instance, people who are less demonstrative may feel manipulated by people who are highly expressive of emotion, whereas those who are more emotionally demonstrative may feel that less expressive people are cold and uncaring.

Generally, the perception in our culture is that Black Americans, Native Americans, and those of Northern European extraction tend to "report" on their illnesses and feelings in a matter-of-fact tone—or won't discuss them at all—rather than show emotion while discussing them. Americans from cultures of the Mediterranean or some Asian groups are reported as being more dramatic and forthright when talking about how they're feeling. Japanese and Japanese Americans, in contrast, often are reluctant to talk at all about disease.

Aside from differences in cultural backgrounds, there are perceptions, exhaustively discussed in the popular press, that females are more expressive of emotion than males.

In short, there can be obstructive differences in the styles of different groups of humans as they confront illness. Keep in mind that any method of expression is simply a trait, not a fault or virtue—that is, each style is adaptive or maladaptive in different settings. For example, keeping a stiff upper lip and trying to be the strong, silent type might be maladaptive when you need to ask for help.

Loved ones

Some families work better as a team than others. It's rare for any team of people to respond perfectly when it comes to dealing with a crisis. We see these lapses often in the workplace, but we are especially hurt when our families fail to respond appropriately.

Owing to the many variations in group behavior, it's not possible to cover in this section all family behaviors with which you might have to contend. Instead, the most common problems and solutions are discussed.

For many people of all ages, a new crisis tends to elicit behaviors that worked well in the past, especially at first. These reflexive behaviors might be arguing, escapism, intellectualizing the problem, or taking control. For children in crisis, we might see a return to the dependent behaviors they had outgrown. The overall impression in a crisis may be that those around us are reverting to immature, maladaptive behaviors. Keep in mind that NHL is a brand-new experience, and that learned coping behaviors can be hard habits to change, especially in a time of great stress.

It may be harder for your loved ones to help you if you don't communicate clearly about your circumstances. With this group, don't be shy or proud. Ask for all the help you need, even if it embarrasses you. Many family members express chagrin at the seeming reluctance of cancer patients to "trouble" them. They in turn hesitate to invade the patient's privacy by prying or being dominant. Consequently, the already upsetting cancer experience can transform into an even larger menace than it is, because nobody will talk about it.

On the other hand, if your family is closely knit, sharing and verbalizing just about everything, the stresses associated with NHL might *appear* to be taking a greater toll than one might see in a family with fewer emotional ties and more independent members. The telling point is the success of your family's long-term adaptation, not any temporary disequilibrium, emotional flotsam, or distancing you may experience.

What you need from loved ones may change as your experiences evolve from diagnosis through treatment. Different relatives and loved ones may prove good at handling different things. Unlike coworkers and casual acquaintances, close family members and loved ones probably won't surprise you too often with their reactions, because it's likely you already know their weaknesses and strengths. You may find yourself occasionally disappointed, but perhaps not surprised.

Neeraj, who has been in remission several years after treatment for NHL/ALL, describes looking forward to his first trip back home to India:

> I completed two years in remission yesterday. I am leaving on Thursday for a five-week-long vacation to India. I will be visiting home for the first time after my cancer diagnosis three and a half years ago. This shall be a special occasion, and is also a family reunion after seven years as my only sister and brother-in-law, who are in Houston, are going too.
>
> I want people to know I had lymphoma because I think people are afraid of cancer. Back home in India, even among the educated, cancer is considered nothing less than a death sentence. (I guess that may be true for anyone anywhere who has not seen cancer from close quarters.) I feel it is important for me to show people that I am as fine as anyone.

Communicating needs to adults

Ideally, communicating with the loving adults in your life about your needs should be relatively easy. Honesty, gentleness, and especially gratitude should serve well. With a couple of exceptions, such as a relative who's mentally ill or otherwise frail, adults who are nearest and dearest should be trusted to handle every aspect, even the worst aspects, of your illness appropriately.

But cancer challenges a family's beliefs and myths about their family unit, and may alter the established dynamics of the family. If the father, mother, husband, or wife has always been a wise and strong provider, for example, the balance of power may shift temporarily during treatment for NHL. If the partner without NHL has developed an untoward reliance on the strong one, it may be a difficult transition to assume control for a while. The partner with NHL may suffer lowered self-esteem when roles shift. It's important to keep in mind that often these shifts are temporary.

Many NHL survivors note that their loved ones become ill, too, while trying to help them deal with treatment and emotional issues. Upper respiratory infections such as sore throats, persistent GI tract problems such as diarrhea, emergence of autoimmune disorders, and worsening of certain other chronic illnesses such as herpes or diabetes often go hand in hand with the extreme emotional stress associated with a loved one's having cancer. At times, though, NHL survivors report that a relative seems to want to be sicker than the person with cancer. This does indeed happen in some families, and if it happens in yours, chances are you've seen this kind of behavior before from that individual. The deciding factor is whether the ostensibly ill person continues to provide help to the best of his or her ability, or uses the illness as an excuse not to help—or even to punish you.

If you find that the adult loved ones in your life are reacting to your needs in unhelpful ways, do ask why. It may be a simple thing to put right. If they seem angry, of course you needn't apologize for having cancer, but it's likely some older, unresolved issues are being forced to the fore by the stress of dealing with NHL. They may feel, for instance, that they owe you little because in the past you were not supportive of them when they needed help. Communication, humility, and open-mindedness may work to break the impasse.

If attempts to communicate don't make much difference, it may be a disappointment to realize that the strength you thought existed in the relationship does not—or at least not for this set of circumstances. Perhaps you could rely on someone else temporarily for what you need. Sometimes loved ones just need some time to settle down and get used to the changes and increased responsibilities that cancer brings.

Avoid asking a third family member to intervene if you have difficulty getting along with a loved one. Triangles such as this seldom succeed because they hint at two against one, and talking behind each others' backs.

If reasonable attempts to get the help you need fail, you might discuss attending family counseling with the person who seems to be acting out of character.

If none of these attempts works, then finding alternate support or finding ways to live without such people, temporarily or permanently, is in your best interest. Because of the seriousness of NHL, your concerns must be put first, at least for the time being. You may be surprised to find that, in spite of NHL, your life is more serene and enjoyable in the absence of such difficult people. A decision not to deal with someone is also a means of dealing with them.

One survivor describes working as one with her husband to find solutions after the shock of diagnosis abated:

> So then we let reality filter back in and started to plan together—who to call first, how to tell them, who not to tell, and so on. And my magnificent husband started to do as much research as he could, bringing me the information as he found it. I also stayed connected to work through a laptop. We tried to be as practical as possible about how this would distort our lives for a couple of months, but kept focusing on when it would be over. That got more and more difficult as the treatments took their toll on me (and indirectly on him), but it was the only goal that mattered, because we assumed this would work and I would come out of this in good shape. Anything less than that might have been dangerously self-fulfilling…I am even more aware of that now that it is behind me and I have had time to really absorb all that happened in such a short period of time.

Communicating with children

Communicating needs to young children has different goals than communicating with adults. While it's true that children sometimes provide major instrumental support if no other family members are available, generally it isn't necessary or fair to expect a great deal of help from children. More often, they can be asked to help with small, safe chores in order to make them feel part of the solution, and to reinforce the honest relationship they've grown accustomed to.

Human children are inclined by biology to think the world revolves around them. Very young infants do not understand, for instance, that Mommy is a separate person who can leave them with Daddy and go grocery shopping, and they may become quite upset when they discover that Mommy is gone. This bonding trait is probably essential to survival for a species whose young have a long and vulnerable nurturing period, such as humans and some other mammals have.

This egocentric thought process lingers well through childhood, though, and causes children to think that the bad things that happen are their fault. They may think that you developed cancer because they were very angry with you when you once punished them, for example. They may even have wished you were dead, and now it appears to be coming true. Depending on their religious upbringing, they may believe that God saw them misbehave and is punishing them.

For many reasons, our children see us differently from our view of ourselves. Lack of experience with emotions, fear of abandonment, or just plain being shorter than we are means their perspective is truly different. Often small children can't distinguish a sad adult face from a grouchy one, for example, and because we are all-powerful from their perspective, unconsciously they hedge their bets by tailoring their actions to forestall anger instead of sadness, which from their perspective is the worse of these two in terms of the consequences for the child.

This difference of perspective may also cause efforts to explain NHL to backfire. If you try to compare NHL to any illness they've had, it may create an extreme fear that becomes obvious when the next normal childhood illness strikes them.

For these and other reasons, honesty with children about NHL is essential.

The following story describes the fear and confusion that Nan, a childhood NHL survivor, experienced after her family excluded her from the truth about her diagnosis, and thus from the emotional cohesiveness and goal-oriented mindset of the rest of the family:

> *My parents didn't tell me that I had cancer when I was a teen. Back then, cancer was the "c" word, and they were petrified. I'd been given three months to live, and mom and dad were determined that by not saying that aloud, we'd all be better protected. So, for five years, I imagined I had "reactive/viral lymph nodes"—until I read my chart upside down in the oncologists office, then looked up "lymphoma" in the dictionary!*
>
> *It was confusing. If all I had was some sort of virus, why couldn't I go to camp? Why was I spending all summer at the Mayo Clinic in treatments that made me violently ill and caused my golden hair to fall out? And why did everyone in line for the experimental radiation look like they were dying? My parents, my source of trust and safety, told me I was okay. My external cues and my own devastating side effects challenged my parents' assurances. Inside somewhere, I knew…*
>
> *Today, I forgive my parents. I know how terrified they were. I also, however, believe in disclosure, and I help others communicate with loved ones about their disease. Doctors need to inform their patients, even children, about the facts. Parents can tell even the youngest kids, with age-appropriate discretion, what is going on. But even the wisest among us needs help, since in our roles as doctor, parent, caretaker, we are not accustomed to creating sadness and fear in those we love.*

Nan was cured of aggressive childhood NHL, but developed low-grade NHL twenty years later. Today, Nan is a licensed counselor specializing in cancer survivorship issues. She offers these thoughts based on both experience and training:

> *Disclosure is linked to fear. So often I hear, "Nan, I can't tell my daughter about my illness. She will be so afraid. And why burden her?" No doubt there is an element of protectiveness. I feel that myself to this day with my kids. But an additional translation might be, "Nan, I can't tell my kids because I am so afraid of their fear. What do I say when they ask me if I am going to die?"*

Others say to me that they want to protect others and not tell:

"Nan, I cannot tell this woman that her tumor has spread. We will simply proceed with the treatment. If she wants to know, she will ask.

"There is no way that you can tell my son he is dying. I won't allow it."

"I am a professional, and it is inappropriate to tell my clients, even if they are cancer patients, that I have this disease."

There are specific circumstances which might create the exception to the "tell" rule: the age of our kids and their emotional stability…our specific patients we work with. But the key question I ask of all who say "no way" is, "What are you afraid will happen if you tell them?" Usually the fears are about us, not them.

Following her second diagnosis with low-grade NHL as an adult, Nan eventually chose to handle the issue very openly with her own children when she recognized their anxiety:

My daughters were three and five when I was rediagnosed with NHL in 1986. I had no visible symptoms and was going for no treatment. I went in for a number of tests, and was working on creating some lifestyle changes, but watch and wait was the tack we were on, so why burden the kids? So I didn't. One day, Lauren, my oldest, overheard me on the phone talking about my lymphangiogram results, and asked me, "Mommy, are you going to die?" Once I started breathing again, I pulled her onto my lap to have our first mother-daughter chat about it. I told Lauren, in five-year-old terms, about my cancer. She wanted to see my lumps, and then, naturally, she wanted to know if I was going to die.

How was I to answer? I saw the fear in her precious eyes and just wanted to scream, "Lauren, it isn't so! I am fine, will live forever, now let's get back to playing house and Legos." I took a deep breath, pulled her close, and committed myself to honoring her questions. "Yes, mommy is a little sick, with a disease called lymphoma. I have lumps in my body that are not supposed to be there. I am working with the doctors to get well, and the reason I am gone a lot and on the phone a lot is because kind and smart people are helping me to get well. Yes, some people have died from this, honey, but they were a lot sicker than I am. We found this problem early, and there is every reason to believe I will be fine."

I also asked Lauren for her help. We talked about the things she could do for me, such as some very important chores. She wondered if backrubs would help me. I told her that I was sure they would. We also talked about death for a few minutes, since she was interested. Next thing I knew, she was part of the solution, thoroughly proud to be involved, and committed to helping me, in her five-year-old way.

A few days later, I received a call from Lauren's kindergarten teacher. She wanted to tell me that Lauren's behavior and attitude had changed. "Uh-oh, here we go," I thought. To my total surprise, she proceeded to tell me that she didn't know what had changed at home, but that Lauren was so much more relaxed and playful, that "our old Lauren is back!" Humbled, I told her the story.

It is tough to talk with children about our vulnerability. We want to protect them. I wanted Lauren to believe I'd live forever. Kids know, however. They respond to what they sense in their environment, not to what we tell them is so. And one of the toughest things for them, as was the case for me as a teen with the disease, is the confusion, the dissonance between what they are told and what their wise, uncluttered intuition tells them.

To this day, I hate giving my children bad news. I do it anyway, and have found out over and over that it invites them to be a part of my team. Their awareness that my NHL has progressed scares them, but we cry together instead of each alone into our separate pillows. We also laugh harder than most, and rally toward whatever solutions I am pursuing. The bottom line is that there are no better teammates in this battle than those daughters of mine. I just had to dare to ask, to notice my fear, but to proceed with heart, in spite of it.

Communicating needs to teenagers

This is a topic on which an entire book could be written. An adolescent trying to break away from the family and become independent is likely to experience quite ambivalent feelings if a parent is diagnosed with cancer. Just at the time in his life when he'd rather avoid talking to any adult, circumstances may force him to become very intimate and empathic with a parent. He must be patient and caring toward one of the people most likely to make him angry by holding him to high standards, enforcing rules, denying him privileges, or restricting his freedom. Some find that teens turn surly or run amok when faced with the physical, emotional, and financial hardships associated with cancer.

Nonetheless, some people find that their adolescent children are extraordinary in their ability to comprehend what's needed, and that they follow through with a maturity that's well beyond their years.

But—even more so than younger children—teens can appear to be knowledgeable and well-adjusted when in fact they are not. This group may have an intellectual maturity that is beyond their level of emotional maturity. A willingness to overlook unexplainable lapses and an honesty that is geared to their level of understanding are wise. Frequent offers to chat candidly are a good tactic. These offers confirm their belief that they can approach you about difficult subjects.

If you have a teen who is developing behaviors that are a danger to herself or others, such as acting out rage, violating laws, or considering dropping out of school, find a counselor who specializes in the adaptation of children to serious illness. Attempts to handle these problems by yourself may risk compounding your health problems, may make of you a psychologically abused parent—and they may fail anyway. A teen may carry "cancer anger" formed during these especially rebellious years well into adulthood.

If you have a teen who is doing housework and assisting with medical care while continuing to carry his academic responsibilities, thank him at least daily.

Mary, a five-year transplant survivor, describes how easily she misinterpreted what her son was thinking and feeling:

> My son was in high school when I was diagnosed. Those difficult years were just beginning. I tried to include him, without giving him too much information, so that he would not feel frightened that we weren't telling him everything. As time and treatment wore on, he withdrew more and more. I thought he didn't understand completely. What I didn't realize—because I was so understandably self-involved, I suppose—is that he was withdrawing in terror.
>
> He visited me just one time in the transplant unit. My husband was careful to wait until I looked somewhat better before bringing him for a visit. At the time, the whites of my eyes were black with blood, and my skin was yellow and peeling all over. I was bloated and bald. My son had

to wash with bacterial soap and put on a gown, mask, and gloves just to enter my room. I was so happy to see him it didn't register that what he was seeing was making it so much worse for him.

When I was released from the transplant unit and home a couple of days, we were sitting in the kitchen together. I was still only up for a few minutes at a time, and we hadn't had any time together before now. I sat smiling up at him as he sat on a stool, and suddenly I realized he was sobbing. I'll never forget the pain that flowed out of him. "Mom, I only had two things to worry about this year: whether or not I got my homework done, and if my mom was going to die."

Good friends

We expect our good friends to stand by us while we're facing serious problems. Close friends can offer us help such as emotional support, occasional running of errands, some cooking, household chores, babysitting, or an escapist night on the town. As with loved ones, we may occasionally be disappointed or surprised if they fail to live up to our opinions of them. On the other hand, many NHL survivors have discovered that good friends earn their wings in heaven by way of loyalty and selflessness, and that some come to mean as much to us as our families do.

Because they usually have a lower emotional investment in the relationship than family members do, good friends can be easier to deal with at times than family. They can be more objective about some of our problems.

This objectivity is purchased with their relative distance. Good friends, in order to remain good friends, may need an occasional vacation from us and our problems. If we give them space to refresh themselves, they are able to return to us with more emotional vigor.

Most people will find that at least some friends or acquaintances will have responses that are disappointing. We can't control how other people react to cancer. Here are the experiences of some people whose friends were disappointing:

When my husband was first diagnosed with lymphoma, I phoned my best friend to tell her. After my call, she didn't phone me for about a week, although we work on the same campus, used to speak about once a day, and usually had lunch once or twice a week. A few years prior, her father had died of acute leukemia. *Several months after my husband's diagnosis, she admitted that at first it was just too difficult to face cancer again.*

Nicole, a registered nurse, finds that her one disappointing experience is understandable:

The only person I felt let down by, I don't blame. A former boyfriend had been trying to contact me while I was being diagnosed. I finally called him back and explained what was going on. I never heard from him again. I don't blame him, though: he had lost his wife to breast cancer a few years ago and didn't believe I could have a positive outcome given the spread of the disease. I think it would have been too painful for him to experience cancer treatment again.

Doris describes how disappointed her very best friends left her feeling after an initial show of support at the beginning of her cancer experience:

One of the most hurtful things that happened to me was when I first came home from all the tests, surgery to put in the Port-a-cath, and my first round of chemotherapy.

Some of my friends came over, and they were wonderful. We had a great talk, lots of sharing. But then they never came back once. When I really needed them—a phone call, card, anything—nothing. All I could think was, "What was their visit all about? Just to find out the gory details?" Some of the people I was closest to never would say a word about it, while people who were practically strangers inundated me with the most personal questions. Go figure!

Mary, a survivor of a transplant for NHL, describes her experiences with friends who couldn't face her:

I had a number of friends disappear. What surprised me were which ones disappeared: I never would have imagined those particular people abandoning me—or anyone—under those circumstances. At first it was very painful. I kept thinking I had done something to offend them. Over time, I realized that, for whatever reason, they couldn't handle my being sick, or my not getting well faster. It didn't really matter because ultimately cancer was a wonderful tool for separating the wheat from the chaff. It was a gift in disguise, because the quality of the friends that stuck it out or surfaced during the crises far exceeds the quality of any of those that left. Maybe that sounds petty or mean, but I don't intend it in a vengeful way at all. It's simply the truth.

Support groups

It would be difficult to say too many good things about the effect of a support group on an NHL survivor. In addition to the personal testimonials from people who feel they found sanity, love, and knowledge from the members of their support groups, research by Dr. David Spiegel has shown that emotional support can extend the lives of cancer survivors.

Support groups are the one place outside of your inner circle of loved ones where you can ask or say just about anything. In some cases, you can ask help of support group members that you would be afraid to ask of family for fear of overburdening or frightening them. Moreover, the setting is sometimes freer than the family setting regarding candid speech, because everyone present understands all too clearly what you're going through.

For some, support groups can be the difference, literally, between life and death. The opportunity to exchange information with those who have already weathered NHL can provide you with the knowledge to question your treatment and seek medical help elsewhere. Support groups are an immeasurably useful way to do this, bringing together a variety of skills, including medical and legal knowledge.

Support groups are offered locally in many areas by groups such as the American Cancer Society, the Wellness Community, or local hospitals. Telephone support groups are overseen by several of the nonprofit organizations dedicated to curing lymphoma. If you have a computer, support groups are also available on the Internet.

Local, telephone, and Internet support groups have their advantages and disadvantages. Many people use several.

Some people are very put off by the thought of talking to others in a support-group setting. Steve, ex-Air Force and a survivor of NHL, describes the complete turnaround in his feelings about support groups:

> *I speak from experience when I say that support groups are a godsend. Thirteen years ago, I was in the middle of treatment, I was depressed, angry, scared, and just about every other feeling you can think*

of. When my doctor mentioned the idea of a support group, I just blew the whole thing off. The way I was feeling, I figured the last thing I needed was to sit around and listen to a bunch of other people whine and cry about how bad they had it.

My wife finally talked me into going to a support group sponsored by the Leukemia Society of America. What I've found over the years is a bunch of folks who have become another family. Whether they're the patient or a family member, each has something positive to contribute to the group. We learn from each other different ways to handle the things that come up, from dealing with sudden baldness to getting through the rough times that inevitably arise. By sitting down for two hours every month with a group of wonderful folks who are in the same boat, I've learned how to take charge of things and how to live with cancer instead of dying from cancer.

We discuss whatever's on our minds at the time. Of course, each individual is usually at a different place in the journey, but we all have the common bond of knowing that, whatever I'm going through now, somebody else in the room has been there, done that, and can help me to overcome it, too. We have people who are newly diagnosed, and those who are long-time survivors (like me). We have some who have had marrow transplants, some who are awaiting transplants, and some for whom transplant is not an option. There are those who sit and "suck up" the energy in the room, seldom speaking out. Then there are those (like me) who don't know when to shut up. But we all come away from each meeting knowing that, when the chips are down, we have someone to talk to who knows exactly what we're talking about.

I go to an oncologist who I believe is the best in St. Louis. (Of course, everybody else thinks the same thing about their own doctor.) He's an expert in lymphomas. He knows the latest protocols, and takes part in a lot of research. He's fantastic at taking bone marrow biopsies, so much so that I had the last two with nothing but the local anesthetic to deaden the skin. He is the epitome of empathy. But he's never had lymphoma or felt the sense of total devastation that comes from hearing the word "cancer" and his name mentioned in the same breath.

My wife is a nurse. She understands and tries to explain to me what's going on with this thing. We've been married nearly twenty-eight years and still deeply love each other. She stood by my side and helped me to become a cancer survivor instead of a cancer victim. She has experienced this whole thing from the vantage point of a family member, and that's its own hell. She didn't know if she was going to have to raise our two daughters alone or not. She's been my rock. But she's never had the disease.

My point with the above rambling is that nobody can relate to having any kind of cancer except somebody who's had it. And that's where the support group comes in. I had just been retired on disability from the Air Force. Like most military men, I was too macho to need all that support crap. I'd work through this my own way. I guess it's just a "guy thing." But I found out it also takes a hell of man to know when to call in the reinforcements. There's nothing like drawing on the experience of others who've already walked the road you're on. Since we don't have a map to show us the way, it always helps to have a guide who already knows it.

And that's what the support group has been for me. They're my guides. Our meetings aren't always totally upbeat, but we do have our moments. Sometimes it turns out to be an evening of silliness and giddiness, especially when a member of the group has some great news to report. Sometimes it's total numbness when we find out that one of our own has lost the battle. But we all know that we're stronger and better people for having known them. If I hadn't found that group thirteen years ago, if I'd tried to go it alone (I come from a long line of hard-headed Germans), I'd probably have either given up years ago or else they'd have me in the proverbial padded cell. When the weight of the burden gets to be too much, let somebody help. And that goes for spouses and family members, too.

Local support groups

Local support groups are useful for those who are able to get about easily, have access to a car, and enjoy face-to-face discussion, even about topics that might be upsetting. If you're in a local support group, you're likely to have a stream of visitors if you're hospitalized, and friends to offer you instrumental support such as help with groceries or babysitting. Often, members trade phone numbers and form deep friendships.

The disadvantages of local support groups are that they usually contain only a small number of people, perhaps ten or less, and only meet at certain times of the week or month. The smallness of the group can affect the quality of the information shared. For example, if no group member has traveled for care, you'll have to make your travel plans with less foreknowledge. Some members of local support groups report that they feel excluded when things take a turn for the worse, as if some group members want to shield themselves from the possibility that similar bad things may happen to them, too. This is less likely to happen if the group is moderated by a trained therapist.

Internet support

Internet support groups offer several hundred friends available at all times of the day. You can communicate at 3 A.M. when you have insomnia, and you can communicate with other survivors even if you have trouble getting around for various reasons. The people you meet will be from all over the country, and in some cases, all over the world, and represent a tremendous amount of experience. Furthermore, if you're a little shy about expressing emotion in front of other people, an Internet group is a good choice because you can write a message and read what you plan to say before you decide to send the message. If you need to cry, you can do so without feeling conflicted about crying in front of other people.

Many of the Internet support groups schedule in-person reunions and gatherings. Often, members form personal friendships and write private email, or trade phone numbers to form even closer friendships. Sometimes members discover that they're living quite close by and become very good friends.

A list of NHL-related Internet support groups follows. Because the Internet is a dynamic resource, this list may not be comprehensive. The number of subscribers given was approximate at the time of writing and will vary over time:

- NHL. Run by Robert Scott Pallack, offering medical discussion and emotional support for all non-Hodgkin's lymphoma survivors. NHL has about three hundred subscribers.

- NHL-LOW. Discussion of medical treatment for those with low-grade NHL. About one hundred seventy subscribers.

- HEM-ONC. Run by GrannyBarb Lackritz, offering medical discussion and emotional support for the hematologic malignancies, including NHL. Several oncologists are subscribed to this list. About eight hundred subscribers.

- BMT-TALK. Medical discussion and emotional support for those who will be having or who have had bone marrow transplantation for any cancer. Several oncologists are subscribed to this list. About five hundred subscribers.

- PED-ALL. Medical discussion for pediatric acute lymphocytic leukemia, which resembles some NHLs. This list was formed in early 1998.

- CLL. Medical discussion and emotional support for chronic lymphocytic leukemia, which can convert into one form of NHL, called small-cell lymphocytic leukemia (SLL). About three hundred subscribers.

- SICKKIDS. A discussion group just for children, but supervised by adults. Find them on the Web at *http://tile.net/listserv/sickkids.html.*

- YAP. A discussion group for young adults age 18 to 25 dealing with their own illness or that of a loved one. This list was formed in late 1998.

The Association of Cancer Online Resources (ACOR) has pointers to all of the hematologic cancer email discussion groups. ACOR offers a handy automatic subscription feature for these and other discussion mailing lists. You can find them on the Web at *http://www.acor.org/.*

The chief disadvantage of an Internet support group is that the loss of a friend is very difficult when we cannot say good-bye in person, when we have no photographs to remind us of them, and no grave to visit. Sometimes group members simply will never hear again from another member, and they never learn what really happened. Some group members deal with their grief by creating a memorial web page dedicated to a lost friend, containing photos and examples of wisdom learned about living with NHL.

Other disadvantages of Internet support groups include cultural differences that cause mistaken communication and needless arguments, heavy mail volumes about topics that you may feel don't pertain to your circumstances, incorrect medical information, a range of social and communication skills, and, of course, the cost of a computer and access to the Internet.

A recent survey has shown that the over-65 age group is among the most active and fastest growing groups on the Internet, seemingly not reluctant to acquire the new skills needed to use a computer.

Telephone support

Telephone support is offered by certain nonprofit groups dedicated to curing cancer and supporting cancer survivors. They offer to act as a clearinghouse for one-on-one telephone contact between those who would like to speak with others in their situation:

- The Lymphoma Research Foundation of America. Call them at (310) 704-2040 or visit *http://www.lymphoma.org/*.

- The Cure for Lymphoma Foundation. Call them at (212) 213-9595 or visit *http://www.cfl.org/*.

- The Blood and Marrow Transplant Newsletter. Call them at (847) 831-1913 or visit *http://www.bmtnews.org/survivor.html*.

- The Leukemia Society of America. Call them at (212) 573-8484 or visit *http://www.leukemia.org/*.

Coworkers

What you can ask of your coworkers depends on the structure and size of your workforce, the level of competitiveness your profession experiences, and the degree to which your work relationships drift into friendships. The minimum we can ask of coworkers is patience and discretion, but frequently they give us much more. Often the feelings your coworkers express and the support they offer are a tremendous reinforcement for your well-being. To know you are needed and missed can be uplifting.

In general, though, we must exercise some caution asking favors of coworkers who are not also friends, because the request may seem out of bounds, or may backfire if we're deemed too sick to perform well after revealing a weakness or need. As with some friends, coworkers may want to know everything about your illness, nothing, or some intermediate subset of information that's hard to define and may change daily.

The good news, though, is that many NHL survivors report that coworkers pitch in and offer assistance without being asked: blood donations, bone marrow donor drives, bake sales, shopping, babysitting, cheering visits, and so on may materialize without your having to ask. Many NHL survivors report that coworkers donate unused sick days to them, or pinch-hit for them if they miss time or feel sick or tired.

This story describes one NHL survivor's mixed experiences with coworkers:

> *At the time I was diagnosed, I had completed some highly stressful work in helping to bring a large local government back from the brink of*

bankruptcy. There had been a lot of turnover, turmoil, and tough decisions. A team of officials (including me) had just gone to New York to make our case to the rating agencies. While there, I knew I was going to see a doctor within the next week or so, but I could not discuss my symptoms with anyone. I was afraid I would be seen as a weakened link through which others would begin to hack.

The interim CAO, promoted from within, was very close to me and tried to be as supportive as possible. Hence the arrangement which allowed me to try to work at home on a laptop as much as tolerable. Given my position, it was not the most optimal arrangement, but I knew it was temporary, though of course I was extremely frustrated by my serious physical restrictions and inability to see people. On the other hand, I did not really want people to see me until I resembled my old self, even though I would never again be my old self.

Given the ever-shifting political winds in this turbulent place and the desires of some whose games of wasting taxpayers' money I had spoiled, I learned that some pressure began to build on this interim CAO to find a replacement for me. She was in a tough spot. She did begin inquiries, as I was told later. Part of her may have been truly afraid I would not survive the disease. I know a number of people thought it was only a matter of time. Part of her may have felt the organizational politics would have made my life miserable anyway if I were to return. I don't know what I would have done in her place, except to stall for time, as I assume she did.

This is not something we have ever discussed, since in the end I made good on my promises to return immediately after my stem cell harvest at the end of my eight-week high-dose chemotherapy regimen. By that time, a new CAO had been hired, and I was able to wobble in, bewigged and befuddled, to meet him the week following the completion of the stem cell apheresis. Things never felt the same, however, for I realized there were people around me who had actually harbored hope that I would die. There were also those who hoped for the best, but who did not know what to say or how to say it once I showed up in person. It was all very awkward. Except for a handful of people, almost everything—positive or negative—was left unspoken.

If some coworkers are reluctant to recognize your illness owing to their own fears or lack of social skills, they might never refer to it, not even to wish you well.

I work with a woman who used to be an RN. Although she knows that my husband had lymphoma, she has never, in eight years, asked how my husband is doing. She left nursing when her son was born because nursing made too many emotional demands on her.

You can feel free to say nothing to the potentially unsympathetic coworker if you choose, but there are disadvantages in not keeping your immediate supervisor informed about your health status. For example, if your supervisor is unaware of problems you're experiencing as a result of your illness or its treatment, you may have difficulty winning a favorable decision if a dispute about your performance arises.

Remember that cancer is considered a disability under the Americans with Disabilities Act (ADA), so negative reactions in the workplace that result in demonstrable emotional or professional harm to you, such as denial of a promotion or censure for using earned sick time, don't have to be endured without legal recourse.

Employee assistance programs (EAP)

Increasingly, employers are finding that it's to everyone's benefit if they offer formal assistance to employees who have special needs at difficult times. Employee assistance programs are designed to help the employee weather life changes and become happy and productive again. If your employer has an EAP, you should ask what it has to offer.

You should be aware, however, that if a health-related dispute over job performance goes to court, employers can subpoena any doctor's records, and so are given access to records that accumulate when you use an EAP. This includes material that most people assume is confidential, such as the notes a psychologist or social worker takes during a therapy session, even if they don't bear directly on your job performance.

If you're seeing a psychologist privately, your employer may not know that you are or who you're seeing. Clearly, this makes serving a subpoena more difficult. But if you use an EAP, the wolf is guarding the chickens, so to speak. In spite of safeguards that supposedly shield irrelevant material from nonprivileged eyes, your employer may become privy to information, for example, about a dependent child who began using drugs after your diagnosis. These confidential documents also may be admitted as evidence into the permanent and public legal record should you have a workplace dispute that is settled in court.

Moreover, the *Wall Street Journal* reported on May 26, 1994, in its "Your Money Matters" column that some less ethical managers put pressure on EAP personnel to open files they have no right to see, in the absence of any dispute in court.[1]

Computerized self-help programs

Although not yet widely used, computerized self-help programs provided by one's employer or health care provider are another means of finding support. The Comprehensive Health Enhancement Support System (CHESS), developed at the University of Wisconsin, is one of the first and most comprehensive of such products. Although currently only available to patients through their health care providers, CHESS is planned to be made available through employers in the future. Web versions of the system are currently being developed. Topic-specific content is available for AIDS, breast cancer, heart disease, asthma, Alzheimer's disease, and alcoholism. The addition of other specific topics is underway.

For more information on CHESS, contact:

CHESS
1120 WARF Building
610 Walnut Street
Madison, WI 53705
Phone (608) 263-0492
http://chess.chsra.wisc.edu/

Social acquaintances

Social acquaintances comprise a wide variety of people, some of whom, such as church or temple members, expect to be asked for help, and others, such as the spouses of coworkers, touch on your life only briefly or occasionally and probably don't expect to be asked to help. Many NHL survivors are pleasantly surprised, though, to find that people they thought were practically strangers pitched in and helped without being asked.

Unlike your family, friends, and coworkers, social acquaintances don't usually have the opportunity to see you doing everyday things, and consequently they may have more misunderstandings about what you're going through. On the other hand, people we choose to see socially may have more in common with us than, for instance, those we have no choice but to work with.

In general, what we can ask of social acquaintances depends on the context in which we know them. If they're fellow Junior Leaguers or Jaycees, we might expect help, as these groups specialize in helping others. If they're the friendly couple with season tickets next to ours at the theater, perhaps not.

Karen Ali, M.S., a caretaker of several family members with NHL and other cancers, offers pragmatic advice on being candid and concrete about the support you need:

> Unfortunately, some people just do not know how to handle this kind of stress, so they run away, or try to minimize what's going on in order to absolve themselves and pretend that they can do nothing to help.
>
> If you have a church family you can turn to—even if you have not been a particularly active member—many do have some resources that might be able to assist you, and all you have to do is ask. Sometimes the social services department of the hospital will be able to help you contact a resource to help you with what you need.
>
> Do you need help with the housework or other tasks of a similar nature? Try to formulate some idea of what it is that you want done. Sometimes it is the vague "I need help" that frightens others from volunteering to pitch in. They might not be able to commit to a long term project, but might be able to do one specific task or job.
>
> Also, priorities may need to be shuffled or standards lowered on some things to get you through the tough spots. Rest when you can. The sweeping and dusting will still be there tomorrow, and I haven't known of a single instance where the good fairies came in and did it during the night!

Organizations that focus on help

Your church, local chapters of the Elks, Rotary, or Shriners, or other civic groups may be able to offer you help ranging from transportation for treatment, to financial assistance, to pitch-in efforts for lawn care and cooking.

Moreover, an enormous collection of nonprofit organizations exist to help you in various ways. Lymphoma-specific groups, those for general needs, for bone marrow transplantation, children's aid, young adults' aid, home care or temporary hospice care, and pain management can be found in Appendix A.

Challenging moments

Almost every cancer survivor has had a verbal exchange with one of the "healthy unaware" that has left him angry, hurt, or speechless.

What you choose to do or say to remarks like these depends on what consequences you're willing to endure. In most cases, the classic reply from Judith Martin (also known as Miss Manners), "Now, why would anyone ask such a rude question?" is right on the mark, but not always socially adroit.

In instances where consequences do matter, you might want to try one of the following replies. These responses are listed only as suggestions—there are no answers that are right for all settings and all personalities. Your style might be completely different, but it's sometimes helpful to know that these kinds of rude questions have been asked of others, and that a few people have found comebacks that were satisfying to them. If someone asks you a rude or outlandish question, there's no rule that says you must be serious in return. Nor do you have to stretch, in your reply, to soothe and comfort the person who asks it, as if his or her discomfort with your illness were the most important issue.

- **The Profound Thought.** A deliberately obtuse reply, perhaps quoting something in a foreign language that sounds impressive, but is meaningless. Latin is a good choice because so few people speak it anymore. How many people know, for instance, the CIA's motto, "Veritas vos Liberabit"? ("The truth shall set you free.") My own favorite reply is, "Nabok sledjze, ba boat yedjze." (Phonetic spelling of a Polish saying, meaning, "Look out, herring. Here comes a boat.") They needn't know you're having fun at their expense. They'll just think that cancer has made you a better person, a deep thinker. And they're right, aren't they?

- **The Escape.** "Gotta go! Time for my bungee-jumping lesson." You can, of course, substitute basket-weaving or yodeling lessons if you think this person might actually be a bungee-jumper.

- **The Sympathetic Noise.** Neutral replies, used by therapists. You can say, for example, "That's an interesting point of view," or "You appear to have given this a lot of thought." These replies give the other party the attention he's trying to get, without committing you to agreement, continued dialog, or revealing intimacy. They're also good transitional phrases for shifting the conversation to a less offensive subject.

If you prefer the head-on approach, here are a few of the most disturbing and least informed reactions that some NHL survivors have encountered, and a few suggested replies, both factual and humorous:

Q: *What did you do to deserve this cancer? (Variation: "Why did you want this cancer?" based on the philosophy of a popular self-help book.)*

A: Many studies have shown no link between lifestyle and NHL, nor between personality and NHL.

A: Maybe because I once ran with scissors? Or because I tore those "do not remove under penalty of law" tags from my pillows?

Q: *They say you develop cancer because of negative thoughts.*

A: That's interesting. Actually, I'm having homicidal thoughts right now, but many studies have shown no link between negative thoughts, stress, and NHL.

Q: *Do you think your smoking caused your cancer?*

A: Studies have shown no links between smoking and NHL, or drinking alcohol and NHL.

Q: *How long does your doctor say you have?*

A: Why?

A: She says I'm still safe buying green bananas.

A: How long does your doctor say *you* have?

Q: *You look so bad/thin/pale/etc.*

A: Actually, I've regained ten pounds, my blood pressure is down fifteen points, and last weekend I walked in the Cure for Lymphoma six-kilometer race.

A: My, what a lovely smile you have! Are those your own teeth?

Q: *What happened to your beautiful hair?*

A: Oh, *this* hair. I borrowed it from a friend.

Q: *You don't look like you have cancer.*

A: Hey, better living through chemistry!

A: Neither do you.

Q: *God doesn't give us anything we can't handle.*

A: My God is too kind to be that petty.

Q: *God must be punishing you for something. (This is a particularly painful question if it's your child who has cancer.)*

A: Fifty percent of men and 33 percent of women will get cancer. That's a lot of people to punish.

Q: *It seems like it always comes back.*

A: It's not possible to make accurate generalizations about this particular form of cancer.

A: Golda Meir lived for almost twenty years with a leukemia that's related to NHL, including the time before and during her years as Prime Minster of Israel.

Q: *Lymphoma is the best kind of cancer you can get! You're lucky!*

A: No kind of cancer is good to get.

A: Would you feel lucky to get it?

Summary

Your experience with NHL may be your most vulnerable, powerless experience since early childhood. Getting the support you need is critical to adequate recovery, especially during and after relatively risky procedures such as bone marrow transplantation.

We humans are imperfect. It's unfortunate but true that if we don't communicate clearly, if old resentments linger, or if altruism dries up, the formidable single problem of facing NHL might evolve into six or seven additional problems.

This chapter attempts to help you get the support you need. While nobody knows better than you how to interact with your family, acquaintances, and coworkers, the past experiences of other NHL survivors may help you spot problems before they arise, or to view old problems in a new way.

The unique characteristics of NHL, and the problems you may face because of them, are discussed in this chapter. Others need to be told of these differences in order to do their best for you.

CHAPTER 14

Insurance, Finances, Employment, Record-Keeping

*Financial ruin from medical bills is almost
exclusively an American disease.*

—Roul Turley

Recovering our health should be all that requires our stamina and concentration after being diagnosed with and treated for NHL. Unfortunately, the side effects of cancer go beyond the physical, impacting our social, professional, and financial well-being. If you're an American with NHL, you're likely to become an instant but unwilling expert on finances, insurance, and workplace issues.

You can ease the nonmedical aspects of your cancer experience in some ways. By becoming familiar with the somewhat harsh business side of cancer, keeping careful records, and anticipating problems, you may avoid hospital billing convolutions, insurance payment denials, employment pitfalls, and financial degradation.

This chapter will discuss some of the more common problems you may encounter, will give tips to avoid problems, and will steer you to up-to-date resources that provide detailed solutions to these problems.

It is not the intent of this chapter to address in detail all issues concerning health insurance benefits, federal legislation such as ERISA, Medicare, and Medicaid coverage, unemployment insurance, and financial issues. In Appendix A, *Resources*, there are many excellent books and other resources which explore each of these topics much more thoroughly. Some issues covered in this chapter, such as estate planning or declaring bankruptcy to protect your house and car, clearly require the aid of professionals such as financial planners or tax attorneys.

Insurance issues

For NHL survivors, problems may arise with health insurance, unemployment insurance, or life insurance. Of these, health insurance is by far the most likely to cause heartache, frustration, and anger, but first, we'll discuss the main impediment to purchasing all kinds of health, life, disability, and care insurance: medical underwriting.

"No medical underwriting"

State and federal authorities have begun to address the problem of health insurance being denied to those with serious illnesses (for which see COBRA and HIPAA, discussed later in this section), but purchases of life, long-term care, and other insurance policies are still impossible or expensive purchases for those with a cancer diagnosis.

The impediment is the medical examination or medical history questionnaire. If the policy is indeed offered to you after the actuaries have examined the statistics for your illness, it may be offered only with very high premiums. Moreover, employers who have no annual open enrollment period may refuse ever to insure you if you did not elect certain insurance options at time of hire, which is their only open enrollment period.

> When my husband changed jobs, we decided to just add his name to my employer's medical policy in order to save money and have one provider. What we didn't realize is that his employer did not have annual open enrollment—the only time he wouldn't be asked about his health was when he was hired.

> After he was diagnosed with lymphoma, I wanted to change jobs. By then, I'd heard horror stories about changing jobs and losing coverage because pre-existing conditions were excluded. I asked him to follow up with his employer to see if he could enroll for their medical insurance. They referred him to the policy's underwriters. (That should have given us a hint of what was to come.) "We will never insure you," they said. This meant I could never leave my job.

> Since then, his employer's policy has been renegotiated for more leniency, and federal laws have been passed to look after the medical insurance needs of people like us. But it was a bitter experience.

If your insurance needs are unmet, you should consider any offer that states that medical underwriting—insurance jargon for a close scrutiny of your health—is not necessary. Some advertisements state very clearly that a medical exam isn't necessary or that pre-existing conditions will not result in refusal.

Note that some medical questionnaires for insurance enrollment ask health questions but do not mention cancer, not even in the section titled "Other." It's always worthwhile to ask for an application form to see just how rigorous the medical scrutiny may be.

Of course, while most of these offers may be aboveboard, a proportion of these policies may be very expensive. The usual considerations for shopping wisely still apply, but if your insurance needs are great, or your estate planning justifies purchasing a whole-life policy that might bypass estate and inheritance taxes, for example, the additional cost may be worth it.

Insurance companies are evaluated by A.M. Best, Moody's, and Standard and Poor. Choose only those with top ratings.

Health insurance

Cancer survivors in the U.S. complain about health insurance problems more than any other issue except cancer itself. The delays and denials of managed care are the most common complaint, but other insurance issues also arise.

If your medical insurance plan is in some way lacking, find out if your employer:

- Offers more than one medical insurance plan.

- Holds an open enrollment each year. Open enrollment is the time period during which you may change plans without a medical examination or questionnaire, that is, without having your pre-existing health conditions held against you.

If so, use the open enrollment period to upgrade to a better policy. Examine all plans closely for what they cover, especially for bone marrow transplantation and clinical trials, treatments likely to be recommended to NHL survivors. Weigh an indemnity or preferred-provider plan, which may trade higher convenience for lower coverage, against a high-coverage HMO requiring referrals and gatekeepers. The indemnity plan may cost more per doctor visit, but may provide you with the freedom to get care wherever *you* think best, without the delay of pre-approval, including out-of-state care within a clinical trial, or at a distant but excellent transplant center.

If you are planning to have a bone marrow or stem cell transplant and your medical insurance company has refused to pay part or any costs, or if they seem to be delaying a decision, contact a lawyer immediately, as some cancer survivors have died while waiting for transplantation to be approved. It's best to use a lawyer who has had experience negotiating for transplant coverage. The Blood and Marrow Transplant Newsletter can furnish you with a list of nearby lawyers who can help you. Call (847) 831-1913 or visit their web site at *http://www.bmtnews.org/*.

If you have been approved for Social Security Disability Income (SSDI, discussed in its own section later in this chapter), you'll be automatically enrolled in Medicare after getting disability benefits for two years. Moreover, Medicare coverage is free for thirty-nine months after returning to work if you're still disabled. If your income is low, your state may pay your Medicare premiums as part of Medicaid benefits. Contact your local Social Security Administration office for more information.

Losing medical insurance coverage if you change or lose jobs is still a problem, but less of a problem than before. In addition to various state laws, two federal laws exist to help you retain coverage:

- HIPAA, the Health Insurance Portability and Accountability Act of 1996, is a federal law intended to prohibit the permanent denial of medical coverage based on pre-existing conditions. HIPAA covers only employers with twenty or more employees. In general, it states that if you have had continuous medical insurance coverage for more than twelve months, your new medical insurance company cannot refuse to pay for medical care for your previous health problems. If your previous health coverage was for less than twelve months, each month you were covered reduces by one month the amount of time your new medical insurance company can refuse to pay for your previous health problems. No medical insurance company, however, can refuse to pay for your previous health problems for more than twelve months. There are loopholes in this law, though, that medical insurance companies are exploiting. In July 1998, President Clinton issued a warning to insurance companies covering federal employees, stating that such denials of payment will not be tolerated.

- COBRA, the Consolidated Omnibus Budget Reconciliation Act of 1985, provides for a continuation of your old employer's medical insurance coverage for a temporary amount of time—from eighteen to thirty-nine months, depending on your circumstances. Always elect COBRA continuation coverage if you lose or change jobs, until you're certain that your new employer's policy will cover expenses associated with your care. HIPAA, discussed above, does not always provide the continuous coverage the law intended, owing to its design and various loopholes.

Some states have older, stricter laws that resemble HIPAA but provide better coverage. Call your state insurance commissioner for details.

An NHL survivor being treated for high-grade disease describes her frustration with the medical insurance and disability insurance industry:

> The biggest problems have been with my insurance company. They love you when you pay them and don't use their services, but as soon as something happens, they turn on you. I cringe every time I open a benefits statement because I know it will be wrong and I'll have to call.
>
> I have decided that I hate managed care. Unfortunately, I can't afford the lesser coverage that nonmanaged care would get me. I will change insurance companies during this open enrollment period; hopefully the next company will be kinder.

Self-insured employers, which generally include very large businesses, are governed by the federal Employee Retirement Income Security Act of 1974 (ERISA) laws that override state laws.

Self-insured employers may hire a medical insurance company, such as Blue Cross, to administer their plan. The insurance information you receive, such as explanations of benefits, may contain the insurance company's letterhead, but your employer is bearing the exact and full cost of your care at the time it is incurred, instead of paying large indemnity premiums in advance.

ERISA was a piece of legislation intended to safeguard employee pension rights, but it has impacted employee health insurance as well, and in confusing ways. For example, owing to the overlap of state and ERISA regulations, self-insured employers cannot be sued in state courts for failing to pay claims. For this and other reasons, disputes about health insurance claims can become very complex and may require the assistance of an attorney.

Medicare and Medicaid

Medicare is not just government-supplied medical insurance for those over age 65. If you have been entitled to Social Security Disability (SSDI) benefits for the past two years, or if you have chronic kidney disease that requires dialysis or organ transplantation, you are eligible for Medicare.

Most frequently we hear of Medicare Parts A and B, but much fuller (and more expensive) coverage may be provided by purchasing Medicare Supplemental Insurance, often called MediGap insurance. Ten versions of Medi-Gap insurance are available, identified as A through J, with J providing the highest coverage.

Medicaid is a health payment program for the financially needy that is run jointly by the federal government and each state government. As such, its rules and benefits vary greatly depending on where you live. Examples of those who may qualify are recipients of Aid to Families with Dependent Children (AFDC), those receiving the Social Security's Administration's Supplemental Security Income (SSI), or certain nursing home patients.

For more information on either Medicare or Medicaid, see the *Mercer Guide*, which is published yearly and is readily accessible in libraries and bookstores.

Unemployment insurance

Always apply for unemployment insurance if you lose your job, are laid off, or if your hours are substantially reduced. Never assume that you're not eligible. Apply even if you have a suit pending for wrongful discharge.

Unemployment law and the granting and calculation of benefits are very complex, and vary from state to state. In order to find information that's appropriate for your circumstances, you'll need to research the laws for your state, either on your own or with an attorney who specializes in these cases.

Life insurance

Life insurance that you buy as an individual is likely to be terribly expensive, if at all available, once you have had cancer. As mentioned in the earlier section, "No medical underwriting," if you have an opportunity to buy a good life insurance policy at a reasonable rate without a qualifying medical examination or other penalty for having a cancer diagnosis, consider the opportunity carefully.

Some employers offer life insurance policies requiring no medical exam with face values in multiples of one's annual salary. Although this usually is term coverage instead of whole-life coverage, it may meet your family's needs very well. Some such policies can be kept even if you leave the company.

Whole-life policies often can be borrowed against, or sold in a viatical arrangement to a company that will buy your policy from you at less than its face value in order to provide you with money now. This is a useful options if your heirs don't need your money, but you do, in order to pay current bills.

Long-term care insurance

Now more than ever, you should consider a long-term care policy as a safeguard against financially crippling nursing-home or nursing-care costs. As with life insurance policies discussed above, however, you're not likely to be able to find or afford a long-term care policy once having had a cancer diagnosis, unless one is offered at group rates with no medical examination required.

One very good option is to ask your children and their spouses if their employers offer such a policy for parents or in-laws as well as employees. This recent trend in employment benefits offerings is an attempt to recognize the increasing responsibilities that families face in caring for their older relatives while trying to work outside the home.

Many long-term care policies are eventually dropped by the client because they are so expensive, and the probability of needing long-term care seems so far away. If expense is an issue for you, you might choose a policy that has a clause that allows you to stop paying premiums after a number of years in return for lower benefits or payments over a shorter time. This compromise, while not ideal, will afford you at least some protection against potentially devastating long-term care costs.

Long-term disability insurance

Employers often offer long-term disability insurance at reduced rates or for free. If you can elect or purchase such a policy, do so. Although the Social Security Administration can pay you long-term disability under some conditions, often it's temporary, and frequently policies available in the private sector pay a better monthly benefit.

Note that most long-term disability policies encourage you to apply for SSDI, and then pay you only the difference between SSA's monthly benefit and the higher benefit your policy authorizes.

Some long-term disability policies can be taken with you if you leave your employer. Choose only a policy marked *guaranteed renewable*, so that your policy cannot be canceled if your health gets worse.

Financial issues

In general, financial issues cannot be addressed adequately in one chapter of a medical consumer's book. Nonetheless, a few issues are discussed in this section to inform you, rather than advise you, regarding problems you may encounter.

Major points

Here's an encapsulation of some fairly prominent issues:

- It may be worthwhile to refinance your home mortgage for a lower interest rate. If the current market rate for mortgages is significantly lower than yours, refinancing may reduce monthly payments, increase equity more rapidly, and ultimately reduce debt.

- Contact the Social Security Administration to see if you, your spouse, or your children are eligible for Supplemental Security Income. Visit *http://www.ssa.gov* on the Web or call (800) 772-1213. (SSI differs from SSDI, Social Security Disability Income.)

- Fundraising in your community or your place of employment can be a very effective way to address debts related to medical care. The Organ Transplant Fund, for example, provides sound help with raising funds for bone marrow or stem cell transplantation. See Appendix A, *Resources*, for a list of other organizations that can help with financial issues such as fundraising.

- Estate planning always should be considered, even for seemingly small estates. Some options, such as a supportive care trust or purchase of a whole-life insurance policy, may preserve some assets for yourself, your spouse, or your children—but may interfere seriously with your eligibility for Medicare. Estate planning is especially important if your spouse or a child has serious health problems of his own, requiring long-term financial support.

- A debt consolidation or home equity loan may be a useful device for reducing debt.

Bankruptcy

The two leading reasons for declaring bankruptcy are excessive medical expenses and credit card debt.

Declaring bankruptcy has changed from a last-ditch, unethical, and humiliating way to escape obligation to an honorable if humble effort to restructure or reschedule debt payment. Of the three forms of bankruptcy that individuals (as opposed to businesses and farmers) may use, only one, Chapter 7 bankruptcy, discharges the debtor of all debt. The others, Chapters 11 and 13, provide for a repayment plan in a hierarchical and agreed-upon way, eliminating or postponing foreclosure on your home or repossession of your automobile. Moreover, once you have declared bankruptcy, your creditors are forbidden by law from harassing or suing you.

Nonetheless, declaring bankruptcy still should be close to your last resort for solving financial problems, and should always be done under the guidance of a professional financial advisor or bankruptcy attorney.

Barbara, a bankruptcy attorney and NHL survivor, describes her perspective on illness, excessive expenses, and bankruptcy:

> As an attorney who has done many Chapter 7 bankruptcies, I always told my clients: filing bankruptcy doesn't say anything about who you are. It's there for people to make a fresh start. And we NHLers don't need the added stress of worrying about how to pay our bills or that somehow filing bankruptcy makes us not good people. In this society we have a lot of baggage surrounding money and how we measure success. As those of us with this disease know, the most important things in life are our friends and families and keeping on keeping on—not how much money we have. There is, as we know, a big advantage to having unlimited funds—ability to find the best treatment and no stress about finances—but in the long run all of us with this diagnosis have to face the same things, and most of us don't have unlimited financial resources. We need to reduce our stress as much as possible in order to fight our disease.

Disability income

Several means are available to replace your income while you are disabled.

Social Security Disability Income (SSDI)

The Social Security Administration may grant disability benefits under the Social Security Disability Income (SSDI) plan to replace lost income for an adult or to provide assistance with caring for a child with NHL.

To smooth the process of applying for Social Security Disability Income, bring all medical records with you, and let your doctors know you're applying, as they will need to give evidence.

If SSDI is denied—and frequently it is on the first application—ask for Publication No. 05-10041, "The Appeals Process." Sometimes just a request to have your case reviewed by the SSA's physicians will speed an approval.

In some cases, it's possible to return to work and continue to collect SSDI benefits. This is possible owing to special incentives the SSA provides to rehabilitate the disabled. The formula used to compute disability benefits while working is complex, but in general, you may attempt a trial work period of nine months, not necessarily consecutively, during which benefits are unchanged. If the trial does not succeed, benefits may continue. Ask the SSA for the publication called, "Working While Disabled...How We Can Help" (Publication No. 05-10095).

Private long-term disability income

If you don't have a long-term disability insurance policy, it's most wise to consider buying one. For those under age 65, the likelihood of long-term or permanent disability is far greater than the risk of death, especially for NHL survivors who, owing to improvements in treatment, now face an illness that is shifting from a fatal to a chronic illness. For NHL survivors who face repeated treatment and aftercare, disability insurance is an emerging need for times when treatment leaves you unable to work. See the section "Long-term disability insurance," earlier in this chapter.

Note that almost all private long-term disability policies will reduce your monthly benefits if you receive other income, including disability benefits from the Social Security Administration:

I've had shocks and disappointments with my long-term disability carrier and the Social Security system. First is the endless forms you have to fill out, with the most inane questions on them. Then there is the frustration I can see in my oncologist every time she gets another form to sign. She has started simply signing them and then handing them to me to complete. The most devastating thing was recently when Social Security approved me. Now, you'd think this was a good thing, right? Well, it turns out that my disability insurance carrier wanted me to apply for Social Security Disability Income (SSDI) so they could deduct the money from what they pay me. To make matters worse, SSDI is almost two months behind in their payments, but the LTD people want to deduct the money immediately, before it is even received! This is the newest challenge that I have to get through. On top of it, my doctor has just pushed back my return-to-work day even further than expected. I hate being broke!

Military (VA) disability income

If you served in Southeast Asia during the Vietnam War and were stationed in or near areas known to be exposed to dioxin (Agent Orange), your subsequent development of NHL is considered by the Veterans' Administration to be related to dioxin exposure. You will likely be eligible for temporary or permanent, full or partial disability income benefits. They will be retroactive to your date of first treatment and will continue as long as any long-term side effect of treatment is present. Such effects might be diminished lung capacity from Bleomycin or radiotherapy, residual neural damage from vincristine, or intractable fatigue.

You can receive partial VA disability benefits while working full time. Note that if you refuse veterans' disability benefits from a sense of pride, it will be almost impossible to reopen your claim later. For instance, if you suffer a heart attack years after being treated with radiotherapy or Adriamycin (doxorubicin) and your doctors are convinced your heart was damaged by these drugs, you will not be permitted by the VA to reopen your case and collect benefits. As damage from treatment may develop years after it's administered, it's best not to refuse a VA settlement if it's offered, no matter how well you feel nor how able to work you may be.

When my husband was diagnosed with lymphoma, we filed a claim with the VA's Agent Orange program, even though we knew they were not covering his type of lymphoma at that time. It was a matter of principle. We wanted to be a statistic to catch their attention.

A few years later, the VA broadened its decision and determined that my husband's cancer was related to Agent Orange exposure. They contacted us, and he received a retroactive payment for one year of full disability. He now receives monthly checks for being, by their ruling, still about 30 percent disabled.

Employment issues

Having and being treated for NHL can disrupt your job attendance and performance. If you're very lucky, you'll have managers and coworkers who accommodate your ups and downs, perhaps holding fundraisers for you, or donating their own unused sick or vacation time for your use. Many of us are not this lucky.

As with finance and insurance issues, you have certain protections under the law. You should verify the details of these laws, as they may change over time.

- The Americans with Disabilities Act (ADA) recognizes cancer as a temporary or permanent disability for which you cannot be penalized by demotion or dismissal. It's also illegal to deny a qualified candidate a job simply because of a disability, but it's difficult to prove this kind of discrimination unless you know intimately every other job applicant and all of their qualifications.

- The Family and Medical Leave Act (FMLA) guarantees you twelve weeks of leave annually for your own healthcare or to attend to a sick family member. During these twelve weeks, your job or a very similar one must be held open for you, and your benefits must be maintained. The FMLA applies only to companies with fifty or more employees within a seventy-five-mile radius. Violations of this law should be reported to the U.S. Department of Labor.

- Worker's Compensation for the development of any cancer is rare because few direct causes of cancer are known, much less those resulting directly from risky job responsibilities. If you develop NHL after developing AIDS following a workplace contamination with HIV, however, you may have a justifiable Worker's Compensation claim, as the rate of NHL among those with AIDS is many times higher than found in the normal population. Consult an attorney who specializes in workplace issues and Worker's Compensation.

Some employers sponsor Employee Assistance Programs (EAP) to counsel employees who are having problems that affect their job performance. A subset of these employers may require participation in their EAP in order to approve payment for benefits for counseling. Please see Chapter 13, *Getting Support*, for the possible drawbacks associated with using EAPs.

Record-keeping

The value of record-keeping cannot be overemphasized. Having evidence in writing of your position is indispensable should disputes or questions arise. Records should be obtained for all treatment, employment, and financial circumstances, and should be kept in some organized way, in a place safe from fire, theft, or flood.

Biopsy samples

A new and very important concern you should address is the permanent storage of your biopsy tissue samples. Owing to the development of new treatment technologies, such as monoclonal antibodies and tumor-derived vaccines, your biopsy samples may be needed years after they are removed from your body.

Yet some hospitals limit storage time for such samples because their storage resources are finite. This means that, lacking instructions otherwise, they may discard your tissue samples after a number of years.

Ask the hospital to keep your samples forever. If they are not able to do so, make arrangements to store the samples elsewhere.

Establish a record trail

Simple though it may sound, getting copies of all medical information, including films, and getting written copies of all tangential records related to employment, insurance, and finance are sometimes overlooked. Here are some tips for obtaining records:

- Request and keep copies of all medical records and bills as you go through diagnosis and treatment. This will establish with the doctor's staff your expectations and set a tone of efficiency, and will permit you instant access to material if you need it for second opinions. Having copies made and mailed after the fact can add five or more days, even weeks, to the time you need to collect records.

- If you're requesting records that must in turn be forwarded to another health center, make a copy for yourself before forwarding the material.

- If you're hospitalized, or if your treatments are done in the hospital on an outpatient basis, ask for itemized copies of bills. General or summarized hospital bills can be astonishingly obtuse, and even an itemized bill can be unclear. Most errors in hospital billing are found only by using an itemized bill's relative clarity.

- Always address financial, employment, or insurance disputes in writing, and keep a copy of what you've written.

- Keep a detailed phone log of all calls made to insurance companies, mortgage companies, and so on.

- Any decision reached verbally to correct errors should be followed by a written confirmation from the company. Ask for this, and if they won't furnish a written reply, write your own reply, stating, "Based on our phone conversation, it is my understanding that the following will happen," listing what you perceive to be true.

- Keep a calendar of appointments. Do not discard it at the end of the year. Keep it as a permanent part of your medical and financial files.

- If space permits, your calendar can double as a log for phone calls, changes in medications or symptoms, blood results, and so on. Otherwise, school exercise books or blank journals, the kind from which pages cannot be easily torn, may serve well.

- Record outgoing correspondence. Send all correspondence that's even remotely important by certified mail, using the return receipt option. Unlike registered mail, which is logged at each stop in the postal system, certified mail does not travel more slowly than regular mail, and isn't much more expensive than regular mail. When the return receipt arrives, staple it to your copy of the correspondence: it is your proof that the mail arrived at its destination. Use fax transmission for speed when needed, but follow up with certified mail. Some examples of uses for certified mail:

  — Correspondence to insurance companies that require thirty days' advance notice in order to review and approve treatment plans such as bone marrow transplantation.

  — All correspondence with the IRS.

- All correspondence with collection agencies, mortgage companies, or automobile loan holders.

- All correspondence with the Social Security Administration.

• Have copies of all original CT and MRI films made for your own files. While copies of the reports that describe and analyze these films are useful, access to films is mandatory for certain kinds of review and decision-making.

• If the original CT or MRI films are loaned to other doctors for second opinions, follow up to be sure they are returned to the central film library or original office.

Organizing the record trail

How little or how much you choose to organize will depend in some measure on how much energy you have remaining, and on your record-keeping habits in general. Don't be surprised if you find yourself, normally a well-organized person, suddenly without energy to file medical reimbursement forms. Others, though, may find that they become more organized as a coping mechanism.

You may find that record-keeping is a task you can delegate to a family member, friend, or neighbor who would love to help you, but doesn't know quite what to offer. Although you may not care to have someone outside your family making phone calls to correct billing mistakes, having someone sort and file bills and receipts on a weekly basis may help you. Sorting mail into stacks for filing is a task that a child might enjoy; scanning and storing documents on a PC might be something that a computer-literate relative might want to do.

Whatever method suits your current needs, do attempt at the very least to store medical and payment records in some way. A minimal technique is to put all records in one place, such as in one or more grocery bags, in case you need access to them in a hurry. If you or your volunteers have the time and energy to do so, you may lean toward a fairly elaborate system of organization that gives you instant access to items by topic, health center, or date.

Summary

There may be the rare person with NHL who relishes a payment challenge from stubborn insurance companies or the character-building experience of financial hardship, but most of us facing these issues along with poor health may begin to feel overwhelmed.

This chapter attempts to highlight the most important and most potentially damaging of these issues, and supplies many references for finding the best and most current information.

Before making irrevocable decisions or expensive purchases, please consider consulting professionals who are familiar with recent changes in the various laws that govern insurance, employment, and finances.

CHAPTER 15

After Treatment Ends

Remember to cure the patient
as well as the disease.

—Alvan Barach

The end of treatment brings a variety of new concerns and plans for NHL survivors. A contradictory mixture of feelings, a changed relationship with the oncologist, perhaps a renewed immersion in one's job, a reassessment of long-range plans, a different physical self—temporarily or permanently, and different behaviors on the part of friends and loved ones all may come about. Your cancer experience doesn't end as the door closes behind you when you leave the clinic; normalcy creeps up on you in the months that follow.

This chapter will discuss the emotional and practical aspects of the end of treatment. We will share with you what others have found difficult, surprising, or exhilarating. First, the emotional aspects related to facing ahead at the end of treatment will be outlined, followed by the physical and medical aspects, and finishing with the social and professional aspects of adjusting after treatment ends.

In some cases, of course, these concerns overlap. For example, it's difficult not to have an emotional reaction to either upsetting or loving things that happen in the workplace.

Emotional responses

Almost everyone looks forward to finishing treatment with feelings of joy, relief, and celebration. Indeed, there are reasons to feel joyous and celebratory. Side effects will diminish, energy will return, expectations of remission are realistic, and life will begin to return to normal.

However, many people also report at least some ambivalence at the end of treatment. Side by side with the expected good feelings can be other, more painful feelings. Here are the thoughts of a survivor of high-grade NHL which reveal quite a mixture of reactions, not at all an uncommon phenomenon:

> *I don't know what the future holds for me. I don't know how long before I have to resume treatments, if ever. I don't know if I'll ever get to return to normal functioning. My diaphragm is still paralyzed; I don't know if it will ever return to normal.*
>
> *I would like to participate in clinical trials if needed, so that something good can come out of this for others, if not for me. My doctor wants me to have a bone marrow transplant if this chemotherapy fails to cure me. This is fine—I just want it to be over with. I don't want to worry every time I cough or feel sick. I want to be able to ignore my health once again. I want to be the strong one.*

The rest of this section talks about feelings that might unexpectedly arise at the end of treatment. These feelings, and all of the feelings described in this chapter, are completely normal. Some of them may not strike you as useful reactions, but they are nonetheless normal reactions for the circumstances surrounding cancer survivorship and should be honored as such. If you decide to join a support group, for example, you'll likely hear many people describing these kinds of reactions, and offering very good ways to turn reactions into useful acts.

Keep in mind as well that many NHL survivors have long periods of feeling happy, sound, capable, productive, and blessed. For many, the positives outnumber the negatives.

The following are loosely defined categories that describe the different kinds of feelings, fears, and reactions experienced by NHL survivors.

Moving on

Almost everyone who has had NHL wants to leave cancer behind and move on to normal living. Some people succeed well with this. Many of us, however, are not that lucky or skilled, or blessed with the right genes or with strong enough faith.

Some people succeed in blocking the experience entirely and immediately submerge themselves in their old life, which is a very healthy and useful form of denial. Some people succeed well in readjusting after their course of treatment, but cannot recapture this serenity if they relapse and are retreated—even if their odds of survival after retreatment, particularly with bone marrow or stem cell transplantation, are better than after first-line treatment.

Many people feel almost like their old selves until it's time for the six-month CT scan, and then very strong fears resurface.

Here are the thoughts of a survivor who has a very strong will to move forward:

> I am male, twenty-six years old, and a citizen of India. I have been in the U.S. for over four years now. Although off school during a year of treatment, I resumed my Ph.D. program once again in January 1996 while taking maintenance chemotherapy. Interestingly, I am majoring in industrial engineering with my focus on—guess what?—the healthcare industry! My specialization is called health systems engineering, which is a mix of business, engineering, sociology, and preventive medicine.

> I consider myself in a unique position of studying the healthcare system both as an outsider and experiencing it as a patient from the inside. After my fight with cancer, I am determined to focus my dissertation and definitely the rest of my research career in improvement issues that would affect us patients directly. My key interests are in improving the quality of care and quality of life of the healthcare industry customers. I am sure all of us would like to get the best out of this courageous fight that we have been putting up with cancer, and I for one am going to use my research opportunities in improving things for us.

Abandonment

Some people fear the end of treatment because they feel that chemotherapy and radiation therapy are all that's standing between them and cancer. Often people secretly feel abandoned by their oncologists and the medical staff at the end of treatment. To the emotionally charged survivor, the medical staff's behavior during a normal wrap-up appointment may seem brusque or emotionally flat. Where are the trumpets, the pat on the back, the teary eyes?

If, on the other hand, the staff was loving and helpful throughout treatment and congratulatory at the end, afterward you may miss the all-pull-together camaraderie that was shared and the special kindness you received.

You may fear the absence of regular and close physical scrutiny given by the doctor. The thought of waiting two or three months to the next CT scan or other reassessment may seem like forever.

Absence of feeling

Sometimes NHL survivors report feeling nothing at all when their treatment ends and their doctor says their chances are good that their survival will be a long one. This numbness may come about as a protective mechanism or from burnout. Most often, feeling will return with the passing of time.

Fear of relapse

Nobody can guarantee that you won't experience a relapse of NHL or develop a second cancer—or that you won't be hit by a bus as you leave the building. In spite of many reassurances, it's human to be afraid. Most cancer survivors have fears of relapse that range from occasional to paralytic. Often the fears can be put to bed for months at time, but they may resurface when it's time for a checkup or when an odd pain manifests, as Marilyn, an NHL survivor, knows:

> I had a strange symptom the past few days, and thought, "This is it," and was mentally preparing for my final farewells when it turned out to be a false alarm. Strange how calm I felt. Ever since the NHL diagnosis, I have worn the world like a loose garment, ready to slip it off at a moment's notice. Actually it's a great way to live, I have found. No one lives forever, and today is all that counts. I think today I really do live each day as if it were to be my last (and the corollary to that is "Plan as if you'll live forever…")

Fear of relapse is normal. Several good ways to reduce these negative thoughts and feelings are by learning all you can about your subtype of NHL, keeping abreast of improvements in treatment, retraining your psyche to focus on the positive, and attempting to enjoy the small, free joys offered by each new day.

Vigilance

Many people experience pronounced, abiding concern about relapse when a new ache or odd body trait is noticed. Fears of relapse are, of course, perfectly normal, and you're to be commended for monitoring your body's reactions and status. You're not a hypochondriac.

Battle fatigue (post-traumatic stress reaction)

Some people may experience insomnia, nightmares about their cancer, fear and avoidance of doctors and hospitals, jumpiness or lack of trust during commonplace interactions with medical personnel such as annual influenza vaccination, or extreme anger or sadness when hearing of someone else with cancer.

Ruminations, doubts

Once the heat of the battle is past, some of us may begin to recall survival statistics we have seen. We may become less than happy with what we perceive our odds of surviving to be. We may begin to second-guess whether what we went through was worth it, whether it was the right treatment choice, whether we'll ever be physically adept again, whether anything else in life is worth doing in comparison to battling cancer. In fact, we would hardly be sentient creatures if these thoughts did not cross our minds at least occasionally.

This survivor of intermediate-grade Burkitt-like lymphoma describes her reassessment of life pre- and post-cancer:

> Since my recovery, I find I am dealing with a new urgency and unresolved issues revolving around why I was so fortunate as to have survived a deadly disease. I am so grateful to be alive. But I am not measuring up somehow. I have not found meaning in my work. Who did I ever think I was in my previous life, anyway? I am not doing enough to help others. Why the hell haven't we found a cure for NHL yet? What am I going to do about that? And so on and so on.
>
> And I know I cannot face death again until I have worked some of this out. Even if I am forced to have a final dance with mortality, I plan to step on a lot of toes.

Diminished coping skills

For such a long time, all that was expected of you was to focus on beating cancer. Now it may seem that the rest of the world expects you simply to pick up where you left off with your normal responsibilities. For those who were not able to continue working throughout treatment, the thought of returning to a full workload of regular responsibilities can be overwhelming.

As you attempt to re-enter your old world, you may notice that things you used to be able to ignore may annoy you, and things that used to annoy you may anger you.

Anger

Now that the time- and energy-consuming process of being treated is behind you, you may find that you're feeling angry about having cancer. You may find that you want to learn all you can about what causes NHL, or that you want to become politically involved to force legislation that favors cancer research or cleanses the environment of carcinogens.

Longing for the past

Some people expect and hope that they'll feel and perform exactly as they did before cancer became a problem, and are disappointed if they cannot. Sometimes the recovery of physical and intellectual stamina is a slow process. At times, you might perceive that all changes or a diminution of performance are cancer-related, when in fact they might be attributable to a number of other things.

Excessive caution

Others feel that the gods would frown on pride if one celebrates at the end of treatment, so they avoid jinxing themselves by celebrating. They may spend years not allowing themselves to enjoy a return of reasonably good health.

Alienation and loneliness

People who haven't had to deal with cancer may strike you now as insensitive or shallow. The vacuous things others say about your cancer experience may leave you astonished or hurt. The topics they want to discuss may bore you. The issues that they view as problematic you may find trivial. You may feel you no longer have anything in common with old friends or even with loved ones. You may begin to consider a job change or a divorce.

Altogether, you may feel out of phase with the rest of the world—until you meet a fellow cancer survivor, and a long, intense conversation follows, during which you're impervious to your surroundings, perhaps sharing funny stories about your experiences that healthy people would find morbid. Suddenly you're aware you're not alone, and that cancer support groups may be a good choice for you.

Watch and wait

Those with low-grade disease have special considerations when treatment ends, because the most common treatments used at the time of this writing for low-grade disease offer long-term, but not permanent, remission. In this respect, survivors of low-grade NHL are always, but not quite ever, in the after-cancer phase.

Nan, a survivor of childhood high-grade NHL which relapsed as low-grade disease twenty years later, says it well:

> Low-grade lymphoma tends to be invisible for most of us. My friends and family, for the most part, know I have NHL, but have no idea that I am "sick." And truth is, I don't act like it and don't like drawing attention to the fact. But the cold reality is that I have a large tumor threatening my life, and that at times, it is hard for me to carry on at full throttle. My environment constantly invites me to sustain my roles as mom of three children, wife, therapist, lecturer, and writer—all passions of mine, by the way. But these are necessarily combined with travel agent (for health-care), insurance agent (the bills are constant and complicated), heart patient (just had open-heart surgery in October, triple bypass and valve replacement, all from side effects of childhood radiation), and scared woman trying to eat healthy and exercise in order to make cancer an unwelcome bedfellow! Whew! So odd, really. Those of us with this disease carry on our regular lives, plus add research for NHL information and support. Thus, with diminished resources, our workload and stress are higher.
>
> Low-grade disease carries an often overlooked challenge for the survivor. How does one know how to take careful care of a body that does not

feel sick or look sick? And, with the lure of wellness, why wouldn't we want to carry on a normal life? If we were unfortunately bedridden with treatment side effects, our friends and family would certainly punt for us. However, more often than not, we are still caring full time for them. Balance is so key, survivors with low-grade disease must champion our own cause. Unlike in the case of those who are more clinically ill, we must advocate for ourselves, whether we look sick or not. We must put ourselves first, become our own best expert, as well as advocate. The lesson is challenging, but as I have humbly learned, life-altering as well.

Anxiety and depression

All of the above, combined with the physical toll of treatment, can result in anxiety or depression for certain people. Anxiety and depression are discussed more fully in Chapter 11, *Stress and the Immune System*, and Chapter 16, *Late Effects, Late Complications*. A counselor who specializes in cancer survivorship can help you with these and other problems.

Medical monitoring

Fifteen or twenty years ago, doctors and patients had few choices for verifying that cancer had gone away and was staying away. Now, we have imaging tools that allow a view—often just a glimpse—of what's going on inside our bodies.

These imaging tools are both a blessing and a curse. While it's true that now we can track progression and regression of tumors much more clearly, there are, for example, instances of both false positives and false negatives from imaging studies that can only be evaluated accurately within the framework provided by additional testing or a second biopsy.

Follow-up tests

As you finish your treatment, your doctor will discuss when to return for follow-up visits. Follow-up visits most likely will include a physical examination, a discussion period for you and your doctor to share concerns, and a series of tests to confirm remission.

Some of the tests used to follow progress against NHL are gallium, thallium, CT, PET, and bone scans; MRI imaging; spinal taps; bone marrow biopsies; and blood testing. Blood tests will always include white cell, red cell, and platelet counts and ratios, LDH levels, and may include beta-2 microglobulin or immunoglobulin level assays. More reliable blood markers for NHL are constantly being sought, which means that your blood may be tested for substances not mentioned here.

It's usual to have imaging studies a few months after the end of treatment, as many anticancer agents continue to have a tumor-killing effect for several months after they're used. Thereafter, imaging studies may be repeated every three or six months for a number of years, then once a year for a number of years.

It's common to have a residual lesion appear on an imaging study where the tumor once was. This might be scar tissue, remaining pieces of dying tumor, disease that has stabilized, or, unfortunately, a relapse of disease. If this lesion is scar tissue or a necrotic (dying) tumor, the lesion may be visible for a year or two after treatment, and then disappear. If this is a remaining active site of disease, depending on your subtype and grade of NHL, it may remain stable for a long time, or it may regrow. Sometimes it's not possible to tell which of these conditions pertain without a biopsy.

It's possible to have new liver lesions appear after certain chemotherapies such as interleukin-2, or suspicious lung spots after irradiation of the chest. These can mimic relapse or spread of disease (metastasis), but PET scanning or biopsy may prove otherwise.

Regardless of the schedule of your follow-up visits, new or returning symptoms must be taken seriously and reported to your doctor immediately. Never assume that they'll think you're worrying too much. It's always better to err by communicating too much instead of too little when it comes to aftercare.

Regression of symptoms and side effects

In general, the lingering side effects and delayed effects you may have experienced during treatment should fade away in the months following treatment.

Certain side effects may take much longer to regress. Recovery of supple veins after vincristine use in the absence of a central catheter, for example, happens slowly over time, if at all. Fertility may improve slowly over months or years following treatment, or it may never recover. Peripheral neuropathy—pain, weakness, or numbness in the hands or feet—may linger for months or years. Fatigue may continue for years after treatment. Blood counts can remain low, or low-normal, for months or years afterward.

When your hair regrows, you may notice that it's a different color, a different texture, thicker, thinner, curlier, or straighter than it was before treatment. These changes are temporary.

You might also notice that old allergies are better or worse, or that you now seem allergic to things you never before were.

In general, but not always, side effects and delayed effects following intense therapies such as those used before bone marrow or stem cell transplantation are more pronounced, and may last longer, than those following treatments utilizing lower doses of chemotherapy and radiotherapy.

For information about delayed effects that drift into long-term effects, see Chapter 16.

Precautions

Certain treatments may result in bodily changes that require long-term prudence, such as avoiding sun and limiting exposure to bacteria and fungi. For example, aspergillus, a fungus commonly found in old buildings and in soil, is released during gardening and remodeling at levels that may be dangerous to those who remain immune-suppressed.

Ask your doctor for special instructions about skin care, physical activity such as sunbathing, gardening, or remodeling that are specific to your circumstances.

Catheter removal

Many people can't wait to have their catheter removed; others prefer to keep it for a while as a talisman against relapse.

If your subtype of NHL is one that tends to relapse after long remissions, as may happen repeatedly with low-grade disease, it might be wise to consider keeping your catheter, especially if additional surgeries with general anesthesia are required to remove it and reinstall it. The wisdom of keeping it to avoid extra surgery should it need to be reimplanted must be weighed against the inconvenience of keeping it clean, and the increased risk of infection it may entail.

Social and professional after-effects

You may be quite surprised to discover that those around you who have never had cancer are totally unaware of the mixture of feelings you're experiencing—that, in fact, they may have a very full agenda of their own feelings, both happy and distressing, to sort out. Conversely, you may find that long-term cancer survivors are a tremendous resource to you in this stage of your adjustment.

Reactions of family and friends

Your closest family members and friends who have seen you throughout treatment have probably adjusted to your circumstances, by the time your treatment ends, in a way that benefits all concerned. Nonetheless, you may find that some family members expect that, almost instantly, you'll be just as healthy and active as you were before. They may even become strident on this point, so strongly does human nature yearn for things to return to normal. You need to communicate clearly with them when you're feeling tired and under par, explaining that many cancer survivors experience long-term after-effects such as fatigue.

Some family members and loved ones may have feelings of anger and frustration that they suppressed while you were being treated. They may now allow these feelings, as well as impatience, to emerge. Candid discussions may defuse these feelings, but if the feelings are directed at you, family counseling may be a good choice.

In some cases, a spouse or partner may decide that this is a good time to end the relationship, now that it's "over," and you're "fine." This is more likely to happen in relationships that were experiencing problems before the cancer diagnosis.

Your children, lacking adult coping skills, might still remain mired in the distress and terror they experienced during your diagnosis and treatment. They might need long-term therapy, or support with social and academic issues.

Getting out and about socially after treatment among those who know you less well can be glorious, fun and invigorating, or exhausting and disappointing. The reactions of coworkers, discussed below, mirror in some ways the responses that you're likely to encounter from the rest of society, but unlike your coworkers, your social contacts may not usually have the benefit of seeing you performing and producing, so their reactions may be more skewed and less informed.

It might be wise to be prepared for a variety of reactions that range from loving and positive to very odd indeed, if you haven't already encountered the entire spectrum of these reactions in the course of being treated. Some NHL survivors report, for example, that friends don't want the survivor to talk about their experiences at all. Others report that friends who avoided them during treatment relax and reapproach them after treatment ends.

With a little forethought and practice, you can defuse negative reactions, reinforce your reputation for tenacity and positivity—or even wax a bit saucy if you're in the mood for humor and not concerned about the social consequences. Some of the negative reactions and questions you'll encounter are simply the result of ignorance or a lack of careful thought, or are a front for competitiveness, spite, or sadism. You're under no obligation to go along with agendas that are not in your best interest, nor to waste a lot of emotional energy answering seemingly serious questions that in fact haven't been carefully thought out.

Barbara, a survivor of mixed low-grade and intermediate-grade NHL, describes the insensitivity of those around her to her experience and her future concerns:

> Everyone around me expects me to be just like a normal person—
> that is, one without cancer. But I'm not. I never will be that Barbara of a
> year ago. I always have to be positive for everyone. I know that in some
> fashion, my low-grade NHL will pop up again, but my friends and family
> don't want to hear me say that. To me, that is not negative thinking, it is
> being realistic… but, of course, it is scary. Also scary is the specter of
> relapse of my intermediate NHL.
>
> I'm tired of not being able to express that to people around me. They
> don't want to hear it—it's too frightening for them, I think.
>
> But I am fragile emotionally, not able to handle the kind of nagging
> stresses I could before my diagnosis. My patience with trivia and annoying people has worn thin. I used to be easygoing and nice to everyone; I
> can't do that anymore. People don't seem to understand that I am struggling every day to remain upbeat and get on with my life knowing I have

cancer...and to learn to live with this diagnosis is an ongoing struggle. Because I am through with treatment for now, look great, feel pretty good (though I tire fast), everyone wants me to be okay all the time—and I'm not.

Re-entering the workplace

Resuming the full complement of professional responsibilities after cancer treatment has ended can be a wonderful experience, a way to occupy the mind with healthy things, a way to reinforce your belief in yourself and your re-emerging health with productivity and creativity.

Often the feelings your coworkers express are a tremendous reinforcement for your well-being. To know you were needed and missed can be uplifting; to be part of a team again can make you feel you've rejoined the human race. Many NHL survivors report that welcome-back parties are planned to greet them, and that coworkers pinch-hit for them if they continue to feel tired. Neeraj, a survivor of NHL/ALL, describes his very good fortune to be working among people who appreciate what he's been through:

> *I work with a research group which develops computer support systems for breast cancer survivors to cope with their cancer, so everyone is very understanding about what I am going through. At the hematology clinic I have been lucky to get the best combination of doctors and nurses, and the doctor who is my primary hematologist is eight years older and is also from India, so he has become almost family to me.*

Occasionally the return to work is less rewarding. If you have been queried over and over throughout your treatment about when you will return, for example, you may feel that your employer thinks you're just a cog in the machinery rather than a human worthy of her concern. If some coworkers are reluctant to recognize your illness owing to their own fears or lack of social skills, they might not refer to it ever, not even to wish you well, or to say they're glad you're back. Very rarely, a cancer survivor will experience horrible reactions from coworkers, such as discovering that, in one's absence, one's desk was sprayed with antiseptic "in case the cancer was contagious," but these extreme reactions from coworkers fortunately are rare.

More often, the reaction will be, "The treatment is over, so now you're fine, right? Ready for a full workload now, right?" If you're still feeling like something Jacques Cousteau would've thrown back, be sure to make it clear that you'll be phasing back in gradually, that you're not feeling up to working a full day or a full week for the first month or two.

Another fairly common reaction among the blissfully healthy is, "Why are you in such a pensive mood? Aren't you glad it's all over?" Your attitude about putting it behind you, or not putting it behind you, might be worth an explanation, but this explanation might meet with limited success with the less perceptive and empathic of your coworkers. American culture, like some other cultures, has a quick-fix or even a superstitious mentality toward many problems, including health problems.

In general, it's nobody else's business how you're coping with the detritus of treatment. You can feel free to say nothing to the potentially unsympathetic listener if you choose, but there are tradeoffs surrounding not keeping your immediate supervisor informed about ongoing problems you may be experiencing. For example, if she is unaware of continuing health problems you're experiencing as a result of your illness or its treatment, you may have difficulty winning a favorable decision if a dispute about your performance arises.

More subtle reactions from coworkers and employers are possible as well, such as denying a promotion to a person who had cancer several years ago, assuming she will never again be able to meet certain challenges.

Remember that cancer is considered a disability under the Americans with Disabilities Act, so the negative reactions that result in demonstrable harm to you, such as the denial of a promotion or censure for using earned sick time, don't have to be endured without legal recourse.

Unused drugs or equipment

Often at the end of treatment you may have drugs and equipment left over. There may be ways to pass these unused drugs along to those who cannot afford them. Although in general federal law prohibits transferring drugs prescribed for one person to anyone else, you might ask your oncologist or veterinarian if there are exceptions to this law.

Nonprescription drugs can be offered to fellow patients and veterinarians.

For donating drugs for use in developing countries with few health resources, contact:

International Aid, Inc.
17011 Hickory
Spring Lake, MI 49456
(616) 846-7490

If you have a wig or any other equipment or supplies you no longer need, such as cleaning supplies for a catheter, many groups, such as the American Cancer Society, accept these as tax-deductible donations to help patients who cannot afford to buy their own.

Summary

Earl Weaver, the long-time manager of the Baltimore Orioles baseball team, used to say, "It's not over until it's over." With NHL, sometimes it's not over *when* it's over. Certain physical, emotional, and social aspects may take longer to realign with the new you.

Most NHL survivors gradually see the cup as more than half full and experience increasingly good health, productivity, and a goodly measure of happiness. Many have occasional or ongoing fears and concerns that time, professional help, or support groups can alleviate.

Dr. Wendy Schlessel Harpham's book *After Cancer: A Guide To Yoiur New Life* is an excellent in-depth guide to meeting the challenges that face us after treatment ends.

CHAPTER 16

Late Effects, Late Complications

We don't consider a patient cured
when his sprain has healed or he's been
restored to a minimal level of functioning.
The patient is cured when he can
again do the things he loves to do.

—Stanley A. Herring

It's difficult to imagine that treatments strong enough to kill NHL would not have an effect on normal, healthy tissue, too. In many cases, these treatments do affect normal cells, but usually these side effects are temporary, disappearing within days or weeks. A few side effects of treatment, though, last far longer for some people, and some late effects do not emerge until years after treatment.

The majority of NHL survivors do not have long-term effects or complications after treatment, or at most they have just one or two lasting effects that may fade away to an inconvenience rather than a problem. A few people, however, have serious long-term effects. Differences among people and their reactions depend on what drugs were given, how they were given, how long they were given, at what dose, what other health problems coexist with cancer, what previous drugs were given, and so on.

At times, it's very hard to accept that NHL's effect on our lives may not end when our treatment ends. This may mean that the discussion that follows is one that you're not ready to read just yet. If you're feeling battered today, put this aside until you feel better, or ask a loved one to read it for you.

Despite our reluctance and fears, it's important for us to know at least a little about long-term effects, for they can be confused with a relapse or can of themselves be life threatening. Often, but not always, they can be addressed and corrected.

This chapter will detail what effects are known to follow certain treatments in some people, and what, if anything, can be done about them. In the summary, we'll discuss why long-term effects can be expected to be less pronounced with newer treatments becoming available. The transient side effects of treatment are discussed in the chapter on side effects.

Late effects are emerging phenomena

Until about twenty years ago, not enough people treated with chemotherapy and radiotherapy for lymphoma and other cancers survived to characterize the lingering problems that are related to treatment or disease. The earliest cancer cures were affected with surgery only, and only for early-stage cancers. The introduction of multi-agent chemotherapy and combined chemotherapy and radiotherapy has saved enough people to make the pattern of late effects at least more obvious, while not yet fully understood. This is particularly so for those who've survived the Hodgkin's lymphomas, childhood acute lymphoblastic leukemia, intermediate- and high-grade non-Hodgkin's lymphomas, and for young males who have survived testicular cancer.

In almost all cases, late effects are more profound for survivors of childhood NHL.

In some cases, combination treatments of chemotherapy and radiotherapy make long-term effects more pronounced.

Terminology

What distinguishes the side effects of treatment from delayed or late effects and complications? The somewhat arbitrary definitions are that side effects of treatment are those that occur within days or weeks of treatment; delayed effects occur within weeks or months of cancer treatment; late effects occur months or years after treatment. Some side effects drift into becoming delayed or late effects, such as unremitting diarrhea induced by abdominal irradiation. The medical community distinguishes between effects and complications by defining effects as expected, and complications as somewhat unexpected.

The following sections, listed alphabetically, discuss specific late effects and complications. For a more detailed discussion of the late effects of cancer, see the book *Childhood Cancer Survivors*, by Nancy Keene, Wendy Hobbie, and Kathleen Ruccione, and Dr. Wendy Schlessel Harpham's book *After Cancer: A Guide to Your New Life*. Dr. Harpham, a specialist in internal medicine, is a survivor of NHL.

For all sections below that mention damage from radiotherapy, see the section called "Radiation fibrosis" for more detail.

Adrenal dysfunction, Cushing's syndrome

Irradiating the kidney can affect the adrenal gland which sits atop the kidney, causing it to malfunction. If the adrenal gland produces too much hormone, Cushing's syndrome can result. If too little, an Addison's-like disorder can result.

Abrupt withdrawal of the drug prednisone can cause a temporary adrenal dysfunction that resembles Addison's disease. Prednisone is a manmade version of the corticosteroid hormone cortisol, normally produced by the adrenal gland. When we add the synthetic version to our body, the adrenal gland, in concert with other glands, senses this, and shuts down production of its own version of cortisol. When we stop taking the drug, the adrenal cannot immediately begin again to make its own. For this reason, if you are taking prednisone for an extended time, the dosage should be tapered to a stop, not stopped abruptly.

Conversely, using the drug prednisone to fight NHL or to control the after-effects of treatment can produce a "Cushingoid" syndrome that mimics overactive adrenal glands. This normally regresses when prednisone usage is stopped, but may result in temporary or permanent diabetes, about which more is said below in the section called "Diabetes."

If you experience weight gain in the abdomen with thin arms and legs, weight loss, moon-face, increased thirst, hair loss, browning of the skin at joints, skin thickening or thinning, and if you are not taking prednisone, ask your doctor to do an ACTH stimulation of the pituitary gland, and dexamethasone suppression testing of the adrenal glands.

Adrenal dysfunction also can be linked to disease of the thyroid or pancreas (diabetes), or damage to brain organs such as the pituitary.

Cognitive and psychological damage

Many NHL survivors report that their memory, concentration, logic, and reasoning skills no longer seem as good as they once were. This is especially so among those who have had cranial irradiation, methotrexate administered to the spine, or the high-dose chemotherapy and total body irradiation that accompanies bone marrow or stem cell transplantation or rescue.

Specific problems mentioned are short-term memory loss, failed word retrieval, reduced math skills, confusing the spelling of words that sound similar (homonyms), moodiness, shortened attention span, and depression.

> *I have definitely suffered some loss of comprehension when I read. It appears to be permanent, but then I'm not dead yet, so you never know. I went right from six months of standard chemotherapy into chemotherapy to prepare me for a bone marrow transplant, and that may be why. I completely lose my vocabulary sometimes, too, as if the synapses get crossed or something.*

> *My memory has also suffered. I used to rely on it for just about anything. Now I rely on my notes.*

There are no known solutions yet for these problems, although interesting research is being done with hyperbaric oxygen treatments to reverse the effects of radiation on the blood supply to the brain.

Post-traumatic stress disorder, depression, and anxiety are recognized sequels to cancer's stress, and can be addressed by a professional experienced in handling the psychological issues of cancer survivorship.

Diabetes

Diabetes can arise temporarily or permanently following treatment with prednisone, which is a synthetic copy of the natural adrenal hormone hydrocortisone, or following radiotherapy of the abdomen or brain.

If you experience increased thirst, weight loss, increased episodes of fungal infection, changed eyesight, slow wound healing, increased urination, and mental confusion or faintness, ask your doctor to test you for diabetes.

Diabetes can arise secondarily as a result of adrenal disorders, and often will recede when the adrenal disorder has been corrected.

Eyes

Radiotherapy or steroid therapy can cause cataracts; radiotherapy can cause "dry eye." Cataracts can be repaired with surgery. Dry eye can be treated with eye drops or prescription drugs.

NHL survivors who remain immune-suppressed may experience a reactivation of cytomegalovirus or of varicella Zoster (herpes Zoster or shingles, about which more is said below), which can affect eyesight. These infections should be treated promptly with antiviral drugs.

Fatigue

The National Cancer Institute reports long-term fatigue as one of the most debilitating long-term symptoms associated with cancer treatment.

For far too long, many cancer survivors weren't believed when they reported fatigue that lasted for years following treatment. The opinion used to be that one should feel tired only while red blood cell counts remained in the abnormally low range.

Now, doctors are listening more carefully to what survivors are saying about fatigue. One study of survivors of the Hodgkin's lymphomas has shown that 37 percent of about four hundred people studied experienced fatigue for as long as nine years after treatment. A study of 125 survivors of bone marrow transplantation revealed that about half experienced chronic fatigue for ten or more years following transplant.

The remaining problem is that medicine often cannot tell us why long-term fatigue occurs or what to do about it, although fatigue seems to increase as the duration or intensity of treatment is increased. Treatments such as tamoxifen or interferon that are spread over a very long time period can cause long-term fatigue. Other causes of fatigue include difficulty breathing, cranial irradiation, damage to the heart, liver, or kidneys, chronic pain, or the worry that accompanies cancer.

A five-year transplant survivor describes her ongoing problem with fatigue:

> I still experience a chronic state of exhaustion. I believe it's just something I have to learn to live with. It has taken a few years to accept it, but now I just plan more carefully. I know that everything I do "costs" energy, and I know that I'll need recovery time afterward. Here's an example:

I wanted to attend a play a friend was in, in my hometown two hours away, with a stop to visit my mother-in-law. I had not slept well the night before, and that little (formerly only inconvenient) fact made all the difference. Even though my husband was doing the driving, by the time we arrived at my mother-in-law's, I could feel the internal shaking from fatigue. When I got up to change my dress for dinner and the play, sweat started pouring. I was nauseated, and visibly shaking. I thought if I could make it to the car, perhaps I could sleep at my friends' house and put dinner off for a little while. We got in the car, but before we had driven two blocks, my husband had to pull over so that I could vomit. We returned to my mother-in-law's, and I lay down with the room spinning. After a tea-and-toast meal and an hour's sleep, the symptoms stopped.

Currently, the only proposed solution for long-term fatigue not attributable to known causes such as low blood counts or organ damage is plenty of rest, good nutrition, a carefully balanced workload, and emotional support.

For an excellent and detailed discussion of postcancer fatigue, see Dr. Harpham's book *After Cancer: A Guide to Your New Life*.

Graft-versus-host disease

The tendency for white blood cells from donor-transplanted bone marrow to attack the body tissues of the recipient causes painful and potentially fatal side effects known collectively as graft-versus-host disease (GVHD).

Some researchers have noted GVHD even following autologous marrow or stem cell rescue (that is, using one's own marrow) if immunosuppressive drugs are administered and then abruptly withdrawn.

At its worst, GVHD may attack skin, liver, or intestine, alone or in combination. Although GVHD may fade away after eight or ten years, many transplant survivors spend years on immunosuppressive drugs to control this phenomenon.

A certain amount of GVHD is desirable because it also confers a beneficial graft-versus-lymphoma effect that lowers the risk of relapse. Thus, doses of immunosuppressive drugs are carefully titrated to achieve a balance between life-saving immunosuppression and a small amount of graft-versus-lymphoma effect.

Growth impairment (short stature, precocious puberty)

Children who have had cranial irradiation, total body irradiation, or brain surgery involving the pituitary gland, may sustain damage to the pituitary and the hypothalamus, two brain organs that interact to control growth.

Growth hormone levels should be monitored, and supplemented if necessary, in childhood cancer survivors. Impaired growth can cause a host of physical problems such as very early adolescence, as well as a series of academic, behavioral, and health problems.

Hair loss (alopecia)

Radiotherapy to the head, armpits, or groin, or treatment with the chemotherapeutic agent busulfan, can result in permanent hair loss. Sometimes the loss is not evident until months later when the existing hair is shed from the follicle, and the hair does not regrow. This is more common following cranial irradiation, high doses of busulfan, or total body irradiation. It is also more common among females or among those suffering from graft-versus-host-disease after bone marrow transplantation.

There is no treatment yet for this disorder.

Heart and vascular damage

Heart and vascular damage can emerge years after treatment with no previous warning symptoms.

Chemotherapeutic agents known to cause cardiovascular damage are:

- Doxorubicin (adriamycin) can cause heart damage if given in high doses or for a long time. The risk of heart damage rises greatly at lifetime doses above 350 to 500 milligrams per square meter of body surface area.
- Vincristine (Oncovin) can damage veins.
- Ifosfamide is also suspected of causing cardiovascular damage.

Radiation to the chest can damage the heart or its pouch-like linings, the pericardium and endocardium, the valves, or can constrict nearby tissues, arteries, and veins, affecting heart function.

If you have any symptoms of heart disease, such as chest pain or tightness, swollen arms or legs, numbness in your arms or hands, difficulty breathing, unusual heart rhythms, or dizziness, see your doctor for an echocardiogram, a stress EKG, or MUGA testing. In some cases, medication or common surgeries can help alleviate heart disease. In extreme cases, a heart transplant may be recommended.

Kidney or bladder damage

Ifosfamide, the nitrosureas, methotrexate, cisplatin, or cyclophosphamide can cause urinary tract damage, although Mesna now is used to protect the bladder from ifosfamide and cyclophosphamide damage, and allopurinol is used to guard the kidneys from the toxins of dying tumors.

Sometimes kidney damage is transient, and sometimes kidney function can be improved or stabilized with dietary changes or dialysis, but sometimes it cannot. In extreme cases, a kidney transplant may be recommended.

Liver damage

Permanent liver damage following chemotherapy is rare, except for that associated with high-dose treatment used as part of bone marrow transplantation. Liver damage associated with graft-versus-host disease following donor marrow transplantation is well known.

Radiation of the entire liver is seldom used for NHL, although involved-field radiation of small parts of the liver may be done. This reduces the risk of liver failure, because the remaining healthy liver, unlike some other organs, is capable of regeneration to replace damaged tissue.

If you're tired, nauseated, or your skin seems yellow or suntanned, call your doctor. Blood tests can detect changes in liver function, and dietary changes or modification of medications and dosages may alleviate the problem. In extreme cases, a liver transplant may be recommended.

Low blood counts

Low or low-normal blood counts can persist for years after treatment, especially following marrow or stem cell transplantation or rescue, owing to the high doses of chemotherapy and radiation used in these procedures. Some drugs, such as fludarabine used for low-grade NHL, do not suppress blood counts greatly at the time they're given, but do suppress the marrow's ability to regenerate blood products over the long term.

Fatigue, infection, or clotting problems can result from low blood counts.

For those with low red blood cell counts, long-term injections of erythropoietin are used to force production of extra red cells if the marrow remains capable of producing red cells. (If it is not, administration of growth factors will not be useful.) Repeated whole blood or red cell transfusions are commonly done, too.

For those with low platelet counts, new drugs still in the testing stage called recombinant thrombopoietins may help produce new platelets if the marrow remains capable of producing platelets—if not, administration of growth factors will not be useful. Repeated transfusion of platelets is commonly done as well.

For those with low white blood cell counts, injections of granulocyte colony stimulating factor (GCSF) or granulocyte-macrophage colony stimulating factor (GM-CSF) are possible. As with red cells and platelets, injection of growth factors are successful only if the marrow remains capable of producing these cells.

Transfusion of white blood cells from a donor are not recommended for those who are not on immunosuppressive drugs, because white blood cells from a donor will attack the recipient's tissue, and white cells from the recipient will attack the donated cells.

Lung damage

Radiotherapy or the chemotherapeutic agents carmustine (BCNU), busulfan, cyclophosphamide, melphelan, bleomycin, or methotrexate can cause lung damage.

> My lung condition resembled both sarcoidosis and NHL that had metastasized to the lung. My CT scans were sent to a specialist, and it was established that I had had an allergic reaction to the methotrexate given pretransplant, and the lung condition had been progressing in the year since. I was treated with prednisone for about three months, and full lung capacity was restored, although I have scarring and pain in my lungs as a result. (Nothing I can't live with!)

Radiation therapy administered to children targeted to the chest may limit the growth of chest structures, causing diminished lung capacity.

If you have chest pain, cough, or any difficulty breathing, or if you have odd swellings under your skin near the chest, stomach, or arms, report it to your doctor as soon as possible. It might be the first symptom of pulmonary damage caused by the treatments you received: symptoms of fibrous scarring in the lung or, rarely, of pneumothorax, which is air that escapes from the lung and settles elsewhere in the body.

Lymphedema

The swelling of body parts owing to lymphatic fluid that cannot move is called lymphedema, and can emerge as late as fifteen or more years after cancer treatment. The lymphatic ducts are delicate vessels that collect fluid squeezed from veins during normal metabolism and bring it back to the veins near the heart. When these vessels become damaged, lymphedema may occur.

The NHL survivor might confuse it with the fluid retention that signals heart, liver, or kidney failure.

If you had radiation therapy, or surgery that might have affected lymph nodes or lymphatic ducts such as removal of pelvic or armpit nodes, and if you were given instructions to follow to reduce the chance of lymphedema, it's very important to follow these instructions for years afterward. Lymphedema can interfere with blood flow and wound healing, and may interfere with the immune response against tumors.

An early sign of lymphedema is a slight impression remaining in the skin when a finger is pressed against it. A sign of more serious lymphedema is a deeper impression following pressure that takes up to thirty seconds to disappear. Symptoms of serious edema are limbs that swell to twice their normal size.

There are many ways to prevent lymphedema, from elevation of a limb to certain hygienic habits or avoiding sun exposure. Ask your doctor about instructions specific for your condition, call NCI at (800) 4-CANCER, or contact the Lymphedema Network, listed in Appendix A, *Resources*.

Lymphedema can be treated with variable success with certain drugs, such as antibiotics and diuretics, but the best cure is prevention.

Mouth, teeth, and throat

Radiation therapy to the head or neck as well as chemotherapy cause many transient side effects, but the dry mouth that may continue long after treatment ends can cause serious problems with dental health, and scar tissue that forms in the throat following radiotherapy may interfere with swallowing or breathing.

If you have dry mouth, you will be at risk for dental problems because the infection-fighting ingredients of saliva are missing. Ask your doctor and dentist for instructions for daily care, such as frequent rinsing with salt water. See your dentist immediately for any redness or swelling in your mouth, or for cracked or discolored teeth, even if you have no pain.

If you are having trouble swallowing or breathing, surgeries to stretch or remove scarred tissue are possible.

Numbness, tingling, dizziness, paralysis, deafness

Numbness, tingling, or pain in the hands or feet—peripheral neuropathy—may persist for months or years following treatment with vincristine or cisplatin. There is no treatment yet for this disorder, although pain management techniques may help.

Treatment with the aminoglycoside antibiotics gentamycin, tobramycin, amikacin, or with vancomycin for infections that arise during cancer treatment can result in temporary or permanent hearing loss, vertigo, dizziness, or ringing in the ears. These disorders can be treated with surgery, drugs, rehabilitation exercises, or noise-blocking devices.

Temporary or permanent paralysis called ascending myelopathy has been linked to the use of methotrexate in the spine, especially in children. If treated promptly with steroids, the condition may improve, but the paralysis also can become permanent.

An NHL survivor who was treated for hybrid NHL/ALL for more than two years describes the effect of treatment on his hands:

> I have been on vincristine for almost two years now, and although I have felt that at times I have slight problems in flipping through pages or typing due to numbness and other effects in the fingers, the effects were

not significant. But today was a rude awakening. I am taking my Ph.D. qualifying exams this weekend, and one of the exams is pretty stressful in terms of the number of questions to be answered in the allotted four hours. So, today I tried to simulate the exam situation and write one answer in the given time and guess what? First, I couldn't write as fast as I used to in my precancer life, and second, since I have not written at the speed required in exams for a long, long time, my wrist and shoulder started hurting within thirty minutes. Finally, I just couldn't grip the pen well enough to write neat and fast and have been feeling dullness in my fingertips since. This is the first time I can feel the effects in this magnitude and the timing is ridiculously bad.

Pain

Pain in various parts of the body, such as the back and legs, can result from bone and nerve damage owing to radiotherapy or from long pressure of tumors on nerve pathways.

Peripheral neuropathy, causing pain in the hands and feet, can result from treatment with vincristine or cisplatin.

If you have chronic, low-grade pain, don't try to ignore it. There are ways to address pain so that it does not become worse or cause permanent damage. Moreover, chronic pain, even low-level pain, has an affect on mood and performance that you might not notice if pain gets gradually worse or if you've been dealing with it for a long time.

If you have persistent pain of any magnitude, you might consider consulting a pain specialist or pain clinic for a multi-modal approach to pain control that may include pain medication, surgery, behavior modification, pain control devices such as implantable nonaddictive morphine pumps or electrical stimulators, ultrasound treatments, or relaxation training.

For pain associated with sexual activity, see Chapter 17, *Sexuality, Fertility, and Pregnancy.* For stress reduction to lessen pain, see Chapter 11, *Stress and the Immune System.* For a lengthy, detailed, excellent discussion of pain and pain management, see Dr. Harpham's book *After Cancer: A Guide to Your New Life.*

All of the following groups offer support or referrals for pain management:

- American Academy of Pain Medicine: (708) 966-9510

- American Society of Clinical Hypnosis: (847) 297-3317

- American Pain Society: (847) 966-5595

- American Society of Anesthesiologists: (847) 825-5586

- National Chronic Pain Outreach Association: (301) 652-4948

- Agency for Health Care Policy and Research: (800) 358-9295

Radiation fibrosis

Radiation fibrosis is the formation of fibrous scar tissue within the body, caused by the immune system reacting to radiation. It unfolds over months or years. This fibrous tissue is knotty and stiff, and interferes with an organ's ability to do its job. For example, fibrosis in the esophagus can cause it to narrow and can cause the muscles for swallowing to be less functional. Fibrosis of tissue in the chest can cause the heart to pump less efficiently and can cause pain upon arm movement. Fibrosis in the sexual organs can interfere with fertility or sexual pleasure. Certain drugs, such as Taxol, when administered along with radiotherapy, can worsen fibrosis.

There is some recent evidence that administering steroid drugs simultaneously with radiotherapy can reduce the body reaction that causes fibrosis, but it appears that not many doctors know of, or believe in, this circumvention yet. Administering steroids after radiation therapy must be done promptly upon noticing the onset of fibrosis, as delay causes steroid therapy to be ineffective.

Recent research with hyperbaric oxygen has shown some promise in reducing the negative effect of radiotherapy on certain tissues such as blood vessels in the brain.

Recall sensitivity

Certain body tissues are permanently affected by chemotherapy or radiation therapy, becoming permanently sensitized, and may react with swelling and soreness if chemotherapy is re-administered months or years later. This is called recall sensitivity. It's a physical, not a psychological, phenomenon.

For instance, if chemotherapy happens to leak accidentally from an arm vein (extravasation) during infusion, the skin into which it leaks may swell and hurt if chemotherapy is administered again—even if it's years later, and even if the other arm is used.

When chemotherapy is administered following radiotherapy, previously irradiated tissue may become sore, even if it's nowhere near the injection site.

Ask your oncologist about precautions that you and she can use to avoid this problem.

Second cancers

One of the most serious risks associated with cancer treatment is the risk of developing a second cancer. These fall broadly into two categories: leukemias and second solid tumors.

Treatment-related leukemias (t-MDS, t-AML)

Certain chemotherapeutic agents, specifically the alkylating drugs such as cyclophosphamide and epipodophyllotoxins such as etoposide are known to increase the risk of subsequent leukemia, with higher doses and longer use of these drugs incurring higher risk. For NHL survivors, these higher chemotherapy doses usually are encountered only in the conditioning regimens for bone marrow or stem cell transplantation, not in the dosage normally found in CHOP, for example.

Some leukemias that follow treatment emerge abruptly and progress rapidly within three years of treatment as an obvious leukemia (t-AML). Some emerge slowly five to twelve years later, perhaps beginning as myelodysplasia (MDS), an imbalance of blood components that often becomes a leukemia.

Radiation therapy does not appear to increase the risk of leukemia unless the spleen is irradiated, or unless all bone marrow is irradiated as preparation for a bone marrow or stem cell transplant.

At this time, the only known cure for treatment-related leukemia or myelodysplasia is bone marrow or stem cell transplantation using donor marrow. Myelodysplasia that is treated as soon as possible with transplantation is more successfully eradicated than the treatment of a frank, rapid leukemia or of myelodysplasia that has advanced to leukemia.

Treatment-related solid tumors (second solid tumors)

Radiation therapy is linked to the development of second solid tumors such as Hodgkin's lymphoma, testicular, breast, kidney, and lung cancers, and certain tumors within the spleen or marrow. Second tumors that arise following radiotherapy almost always arise in or near sites of previous irradiation, called radiation ports. Rates of radiation-induced tumors begin to rise about fifteen years after treatment. Radiation-induced tumors are more likely among childhood cancer survivors than among those treated as adults.

The chemotherapeutic agent cyclophosphamide has been linked to the subsequent development of bladder cancer. Co-administration of the drug Mesna may protect the bladder from this risk.

One study of Japanese patients noted a link between cirrhosis that develops following radiation therapy or chemotherapy and subsequent primary liver cancer. This kind of tumor may be more likely to occur among Asians harboring the hepatitis C virus.

Sexuality and fertility

Long-term damage to sexuality and fertility is possible when NHL is treated with certain chemotherapies or with radiotherapy to the pelvic organs. Difficulties such as failed ovulation, failed conception, irregular menses, inability to achieve or maintain an erection, and pain during intercourse are possible. These problems are discussed more fully in Chapter 17.

Shingles

All who had chicken pox as a child, and cancer survivors who receive marrow from a donor who had chicken pox, harbor within their nerve cells a herpesvirus called varicella Zoster, the virus that causes chicken pox and shingles, two manifestations of the same illness.

There are many human herpesviruses; varicella Zoster is just one. It should not be confused with the genital herpesvirus that is transmitted sexually.

When the immune system becomes suppressed or dysfunctional, varicella Zoster may re-emerge from nerve endings, causing quite terrible pain and blisters called herpes Zoster or shingles. Immune dysfunction is common among those who have lymphoma, leukemia, myeloma, AIDS, or those on immunosuppressive drugs following a transplant. The virus can affect any or all nerve endings within the entire body, but it is most likely to appear along the side of the face, neck, arm, or side of the body. Although 10 to 20 percent of those with shingles may never produce blisters, they will still experience itching or pain, or both. The blisters tend to appear in a line, following the path of nerves.

Shingles that affect the eye can cause temporary or permanent blindness.

As soon as symptoms appear, call your doctor. An antiviral medication such as acyclovir, and perhaps pain medication as well, should be started promptly. It is not unusual to require codeine or even morphine briefly for severe shingles episodes.

Shingles normally heal within four to six weeks, but some patients experience lingering pain for years afterward. If this happens, a procedure called a nerve block or glycerine block can be performed by a neurosurgeon. It should alleviate pain for several months and can be repeated if needed.

Shortness of breath

Shortness of breath can be caused by a number of treatments used for some NHL patients. See the sections regarding heart damage, lung damage, low blood counts, or radiation fibrosis.

Skeletal damage

Radiation therapy can damage bone, causing pain, fracture, and asymmetric growth, such as curvature of the spine.

Long-term high-dose steroid therapy with drugs like prednisone can damage bone, causing avascular necrosis of bone, a painful condition that can be treated with joint replacement.

> I have extensive bone damage from prednisone which I took during first-line treatment and then again after my bone marrow transplant for a lung condition. I have bone infarcts on my sacrum, femurs, and tibias, as well as osteonecrosis in my hips, sacrum, and knees. I have considerable pain and take narcotics daily to function.

Recently developed drug treatments for myeloma such as Pamidronate (Aredia) eventually may be used to rebuild bone among those suffering from other illnesses, but in some cases, joint replacement or prosthetic implants to provide skeletal support may be necessary.

Skin

Many causes are found for skin problems that follow NHL treatment, from garden-variety dry skin, perhaps owing to altered absorption of nutrients, to radiation- or chemotherapy-induced thinning and scarring. Other problems include re-emergence of autoimmune disorders such as psoriasis, and graft-versus-host disease following a transplant. Rarely, immune-suppressed survivors of NHL may contract mycobacterial or fungal infections that resist treatment.

If you can't find relief easily, ask your oncologist to refer you to a dermatologist who has experience in treating cancer survivors.

Stomach or intestinal distress

Long-term damage from irradiation of the abdomen may appear as diarrhea, or as constipation from narrowed, tightened intestines or damaged nerves. Medication for diarrhea may help the former, and surgery may correct the latter.

Constipation from immobility or from use of pain medications may also be a lingering effect. Exercise, stool softeners, or a switch in pain medication may ease these effects.

Nausea related to liver damage from chemotherapy may occur. Changes in medication or diet to improve liver function may reduce nausea. In extreme cases, liver transplantation may be recommended.

Pain and constipation may result from the use of chemotherapy drugs that damage nerve cells, such as vincristine.

Surgical complications

A number of late effects linked to prior surgeries are possible owing to the development of scar tissue called adhesions, unavoidable damage to nerves, or use of improper surgical technique. Ask your doctor about any symptoms you're having that you suspect may be related to a prior surgery. Adhesions, for example, can be corrected with follow-up surgery.

Swollen arms, legs, hands, feet

Swollen extremities can result from several of the treatments used for NHL or can be caused by lymph node removal during diagnostic surgery. See the sections above on heart, liver, or kidney damage, or lymphedema.

Thyroid dysfunction

The thyroid gland is a butterfly-shaped organ that wraps around the trachea. When it has been damaged by cancer treatment, it may become underactive, overactive, or cancerous.

Irradiation of the head, neck, or chest can cause the thyroid gland to fail during or after therapy. Irradiation of structures near the thyroid can affect the thyroid because radiation scatter, a ricochet effect among body organs, is difficult to control.

Certain chemotherapies, including some of the interferons or interleukin-2, can cause the thyroid gland to fail during or after therapy

Symptoms of an underactive thyroid (hypothyroidism) may include lethargy, dry skin, numbness in hands or feet, weight gain, mental slowness, sleepiness, depression, immune suppression, intolerance of cold, and loss of hair or altered hair quality. These symptoms also resemble the side effects of many cancer treatments, but thyroid blood levels can be tested to distinguish low thyroid function from transient side effects. Hypothyroidism that is not caused by a tumor is safely and quickly remedied by replacing the missing thyroid hormones using thyroxine, an oral medication.

Symptoms of an overactive thyroid (hyperthyroidism) may include weight loss (or, rarely, gain), excessive appetite, irritability, intolerance of heat, insomnia, rapid heartbeat, high blood pressure, protruding eyes, stroke, and loss of hair or altered hair quality. These symptoms resemble the side effects of prednisone use, but thyroid blood levels can be tested to distinguish overactive thyroid function from the transient side effects of steroid use. Hyperthyroidism that is not caused by a tumor can be treated with drugs that block thyroid hormone activity, such as Tapazole; with high blood pressure medicine to control symptoms temporarily; via surgery to remove the thyroid; or by injections of radioactive iodine-131 to destroy overactive thyroid tissue.

A malignant tumor of the thyroid gland may produce a mixture of the above symptoms. Surgical removal of half or all of the thyroid gland is used to cure thyroid malignancy. This surgery is very safe, and is curative in over 95 percent of cases, depending on tumor stage and histologic subtype.

Thyroid disease also can be linked to dysfunctions of the adrenal gland that resemble Addison's and Cushing's diseases, or to damage of brain organs such as the pituitary.

If you suspect thyroid disease, your doctor will order imaging studies. Tell all medical personnel involved, especially the radiologist who will read your scans, that you are an NHL survivor, because relapses of certain NHLs such as the MALT NHLs can occur within the thyroid gland.

Summary

The delayed and long-term effects and complications of NHL treatment are not common, but they can be serious. It's useful to be acquainted with them, particularly with those that can emerge years later with no warning or those that can mimic a recurrence of NHL.

Many, but not all, of these effects and complications can be corrected, stabilized, or lessened.

The likelihood is that undesirable long-term effects will become fewer as newer treatments are developed. The medical community is keenly aware that many cancer survivors pay a high price for their survival in reduced quality of life. One goal in the development of new treatments is reduced toxicity.

One trend today is to design new treatments that specifically target the parts of the tumor that are different from normal cells. This means that more healthy tissue will be spared, and that such therapies might be used many times without cumulative toxicity.

CHAPTER 17

Sexuality, Fertility, and Pregnancy

*Any scientist who has ever been in love knows
that he may understand everything about sex
hormones, but the actual experience is
something quite different.*

—Dame Kathleen Lonsdale

NHL and the treatments used for it today may affect male and female sexual development, libido, fertility, and the success of pregnancy. For some of us, sexuality, fertility, and pregnancy take a back seat during the cancer experience, but for others, these are very emotional issues—almost as emotionally charged as cancer itself.

Be sure to bring sexuality and fertility issues to your oncologist's attention if he does not mention them, especially if you or your partner are at the high end of the childbearing years. Avoid having your doctor's assumptions about your age, family planning, or sexuality place your fertility and sexual function at risk.

Because of the possibly deleterious effects of treatment on fertility, you should consider harvesting sperm or ova for future use if you are facing chemotherapy or radiotherapy for NHL. Even those who believe they will never want children should consider taking the precaution of preparing for future fertility needs. A diagnosis of cancer can cause profound changes in outlook for most survivors, and your perspective on becoming a parent may well change after spending some time facing survival issues and weathering successful treatment. Exceptions exist, of course. For example, those who have already raised a family may feel that harvesting sperm or ova is unnecessary.

Ways to recognize, prevent, correct, or adjust to issues of sexuality, fertility, and pregnancy are discussed in this chapter. The opening section consists of the insights of a cancer counselor on issues of sexuality and fertility. Next, specific issues of sexuality are discussed, as well as fertility issues such as harvesting ova and sperm, fertility treatments, and how chemotherapy, radiation, and surgery can impact fertility. Males, females, and children are discussed separately. Then we turn to pregnancy, both pregnancy during NHL and pregnancy after NHL. Finally we look at how treatments can affect the sexual development of children who have been treated for NHL.

A full discussion of techniques to enhance sexuality and fertility after treatment for NHL is beyond the scope of this book; only certain techniques are mentioned in the text that follows. References have been included in the bibliography and in Appendix A, *Resources,* so that you will be able to verify facts or do further reading, if you choose.

An educated opinion

These thoughts are from Nan Suhadolc, M.S.W., L.C.S.W., a survivor of both aggressive childhood NHL and of low-grade disease which returned twenty years later. Nan has devoted her life to counseling cancer survivors:

> Each of the cancer support groups I facilitate has its trademark characteristics, but one of the most wrenching is the one for young adults, ages 18 to 30. The reason is the issue of fertility, since bone marrow transplants and other aggressive chemotherapy regimens can cause both infertility and impotence.
>
> Men and women, either entering or in their childbearing years, often face the side effect of infertility as they enter treatment for life-threatening illness. In my own case, as a teen with cancer, I was more concerned about my hair falling out and possible infertility than about survival. Foolhardy? Depends on your priorities. Many women define themselves by their ability to bear children and by their role as mother. To take that away threatens the core of their life, and in many cases brings the young women to the question, "Would I rather have children than live long?"
>
> Men face similar but underrated challenges. My best friend, Michael, underwent a bone marrow transplant in the early stages of his life with NHL. The consummate Olympic shot put athlete and Harvard lawyer, he prided himself on his masculinity, expressed as head of household, father, and provider. The doctors outlined the usual side effects of chemotherapy

and transplantation, but nobody mentioned impotence. Post-transplant, the most heart-wrenching call I received from Michael came at 2 A.M., when he finally had to talk about it.

"Nobody told me!" he shouted. "They never said I couldn't make love with my wife. I'm not sure I'd have done the damn thing if I had known I'd never make love again!" More important than whether he'd have gone ahead is the fact that the doctors chuckled at his outrage. "We saved your life, and you're upset about this?"

The situation isn't hopeless. One can endure aggressive treatment and often still bear children. I live with heart damage and experienced two high-risk pregnancies, but I later gave birth to two beautiful daughters, twelve years post-treatment. After our second was born, as a preventive measure I had a tubal ligation. Nonetheless, I am the proud mother of yet another daughter, whom we adopted at birth. The keys to this and other such self-conscious issues of survivorship:

Hope. Never say die, just keep going until you know all the options.

Ask questions! Ask your doctor about infertility. Can you store eggs or sperm for later use? Is there a chance of losing your fertility? If so, is treatment necessary now, or can you have a baby first? Don't let a fear of death inhibit the questions that might offer you a reason to live!

Support. Fellow survivors can offer incredibly valuable suggestions, in personal groups, or via the Internet, and nine times out of ten you will find your way to the best help there is, armed with all the necessary questions.

Finally, there are other ways of parenting children. Adoption is a wonderful alternative, as are the various ways one can now save eggs and sperm for later implantation. The saddest experience is one where the young adult accepts that fate has dealt a childless hand, when there are so many options and so much valuable support available.

The following sections first discuss sexuality, then fertility, and finally pregnancy.

Sexuality

It's not at all unusual for cancer survivors to report decreased or frustrated sexual desire during and months after treatment. Indeed, some report these problems for many years following treatment. Fortunately, issues of sexuality during and after cancer treatment are common and treatable. If you're unhappy with your sexuality, discuss with your oncologist a referral to a gynecologist, urologist, or andrologist who specializes in postcancer care, and consider consulting a sex therapist if you feel it's warranted.

Many good medical solutions are available today for those who suffer neurological or other physical impairments from cancer treatment. Various therapies are available, for instance, to sustain erection and to relieve vaginal pain. If sexual hormones are out of balance, sexual pleasure and satisfaction may improve with hormone replacement therapy. In addition, an extraordinary array of medications and devices is available to help those with sexual side effects from cancer or its therapy.

As a survivor, you need to be aware, however, that separating the psychological effects of disease from the physiological effects of treatment may be difficult or impossible. Moreover, it's important to bear in mind that most sources of support for sexuality after cancer deal with *all* cancers, and that subtle neuropathologic problems may remain after specific neurotoxic therapies for NHL, such as vincristine or cisplatin, problems perhaps undetectable using the equipment available today. Consequently, your efforts to find help may have to target multiple resources. For example, your libido may suffer when treatment-related chronic fatigue or chemically induced depression are present.

Purely emotional perceptions and misconceptions regarding sexual drive and satisfaction are always a possibility, of course, but they may be compounded by frank physical damage causing dry ejaculation, impaired valve function that causes ejaculation of semen backward into the bladder, difficulty maintaining an erection, vaginal and vulvar pain during intercourse, vaginal ulcers, and surgical sites that ache or are numb for up to a year after surgery. This means that, should you decide to seek help *only* from a sexuality counselor, it's possible for physical difficulties to be misdiagnosed as psychological problems. Medical history is full of such errors, such as the "Fakers' Disease" of the nineteenth century, which we recognize today as the autoimmune disorder multiple sclerosis. In short, if you're convinced that your problems have a physical basis that outweighs any psychological component, avoid those who attempt to label you as emotionally ill and seek help elsewhere.

Several sources of information are available to you in dealing with decreased or unsatisfactory sexuality after cancer treatment:

- Your family doctor or oncologist
- Counselors who specialize in issues of sexuality
- Support groups
- Various books

Each is discussed below.

Your doctor can be a source of basic information regarding how cancer and treatments are affecting you physically and how those physical changes are impacting your sexuality. Your doctor might not be able to address all your concerns, though. She might lack knowledge in this specialty; she might have less time than you need for discussion; she may incorrectly interpret what's important to you unless you're very clear when communicating. She might feel uncomfortable discussing sexuality, or she may feel it's "just a psychological problem." She should be able to refer you to counselors, however, who can guide you in separating the physical and psychological components.

Purely psychological discomforts may be more difficult to address, and success in this area may depend on one's access to good counselors. The best choice is a sexuality therapist who is familiar with both the physical and psychological effects of serious illnesses such as cancer. Large urban centers are more likely to have specialists in sexual counseling than rural areas.

Support groups, either those focused on cancer or on the sexual problems following other illnesses, are an excellent way to discover tactics, insights, and clinical information regarding sexual problems after cancer.

Several of the larger books about cancer that contain chapters on sexuality are listed in Appendix A.

An extraordinarily good resource that deals with these issues in a sensitive, fair way is Leslie Schover's 1997 book, *Sexuality and Fertility After Cancer*. Especially impressive is her sensitivity toward those over age 65, whose sexual needs sometimes are neglected by the medical community. As those over 65 are well aware, people remain sexual beings for their entire lives.

Dr. Schover describes the techniques and technologies available for sustaining erection, reducing vaginal pain, getting pregnant, and many other problems that are all too often borne silently. She discusses sexual adaptation for those minus genitals, breasts, and those living with an ostomy and scarring. Childhood cancer survivors and their unique adaptations are covered. Her discussion of the possible divergence in sexuality caused by cancer is grounded in a thorough introduction to sexual function in the absence of cancer.

A word of caution about Dr. Schover's book is in order: she mentions that young males are less susceptible to radiation-induced sterility than older males. Some studies of the lymphomas have found otherwise.

Although full coverage of sexuality after cancer is not possible in this brief chapter, a few of the points made by Dr. Schover and others are worth mentioning specifically:

- Communicate about sex. Communicate not just during or after attempting sex, at which times emotions are too highly charged, but always. In particular, tell your partner if you're experiencing pain.

- Cuddle, touch, and be affectionate, even if you're temporarily not up to sex as you used to know it. A sexual relationship based on love can be described as one of continual foreplay. Just walking side by side, touching, can be an act of lovemaking.

- If you're a female who has had pelvic irradiation, the scarring of radiation fibrosis can develop over several years. It's important to use the vaginal dilator the doctor recommended or have frequent sexual intercourse to prevent this scarring. Use these techniques three times a week or as your doctor recommends. Not only will sex be less painful, but the gynecologic exams that you must have as follow-up for cancer care will not become more excruciatingly painful over time.

- If you're male, bear in mind that male orgasm without erection and without ejaculating is possible. Moreover, many partners consistently report sexual pleasure that does not require penetration by an erect penis. Good options for achieving an erection, such as medication or hydraulic implants, exist if failure to obtain or maintain an erection continues to be a concern.

- Be patient, expect new sensations, and keep an open mind about new experiences. Sex may be very good after cancer, but it might not be exactly the same as it was before cancer.

- Ask your doctor if the partner being treated should protect the other partner from chemotherapeutic drugs that may persist in sperm or vaginal secretions. The amount of chemotherapeutic agents present in body fluids is likely very low, but it may be best to be careful (radiotherapy poses no similar risk). Wearing a condom or vulvar shield might be recommended.

- Cancer cannot be "caught" during sex, although some viruses that may cause certain cancers can. In addition to HIV, human T-cell lymphotropic virus I (HTLV-I) is transmitted by sexual contact, as is the papilloma virus thought to be linked to most cases of cervical cancer.

- The endorphins released during sexual pleasure reduce pain elsewhere in the body.

A male survivor of NHL/ALL described how frustrating meeting women and dating can be after a cancer diagnosis:

> It's very difficult being my age (29) and being an unmarried male cancer survivor. I have difficulty at times just meeting women or strengthening new relationships, as my academic workload requires so much of my attention and energy. I'd like very much to have a serious relationship, to get married and start a family with a woman who either has had cancer or who has had experience adjusting to another serious illness.
>
> Although I would ideally prefer to marry a woman from India, who has been brought up in the same culture, my experience with cancer has made me a member of a community that transcends barriers of race and nationality.
>
> I have met such wonderful people (via Internet discussion lists hem-onc and bmt-talk) from various countries that the meaning of my culture has changed. Today the most important characteristics in my life partner would be her value systems, attitude, and approach to life first, and nationality second.

A female survivor describes how painful intercourse has become because she was never instructed to tone vaginal tissue with a stretching device:

> One of the totally preventable side effects of my chemotherapy and pretransplant treatment was the loss of tone in my vaginal tissue at age 38. My body changed so much during chemotherapy that my husband and I were not very active sexually. Then, two months after my

chemotherapy stopped, I was admitted into the transplant unit. I was quite ill for months, and for the year after, sex was not even an issue. When I was feeling able to become physically intimate again, there was a great deal of pain. It was not until I saw a physician for this specific problem that I was informed that, during what had resulted in a long period of abstention, I should have been keeping my vagina stretched. It never occurred to me that this could happen, and no doctor had warned me that it might.

In the five years since my transplant and this discovery, I have attempted to stretch the tissue using a series of dilators provided by the hospital. Had I used these dilators during my chemotherapy and recovery from the transplant, I would still be intact.

My husband is very patient and understanding, fortunately, and we love one another deeply. But our intimacy has changed. I have not been able to stretch the tissue much. Intercourse is difficult and unsatisfying. As much as I grieve for myself, I feel even angrier that my husband suffers because of it. This was an important part of our lives. We have lost something precious because of an oversight by my doctors. So much of what transpired could not be helped, and certain indignities cannot be avoided, but this loss, which affects our lives so profoundly, was completely unnecessary.

Fertility

If you were treated for NHL as a child, or were treated for NHL as an adult and are still in your reproductive years, you may experience temporary or permanent fertility problems such as cessation of menstruation or sperm of poor quality. Treatments to boost fertility and aid in conception are available.

The medical literature contains relatively little information about NHL, fertility, and pregnancy compared to other cancers such as Hodgkin's lymphoma and childhood acute lymphoblastic leukemia (ALL). These latter illnesses occur primarily in children and adolescents and are successfully treated, which means that many are now long-term survivors who have experienced subsequent fertility problems.

Some of the drugs used to treat these cancers and NHL are identical, and radiation sites and dosage may be similar. This means that certain comparisons can be made between the findings of the more plentiful fertility studies following those cancers and NHL, particularly for children with NHL treated via protocols similar to those used for ALL. Nevertheless, owing to the scarcity of information regarding fertility directly related to NHL, and to the ongoing development of new treatments for NHL, you should discuss with your oncologist the potential risk to fertility that your specific treatment may entail.

Harvesting sperm, ova, and stem cells

Harvesting of sperm or ova is highly recommended for many about to be treated for NHL. Even if you feel you'll never want to be a parent or that your family is complete, you should consider harvesting sperm or ova because you may change your mind. However, do not expect the oncologic medical staff to be forceful, convincing, or even forthcoming on this issue.

Ova are harvested by inserting a fine needle through the abdominal or vaginal wall, guided by an imaging tool such as ultrasound. In some cases, hormones that stimulate egg production are given in advance so that many eggs will mature simultaneously. These abundant eggs are then harvested in one procedure and frozen (cryopreserved). This is usually an outpatient procedure for which you'll be given anesthetic and sedation.

It may be difficult to find a center that freezes ova that are unfertilized, as the technology to successfully fertilize ova (also called oocytes) after thawing is fairly new. Most centers prefer to harvest ova, fertilize them, and freeze the resulting embryos. Ask your doctor about this before the procedure if you don't have a partner or sperm donor, or ask the center to proceed with freezing anyway, assuming the enhanced fertilization techniques will be readily available when you decide to use the oocytes you've stored.

Sperm can be harvested in several ways. The simplest method is the collection of ejaculate either following masturbation or following sexual intercourse during which a special collecting condom is worn. Harvesting via masturbation or sexual intercourse usually must be done in a private room in the sperm banking facility, not at home. Because sperm die so quickly, they must be frozen immediately.

Some recent studies are examining the ability to harvest and store testicular stem cells, the cells from which sperm arise. In theory, after treatment for cancer these saved stem cells could be reimplanted into the testicle that was so heavily treated that all remaining stem cells were destroyed. This is usually an outpatient procedure for which you'll be given anesthetic and sedation.

In the past, males with certain cancers such as testicular cancer or lymphoma were thought to produce sperm of such poor quality owing to the cancer itself that harvesting and storing sperm was thought to be useless. With newer fertility techniques, however, even sperm reduced in number or of lesser quality can be used to produce a pregnancy. You should consider harvesting and storing sperm in spite of its quality or quantity.

Chemotherapy and female fertility

For females, having been treated with chemotherapy for NHL appears to entail a not yet fully quantified risk for subsequent infertility. Alkylating agents such as procarbazine and cyclophosphamide have been shown to damage ovarian function, but less severely than they damage testes in the male. Some studies have shown that females treated with chemotherapy are indeed able to conceive and bear children, while other studies have shown at least partial impairment of fertility, impairment of the ability to retain a pregnancy following chemotherapy, or the development of early menopause.

For those able to conceive, carrying pregnancy to full term and giving birth to a healthy baby who develops normally appears likely for women who have been treated with chemotherapy. There appears to be no increase in cancer or other health problems, nor in cognitive problems, among the children of women treated for NHL with chemotherapy.

One study has shown that pretreatment of women about to have chemotherapy with gonadotropin-releasing hormone agonists (GnRH-a) appears to protect the ovaries from chemotherapy.[1]

Chemotherapy and male fertility

For males, chemotherapy regimens that contain alkylating agents such as procarbazine or cyclophosphamide may affect fertility permanently.

Some studies have found an increased risk of outright sterility to be related to the dose of drugs such as cyclophosphamide, with lower doses entailing lower risk.[2]

Other studies have found that the testes of males not yet in adolescence are less likely than those of mature males to be adversely affected by chemotherapy. Still other studies have found that the testes of mature males can be protected from the deleterious effect of chemotherapy by simultaneously administering testosterone, but information on this protective effect conflicts.

Finally, some studies have shown a very slow return of male fertility over a span of years after treatment with these drugs.

There is no conclusive evidence that young boys will enter puberty earlier than normal following chemotherapy, as do many girls.

Radiotherapy and fertility

Radiation therapy generally is without risk for future infertility unless the brain, pelvis, abdomen, or testes are irradiated.

Radiotherapy is clearly harmful to the ovaries, testes, and associated reproductive structures, with demonstrated dose effects such that low doses cause subtle damage and increasingly higher doses eventually cause outright sterility.

If an ovary or testis is the site of the NHL tumor or the site of likely spread, treatment with radiation therapy may be essential for survival, and fertility may have to be sacrificed. In this instance, harvesting and storing sperm or ova in advance of treatment is clearly the best and perhaps the only option for preserving fertility.

Radiotherapy and female fertility

Following radiotherapy, older females are more likely to experience loss of fertility than younger females owing to the decreasing number of viable ova within the ovary as females age.

In addition to outright sterility following radiation therapy, subtle damage among ovulating, menstruating women who appear to be capable of conceiving a child may include compromise of the blood supply to the uterus and changes in uterine size. Structural and functional changes such as these may make conception and implantation more difficult and miscarriage more likely.

Ovarian function that has not been totally destroyed by radiotherapy may return to normal levels in the years following treatment. This can be tracked indirectly by following blood levels of pituitary follicle-stimulating hormone and luteinizing hormone (FSH, LH), two substances that act as messengers from the pituitary to the ovary to stimulate egg growth. In some instances, even seemingly inadequate ovulation, as indicated by abnormally high values of FSH or LH and the absence of menstruation, nevertheless may produce a pregnancy.

Cranial irradiation can interrupt the function of the pituitary and hypothalamus. Because these two organs within the brain control overall growth as well as the function of ovaries and testes, there can be a corresponding disruption of the production of growth and reproductive hormones when the pituitary and hypothalamus are affected. This may result in failure to ovulate or menstruate in adolescent females.

Methods to protect the ovaries from radiation, such as surgery to temporarily or permanently move the ovaries out of the radiation field (oophoropexy), are available to preserve fertility and are generally successful, although temporary or permanent infertility may result in spite of these precautions. In some instances, a second surgery to restore the ovaries to a position realigned with uncontorted Fallopian tubes is necessary. Lead shields can be constructed to protect the ovaries from almost all of the radiation administered, but internal scatter—an echoing of x-rays among internal organs—still may affect the ovaries adversely.

Radiotherapy and male fertility

In addition to outright sterility, subtle damage in the male may include ducts within the pelvic reproductive array that are constricted or totally blocked, cells in the testes that can no longer produce sperm, or sperm that are decreased in number, are misshapen, or have impaired motility. The blood supply to the penis that is responsible for erection may be compromised if the veins are constricted from the scarring that can follow radiotherapy.

Some studies have found that the fertility of young males is affected more strongly by radiotherapy than that of older males; other studies have not.

Testicular function that has not been totally destroyed by radiotherapy may return to normal levels in the years following treatment. As with women, this can be tracked indirectly by following blood levels of pituitary follicle-stimulating hormone (FSH), although in some instances even seemingly inadequate production of sperm, as indicated by abnormally high values of FSH, still may produce a pregnancy.

As with females, cranial irradiation can interrupt the function of the pituitary and hypothalamus in males. Because these two organs control overall growth as well as the function of ovaries and testes, there can be a corresponding disruption of the production of growth and reproductive hormones when the pituitary and hypothalamus are affected. This may result in impaired production of sperm.

Similar to the ovaries, the testes can be shielded from most pelvic radiation using lead shields, and surgery to displace the testes out of the path of radiation, called orchidopexy, is possible. Damage owing to scatter may still occur, though, as the testes cannot be shielded from all other internal organs or from all angles.

Surgery and fertility, male and female

Various surgical procedures can cause subsequent problems with fertility in the female or male NHL survivor. Scar tissue (adhesions) can immobilize and constrict the reproductive organs and limit the blood supply to the sexual organs, a blood supply necessary for erection and for nurturing the growing fetus.

For females, the path from the ovary through the Fallopian tube to the uterus must remain open for a successful conception and implantation, and the end of the Fallopian tube nearest the ovary must be free to move in order to channel the fertilized egg into place. If this path has been blocked by scar tissue, a second surgery later in life may be necessary to remove adhesions and straighten or reopen these pathways.

For males, certain surgeries or the adhesions of the healing process can bind or damage the vas deferens, part of the network of sperm production and transport. In addition, those needing to have lymph nodes within the pelvis biopsied are at risk for neurologic damage that may make ejaculation incomplete or impossible. Nerve-sparing surgery can be used to avoid this problem. For those suffering this damage who wish to father a child, techniques such as stimulation of ejaculation with electricity or microsurgery to retrieve sperm from within the testes are possible.

In addition to careful surgical technique such as maintaining adequate blood flow to tissue and avoiding the introduction of foreign material into the abdominal cavity, synthetic materials are available to the surgeon that can be laid between the pelvic organs during surgery to prevent adhesions from forming during the first critical days following surgery. These materials eventually dissolve within the body.

Fertility treatments

A full discussion of techniques to enhance fertility is beyond the scope of this book, but several general methods are discussed.

Infertility that occurs after chemotherapy or radiotherapy may be treatable by fertility specialists, called reproductive endocrinologists, using techniques such as hormonal stimulation, harvesting of sperm and ova, concentration of sperm, selection of healthy, motile sperm, detection of sperm within urine, assisted penetration of the ovum by sperm, ex vivo fertilization and reimplantation, or microsurgery to correct blocked ducts.

If harvesting of sperm is being attempted following NHL treatment that has impaired ejaculation or damaged the testes, in certain survivors sperm can be collected from the testes via fine-needle aspiration or microsurgery.

A few studies have shown that certain hormone stimulators called gonadotropin-releasing hormone agonists may aid in the regeneration of sperm from damaged testes.

Pregnancy during NHL

Perhaps one of nature's cruelest tricks is the development of cancer during a pregnancy. For the mother diagnosed with cancer, grave concern for the well-being of the unborn child exists amidst terror for herself. For the father diagnosed with cancer, concern about the heritability of cancer may exist along with fear that the unborn child soon may be fatherless.

It is rare for any cancer to arise in the mother during pregnancy, and rarer still for one of the NHLs to develop during pregnancy. You should discuss with your oncologist how your treatment might affect your unborn child, and what options are available to you. When a cancer does arise, the mother might opt to defer treatment until after the child is born, if the NHL is not an aggressive one. An early induced delivery may also be possible, allowing cancer treatment to begin more quickly. It might be wise to prepare for the fact that some oncologists suggest termination of pregnancy to save the mother's life.

Most NHLs that arise during pregnancy occur in one or both breasts and manifest as a localized swelling or as an enlargement of the entire breast. Breast lymphomas are diagnosed with mammography, needle biopsy, and tissue biopsy. There is evidence that the hormones of pregnancy may hasten the development of a pre-existing microscopic breast lymphoma. There is no evidence that the hormones of pregnancy can cause a breast lymphoma to develop when no underlying disease existed before pregnancy.

There is disagreement among researchers regarding classification of certain pregnancy-related NHL breast tumors. Some are lymphomas of mucosa-associated lymphoid tissue (MALT), but others, or perhaps even most of the breast lymphomas associated with pregnancy, are Burkitt-like NHL. Still others masquerade as the more common tumors of the breast, adenocarcinomas, most often seen in women who are not pregnant.

NHLs may occur during pregnancy in other areas of the body, such as the placenta, but this is rare.

Chemotherapy during pregnancy

The thought of treatment for cancer during pregnancy causes most people anguish. They intuit that the treatments that are so effective against the rapidly dividing cells of the tumor must surely harm the rapidly growing child in the uterus. The facts, however, are more complex.

For aggressive, riskier NHLs that may not permit one to postpone treatment, certain chemotherapy regimens are considered safe for the developing child by some doctors, but reports of successful pregnancies simultaneous with chemotherapy conflict. It appears that the placenta may be an effective filter that prevents not only pieces of the mother's tumor (metastases), but also the chemotherapeutic agents commonly used today for treating NHL from reaching the fetus, but other requisites of pregnancy, such as the greatly increased blood supply to the developing child, may be compromised by certain drugs.

What this amounts to is that, while some studies report miscarriage during chemotherapy for NHL, other studies report successful full-term pregnancies producing children of sound health. Owing to the scarcity of information directly related to NHL and to the ongoing development of new treatments for NHL, you should discuss with your oncologist the potential for damage to the fetus that your specific treatment may entail.

If treatment continues after the birth of the child, breast-feeding may be dangerous to the newborn child owing to chemotherapy drugs in breast milk. Verify this possibility with your oncologist.

Radiotherapy during pregnancy

Irradiation of the abdomen or pelvis for either diagnostic testing or treatment must be avoided to protect the fetus. Irradiation of other organs may be possible if the developing fetus can be properly shielded.

Treatment of side effects during NHL pregnancy

Many drugs are available to relieve the side effects of chemotherapy and radiotherapy, but you should consult your oncologist and pharmacist regarding the safety of any prescription or over-the-counter drugs you plan to use. Be sure to tell your pharmacist and all medical personnel who prescribe drugs for you that you are both pregnant and being treated for NHL.

Pregnancy after NHL

If you are an NHL survivor who becomes pregnant, your chances of carrying a baby to full term and giving birth to a healthy child are very good. However, you should be evaluated as a possible high-risk pregnancy. Ask your oncologist for a referral to a gynecologist/obstetrician who is experienced in treating cancer survivors and has a subspecialty in fertility techniques and high-risk pregnancies.

Children's sexual development

The cure of cancer in children using the treatments available today is in many ways the beginning of a new set of problems.

Children and adolescents who are treated for NHL are susceptible to early, late, or absent puberty or, for females, very early menopause in their twenties. Their cases should be followed carefully for years by a pediatric endocrinologist and, when warranted, given growth hormone, estrogens, or androgens.

Early puberty can be caused by cranial irradiation or, at least for girls, by chemotherapy. Children with inadequate levels of growth hormone owing to pituitary damage following cranial irradiation may enter puberty much earlier than their peers. Broadly speaking, the lessening of the pituitary's chemical growth signals within the brain trigger the beginning of puberty. This can result in very short stature and an array of behavioral problems. For girls, both chemotherapy and radiotherapy are risk factors for early puberty. For boys, no conclusive evidence exists that chemotherapy can cause early puberty, but cranial irradiation may.

Children lacking estrogen or androgen from compromised ovaries or testes, or from inadequate pituitary signaling to the ovaries or testes, either fail to enter puberty at all or adolescence begins far later than it does among their peers.

Female children treated for NHL in protocols that resemble those for childhood acute lymphoblastic leukemia are at increased risk for obesity in adulthood.

Summary

Issues of sexuality during and after cancer treatment are common and treatable. Take advantage of the resources available by finding a gynecologist, urologist, or andrologist who specializes in postcancer care, and consider consulting a sex therapist if needed.

Regardless of your feelings about possibly becoming a parent, you should consider addressing the preservation of fertility before treatment begins, as the effects of some treatments on fertility, when combined with multiple factors such as patient age and site of tumor, are not completely understood. Harvesting of sperm or ova should be considered even if you feel you'll never want children.

Temporary or permanent fertility problems such as cessation of menstruation or sperm of poor quality may arise if you were treated for NHL as a child, or were treated for NHL as an adult and are still in your reproductive years. Very effective treatments to boost fertility and aid in conception are available.

The preservation of the health of the fetus and the health of the mother when treatment for NHL is necessary during pregnancy is the topic of ongoing scientific review. Some chemotherapy regimens appear safe, but the fetus must be shielded from radiotherapy. You should discuss with your oncologist how your treatment might affect your unborn child, and what options are available to you, such as delaying treatment, early induced delivery, and avoidance of radiotherapy.

CHAPTER 18

Relapse

*We do not know what we mean by cure
because there is a great difference between
cure and long-term survival.*

　　—Arthur Holleb

Fear of relapse is a nightmare that all of us experience at one time or another. Unfortunately, for some of us there comes a day when the nightmare is still there when we awake.

Depending on the subtype of NHL we have, and what we've learned about it, we may be well prepared intellectually and emotionally for relapse, perhaps with a new treatment plan already selected. Others among us may be utterly broadsided by the news.

This chapter will begin with a definition of relapse, and then will describe who is likely to relapse, how relapse is detected, in what areas of the body relapse may occur, when it's most likely, and why it occurs. There are indeed instances of test results mistakenly being interpreted as relapse—and we'll discuss what findings may constitute equivocal results—but chiefly this chapter will focus on true relapse. A discussion of the difficult emotional issues that arise upon relapse, which often are different from those we encounter at first diagnosis, will follow.

Treatment of relapse is discussed in Chapter 6, *How the NHLs Are Treated,* and Chapter 19, *Clinical Trials.*

What is relapse?

Relapse is the return of disease in a patient who had achieved and maintained a complete remission—defined as the disappearance of all disease—for longer than thirty days after treatment ended.

If signs of disease recur in a survivor who achieved a partial remission—greater than 50 percent reduction in tumor size—the return of disease is called disease progression, rather than relapse, because full remission was never realized.

If signs of disease return within thirty days following treatment, then by definition no remission was achieved, regardless of the amount of tumor shrinkage observed during treatment.

Tumors that shrink, but neither disappear nor regrow, are categorized as a type of partial remission called stable disease.

It's possible to mistake the after-effects of treatment for symptoms of relapse. It may relieve you of some anxiety if you review Chapter 16, *Late Effects, Late Complications*, which describes most of these physical changes.

Why does relapse occur?

The most widely accepted theory for relapse is that not all lymphoma cells were killed by the original treatment. Other theories hold that genetic predisposition, continued or recurrent exposure to environmental toxins, or unabated or repeated exposure to an infectious agent are responsible for relapse. Interesting research has been done showing that cancer cells can acquire resistance to chemotherapeutic drugs by turning on genes that block the cellular intake of certain drugs and others related to them, a phenomenon called multiple drug resistance (MDR).

Nonetheless, successes with high-dose treatment followed by bone marrow transplantation or bone marrow rescue suggest that the lingering cancer cell theory is correct.

How is relapse detected?

Some NHL survivors detect swollen nodes, or experience old, familiar feelings of malaise, or notice other recurrent symptoms. These very frightening findings trigger a visit to their oncologist. Other survivors note entirely new symptoms that they wouldn't normally think of as related to NHL, but somehow they know that things just aren't right. Still others may be feeling fine, yet a routine imaging study, blood test, or marrow biopsy shows a return of disease.

It's likely that your oncologist will order one or more tests if either you or she notices anything that hints at a return of disease. Many of these tests, such as a CT scan, bone scan, or gallium scan, will be familiar from your experiences during your initial diagnosis.

Clinical relapse

When symptoms or signs of returned disease are noticed by the survivor, a loved one, or a medical professional, and the return of disease becomes unquestionably apparent during a subsequent physical examination or imaging study, it's called a clinical relapse.

If you have symptoms of recurrence many years after successful treatment, you should consider requesting a re-biopsy of the suspicious area to determine whether this is a relapse, a second primary cancer, or a benign side effect of earlier treatment.

Cytogenic relapse

Cytogenic relapse is relapse detected by one or more tests on the cellular level in the absence of physical symptoms.

Various blood tests, for instance, may detect the spread of NHL from the lymph nodes into the blood stream. Fluorescence in situ hybridization (FISH) and flow cytometry detect cell surface antigens produced by cancerous cells. A bone marrow aspiration or biopsy may detect irregularities in cell appearance or in genetic material that are associated with relapse.

Who relapses?

Very broadly, and only in the context of today's treatments, one can say that low-grade disease relapses more often than intermediate- or high-grade disease, and that, for intermediate- and high-grade disease, those who were diagnosed in the advanced stages of illness are more likely to relapse than those diagnosed in early stages.

With many new treatments being developed for NHL, however, it's not wise, correct, or ethical to adhere to generalities without continually revisiting the progress of research and without noting exceptions. Certain subtypes of NHL, for example, respond very well to treatment and are less likely to relapse than others. Chapter 4, *Prognoses*, discusses these exceptions in detail.

When am I safe from risk of relapse?

For intermediate- and high-grade disease, the longer you remain in remission, the less likely you are to relapse. As with other cancers, you may be considered cured once you have been in remission for five years. Although there is no guarantee that NHL will not re-emerge many years later, it's far less likely as time passes, and indeed, a recurrence at a much later date should be fully evaluated, including re-biopsy, for the possibility of a second primary cancer rather than a relapse of NHL.

For low-grade disease diagnosed at stage III or IV and treated with protocols available at the time of this writing, both long-term stable disease and remission for five or more years is likely to be followed by relapse or disease progression. The exception is low-grade disease treated with bone marrow transplantation, the results of which are too new to evaluate for long-term success.

Where does a relapse occur?

The various subtypes of NHL behave differently. Some types may relapse at the original site of disease; others may relapse at quite different sites. If you are HIV positive or immune-suppressed, you may experience a relapse in the central nervous system. Disease that was not originally found in bone marrow may relapse there, causing pain.

Transition to another grade

Occasionally a relapse is accompanied by a transition to another grade of NHL. Usually the transition is from low-grade disease to a higher grade, but it's also possible for a high-grade NHL to return as a lower grade, although this is less common.

Sometimes biopsied tissue will reveal two grades of NHL in the same patient, in the same lymph node, or in two different organs. When this occurs, usually the treatment is geared to eliminating the higher-grade NHL because it may become rapidly aggressive.

Transition to another lymphoma

Occasionally, a relapse of NHL will, upon biopsy, reveal a mixture of NHL and one of the Hodgkin's lymphomas, or a mixture of B-cell and T-cell NHL.

This may be either a reflection of our still imperfect classification systems or a true instance of multiple tumor types.

Gray areas

In the last ten or fifteen years, we have benefited by the tremendous progress made in medical science's ability to detect cancers at much earlier stages than in the past. Nevertheless, we forget at times that our sophisticated imaging tools still provide just a glimpse into the body's complex workings. Consequently, imaging studies sometimes yield equivocal results that must be qualified with additional testing or even with a second biopsy.

Following some types of chemotherapy, for example, fatty lesions can form in the liver. These benign lesions may appear upon CT scanning as liver metastases. Positron emission tomography (PET) scanning can distinguish these lesions from NHL that has spread to the liver.

At times, nodes will appear much smaller after treatment without fully disappearing. They may remain the same size for years, and then disappear. It's thought that these nodes may be scar tissue. Some types of lymphomas are more likely than others to scar (sclerose); ask your doctor if your subtype of NHL may exhibit this characteristic.

Odd lesions on the lungs are sometimes seen on imaging after treatment has ended. If you had radiation therapy targeted to your chest, these lesions may be fibrotic tissue arising from an immune system reaction to radiation therapy.

Treatment options

How your relapse will be treated depends on how your first appearance of disease was treated. Often, oncologists assume that the drugs you were given as first-line treatment will not be the best choice for treating relapse. The thinking is threefold:

- If they were very effective, you would not have relapsed.
- NHL cells can become resistant to drugs, making them ineffective.
- Some drugs are toxic to various organs, and their lifetime dose must be limited.

Upon relapse, it's usually the case that a second drug, a series of drugs, or radiotherapy will be attempted. Because NHL treatments are evolving continually, any attempt to describe herein the specific treatments your doctor might suggest would be quickly outdated. See Chapters 6 and 19, and Chapter 23, *The Future of Therapy*, for information on treatment of relapse.

If you didn't familiarize yourself with clinical trials during your first experience with NHL, now is a good time to do so. Clinical trials are a good way to gain access to new treatments before they are made available to the general public.

Emotional issues

Clearly, relapse is an emotional lowland for almost anyone affected by NHL, including the survivor, the family, friends, and the oncologist.

The emotional issues faced at relapse are different in quality and scope from those encountered at first diagnosis and endured during treatment. What follows are some of the reactions that many NHL survivors describe having.

Fear and terror

Feelings of fear or raw terror may overcome you, even if the odds remain in your favor. A sense that your options are narrowing may grow stronger, even if they are not. Thoughts of death that you may have been able to put aside during and after treatment crowd back in, even if you know that there are still treatment options open to you. Fear of different, stronger treatments may emerge.

Abandonment

There may be a sense that you fought the good fight, and now you deserve peace, contentment, and normalcy. Not only are you not getting these just rewards, you're getting something that could hardly be worse. You may wonder why unethical, unkind humans go about happy and healthy. You may find yourself wishing that certain particularly unpleasant people would get cancer, too.

Anger

Anger over life's unfairness, perhaps kept in check or rationalized during the first round of treatment, may now emerge and may cause you, and those around you, much discomfort. What psychological adjustments you may have made to your illness may go out the window, seeming to be a waste of time. Anger may manifest as rage, irritation, cynicism, or depression.

Grief

Many people grieve from the moment of diagnosis. They grieve for lost health, energy, and diminished opportunities of many kinds, from career opportunities they had to forego to have treatment to loss of fertility or ruptured relationships.

Not surprisingly, an expanded sense of grief may emerge upon relapse. Some people can't help but remember having heard that, for many cancers, failure of first-line treatment entails a poor prognosis. Although you may know that this generality does not apply to all of the NHL subtypes, it's still a frightening thought that makes some people grieve for the life they may lose.

Despair

The initial diagnosis of NHL and first-line treatment often are addressed with a can-do attitude that may be difficult to sustain at relapse, even if your chances of long-term survival are just as good after an additional therapeutic regimen that achieves a solid remission. There's something about facing the battle all over again that might make you weary at the very thought of it. You may feel that the difficult treatment you've already endured was a waste of time. You may question the quality of your life. You may contemplate suicide.

Loss of trust

You may lose trust in the medical system in general or in your oncologist in particular. If a strong faith sustained you during diagnosis and first-line treatment, you might find yourself questioning this faith now. You might lose confidence in your own ability to meet physical and emotional challenges.

Low-grade disease: one person's story

What follows is a description of Nan's emotions surrounding her experience with NHL that was initially high-grade, but relapsed years later as low-grade disease:

> Each type of lymphoma has its idiosyncrasies, a different sense of the particular stakes, and of the nature of the journey. I had high-grade lymphoma as a teen, and experienced that urgency, that sense of "must treat or die" that accompanies aggressive diagnosis. I was given three months to live; treatment was necessarily swift and aggressive. And I got lucky. Big stakes, harsh treatment, near-death experience, and the gift of cure.

> My survivorship experience with low-grade NHL has been entirely different. Diagnosed in 1986, a nasty test called a lymphangiogram showed that all of my nodes, from my neck to my knees, were both enlarged and abnormal in architecture. The horror I felt plunged to the core of my being, as my poor oncologist, also a friend and colleague, gave me the news. I might look for six years' survival, he said, and he'd do his best to help me.

> The glitch however, was that that "help" was to take the form of nothing. Nothing to do! How could that be? My precious daughters were only four and six years old—what good was "maybe six years"? Indeed, Dr. Saul Rosenberg had discovered that for low-grade, nonsymptomatic NHL, the best course was watch and wait, which meant "go home, Nan, and live your life while you wait for the beast to transform into its more aggressive form so we can take our best shot."

> This phrase "watch and wait" really pisses me off. I hate it for myself and for the patients I work with. Oncologists tend to agree, but aren't invested enough to actually change the established vernacular. It is a dangerous phrase. Inherent in those three words is the assumption that the disease will come back, will transform to a more aggressive cell type, and will need treatment later. Why would anyone want to assume this? Haven't we discovered the power of words? Even science has begun to study support groups and the impact of hope—not only on an individual's quality of life, but on actual length of life. Where is there hope in telling me that I am to wait until the predetermined worst happens so that I can then do something?

Let's rewrite the speech, shall we? "Nan, you have low-grade lym-phoma, which is one form of non-Hodgkin's lymphoma. This type of NHL tends to have a personality of its own, it waxes and wanes, comes and goes, and nobody is certain at this time what sets it off or puts it back. What has been documented is that those in your situation fare equally well without aggressive treatment as with it, sometimes better. There are individuals your age and stage who have lived for years and years with-out treatment, who continue to live well. Others' NHL becomes bulky or perhaps develops symptoms, at which time we would recommend any number of treatments, from low-grade chemotherapy to trials with mono-clonal antibodies and the like. There is every reason to believe you can live long and well with this disease. We must know that wellness is key, and believe that it is just as likely that your nodes will recede—wane—as it is that they will grow or wax. My suggestion today is that you take some time to get used to the diagnosis, then we can explore your options. Here is some reading material, get acquainted with this disease, it's less scary that way. And at the very least, let's consider what you can do to bring your body to its optimum state of wellness, so you are best able to fight the NHL, and to offer you the most quality of life."

Family and friends

The reactions of friends and family may be completely supportive, positive, and loving, or particularly inept. Unless they're kept well informed about your illness and its likely patterns, they may give up on being sustaining, instead treating you as if you have one foot in the grave. They may mourn prematurely; they may practice living without you emotionally. One way to forestall these negative reactions is to inform them from the beginning that NHL can be treated very successfully at relapse.

Employers may begin to lose patience with you at the prospect of yet more absenteeism. Your children may once again exhibit earlier, less adaptive behaviors that they had outgrown, such as aggression, bedwetting, or tem-per tantrums.

Getting help

Support groups are an inestimable resource for regaining emotional footing and a balanced outlook. If you didn't examine options for finding support during your first experience with NHL, it would be wise to do so now. It's not an overstatement to say that you'll be overwhelmed by feelings of hope and energy when you discover how many other people have gone through what you're experiencing, and came through it in good shape.

Many forms of support are available for cancer survivors in general and NHL survivors in particular. Chapter 13, *Getting Support*, details these options.

Summary

Relapse of NHL is an extremely difficult time for most of us. Fear, hopelessness, anger, and overwhelming sadness are common feelings.

Relapse is not a death sentence. There are good options available for retreatment, and many people report feeling very much better after they familiarize themselves with the options available.

CHAPTER 19

Clinical Trials

*"Come to the edge," he said. They said: "We
are afraid." "Come to the edge," he said. They
came. He pushed them...and they flew.*

— Guillaume Apollinaire

Why would anyone choose an experimental therapy over standard NHL treatments that have well-known risks? Aren't clinical trials of new treatments dangerous? Aren't these experimental treatments just for people who have no other choices left? And why are they called clinical trials?

Luckily for us, non-Hodgkin's lymphoma is the subject of a great deal of very promising research. Because NHL is a cancer of the immune system, the research for it and the treatments arising from this research are unique, and in some cases represent the leading edge of what well may become treatment for all cancers. These new and possibly better treatments are available to NHL survivors in carefully controlled settings called clinical trials.

Many of the treatments now in the pipeline are of very low toxicity, unlike some traditional, standard chemotherapeutic agents. Many experimental treatments, such as monoclonal antibodies and interleukin-2 treatments, use natural cancer-fighting body products that are amplified outside the body and then reinserted. Others, such as idiotype vaccines, use our own white blood cells that are retrained to attack tumors. Other treatments are of substances that force immature cancer cells to mature; others aim for and destroy the parts of the cancer cell's chromosomes that make cancer cells immortal.

Critical information on clinical trials will be shared in this chapter. We'll discuss the structure of clinical trials, and how they're run. Their advantages and disadvantages, safeguards for the patient, and the patient's rights are outlined. We will show you why it's often to your advantage to do your own searching instead of relying on trials your doctor may recommend, and how to evaluate different trials. What to expect and what to do when you're finally enrolled are explained.

This chapter focuses on finding and evaluating clinical trials for treatment, not on trials for support, prevention, or detection. For the sake of readability, we will use the word "substance" throughout this chapter, with the understanding that either new substances or new methodologies can be the objects of testing.

Who should examine clinical trials?

The National Cancer Institute recommends that, if you have low-grade NHL, or if you have intermediate- or high-grade NHL that has not responded to standard treatment or that has relapsed, examination of clinical trials may be very much worth your while. The factors that contribute to this statement are discussed at length in Chapter 4, *Prognoses*.

Nonetheless, all NHL survivors should become familiar with methods for finding trials, and with the general structure and function of trials. If you wait until you need a trial to attempt to learn these things, you may run out of time.

What are clinical trials?

Clinical trials are the tests by which new treatments are evaluated to see if they offer more benefit than existing treatments. Success of a new treatment in the highly structured, controlled environment of a clinical trial is required by the U.S. Food and Drug Administration (FDA) before treatment can be approved for wider use by doctors and patients in less controlled settings. When clinical trials show that a new treatment is better than older standard care, and these results are verified by objective third parties, the treatment that was used in the clinical trial becomes the new standard for care.

Clinical trials are tests run in the clinic or—more clearly stated—on humans. The word "clinical" distinguishes these trials from tests done on tumor samples or on animals. Clinical trials are not started on humans until a substance has shown promise when tested first on human tumor samples, and then on animals, usually mice.

There are many kinds of clinical trials. The ones that usually interest most NHL survivors are the ones that focus on treatment, but trials also exist to improve cancer support, detection, and prevention. A clinical trial can test either a new substance, or a new method for administering treatment.

Usually, clinical trials will not admit cancer survivors unless they have already tried standard treatments without success. There are a few trials, however, that admit only those whose cancer has never been treated.

Clinical trials are designed and structured such that the results can withstand the minute and critical scientific scrutiny necessary to determine if a new treatment is effective. By the time a new substance is being used as part of a phase III trial (explained below), the group of patients receiving the new substance is so closely matched on so many characteristics that any difference in their progress against cancer can be attributed with a good deal of certainty to the new treatment, and only to the new treatment. Three study designs that aid in ensuring that the results of treatment are attributable to the new agent and not to chance or confounding factors include randomization, blinding, and double-blinding:

- A randomized trial is one in which patients closely matched on various characteristics—disease stage, prior treatments, health, age, sex, and so on—are assigned via computer to receive either the new treatment, or existing, standard treatment. This means that you might not receive the new substance at all. Randomization is used to demonstrate as clearly as possible that a group of patients very closely matched in all respects to a second group did either better or worse, and that *only* the treatment given explains the difference in outcome.

- A blinded trial is one in which not only are patients randomized, they also are unaware of which treatment they're being given. This is considered necessary to rule out the *placebo effect*, defined as the ability of the human body to respond differently to treatment in measurable, physical ways, based on complex psychological and motivational factors experienced by the patient. Some patients might respond better to a treatment, for example, simply if they know they're getting a new treatment as opposed to an older one. Passive, compliant patients might report responses that they think will please the doctor and staff. The placebo effect is the subject of some controversy, with some researchers maintaining it's truly measurable, while others believe its supposed effects can be attributed to other phenomena, such as inaccurate metrics or patient subjectivity.

- A double-blinded trial is one in which neither the patients nor the medical staff are aware which substance is being given to whom. Double-blinding is used to eliminate the possibility that subtle factors, such as motivation and mood on the part of the doctor or nursing staff that might be sensed by the patient, could account for differences seen in the progress of the group receiving the new treatment compared to those receiving the old—see the placebo effect, described directly above.

In these respects, clinical trials differ from less rigorous tests designed and administered by doctors and researchers working independently on new substances. Independent researchers often lack complete records and consistent evidence that can be verified by impartial observers, and often their patients are not subjected to the necessary long-term evaluation—five years or more—that determines whether the new treatment truly made a sustained difference in tumor regression.

In general, if trials are run by a university, an NCI-designated regional cancer center, or a pharmaceutical company adhering to NCI and FDA guidelines, the chances are very good that safeguards for the patient are part of the design, and that the substance being tested has been reviewed and approved for use by a committee of responsible and knowledgeable researchers. Therapies offered by independent researchers in their own for-profit clinics, especially those that involve ingesting or injecting an untested substance, should be avoided or, at the very least, approached with extreme caution.

Why use clinical trials?

Aside from the altruistic aspect of participating in a trial in order to benefit others—an aspect that may or may not motivate you—clinical trials offer you a good chance to receive more effective treatment, and perhaps a cure, years before it's available to the general public. For example, the recently approved monoclonal antibody treatment for low-grade NHL, Rituxan, has been available for several years to those with low-grade NHL who were willing to enroll in clinical trials testing this substance. Intron-A, a manmade version of interferon-alfa, a human body product that fights infection and cancer, was approved by the FDA in December 1997, but was used by patients in clinical trials for years beforehand.

Steve Dunn is a nine-year survivor of metastasized kidney cancer. Below is a brief retelling of his difficult experience with this cancer, which, prior to the availability of interleukin-2 therapy developed at the NCI, had five-year survival statistics in the 2 to 3 percent range. Like most of us, Steve started at ground zero with no medical background or insider information to assist his search.

Steve's full story is available at the web site listed with the following excerpt, one of the best cancer sites on the Internet. His personal story alone is probably enough to convince most people of the benefits of finding the best clinical trial for their circumstances. Moreover, his advice to patients for locating, examining, and choosing a clinical trial is unparalleled in the scientific and lay literature.

Here's an excerpt from his story, told at Steve Dunn's CancerGuide, *http://www.cancerguide.org/*.

> *I was diagnosed with advanced kidney cancer in late 1989, at the age of 32. Only a month after surgery, it was discovered that my cancer had spread to both lungs and nine bones in my spine. At this point the situation was desperate with no standard treatment and dismal long-term statistics. Early on, some incidents with my doctors and some help from a friend convinced me that if I wanted the best treatment, it was up to me to find it. I bumbled and stumbled my way through researching my options and through the system, but ultimately, through finding the latest data and close collaboration with my physicians, I was able to make a good choice of a promising experimental therapy, high-dose interleukin-2 combined with interferon. To paraphrase Stephen Jay Gould, I found the right information, asked the right questions, and enrolled in the right trial, and it saved my life.*

Won't I be just a guinea pig?

In the U.S., the long and not altogether honorable history of the clinical trial process has resulted in laws, procedures, and methods that safeguard the patient. For example, each clinical trial has a lengthy plan, called a protocol, that will be given to you if you ask for it. The protocol describes what will be done, when, and what action will be taken if certain undesirable effects occur. You should always ask for, and read thoroughly, a copy of the full protocol.

Informing the prospective patient and obtaining consent from the patient are time-consuming and repetitive processes done to ensure that all risks and benefits are made clear. For example, the patient should be made aware that she can drop out of the study at any time, and that care cannot be denied her if she does so.

Unfortunately there still remain cases of patients being pressured to sign clinical trial consent forms without full information or at the last minute without time to consider other options. Remember that very few lymphomas progress fast enough to require a same-day, or even a same-week, decision.

- Always ask that the consent forms and the protocol be sent to you well in advance of your scheduled visits.

- Do not sign a consent form until you have received and read a copy of the full protocol, and have considered all other clinical trials for which you might be eligible.

Only institutions funded by the federal government or governed by pertinent local laws are required to abide by consent guidelines. If you're being treated in a for-profit hospital that receives no government support, it's possible for you to be treated in a study without your knowledge or consent, thinking that you're getting standard treatment. Ask your doctor if your treatment represents state-of-the-art treatment as defined by the NCI or if you're being treated in a study. In addition, phone your state health department to determine if your state has its own laws regarding consent issues.

Placebos

For cancer clinical trials, true placebos are almost never used. A true placebo is a drug or treatment that has been made to look exactly like the active substance or the effective procedure, but it has no active ingredients. In clinical trials of antihistamines, for instance, the placebo used most often is a sugar pill.

For randomized cancer treatment trials—usually phase III trials, of which more is said below—the new treatment is compared to existing, accepted treatment, not to a placebo. Exceptions to this ethical policy are new treatments for which no corresponding previous treatment exists, such as trials of the earliest efforts to purge bone marrow of cancerous cells prior to bone marrow transplantation. In that instance, standard care was represented by reinfusion of unpurged marrow, and the test treatment involved reinfusion of marrow purged using an experimental technique.

How are clinical trials run?

Clinical trials are organized into three stages: phase I, phase II, and phase III. Each phase attempts to address different and increasingly complex issues concerning the success of the new treatment. Some drugs are tested in trials that are a combination of two phases, such as phase I/II or phase II/III. Usually this is done if some knowledge of the new treatment's effect on humans is already known so that its development and testing can be expedited.

There may be clinical trials in which you can participate locally on an outpatient basis, but many require travel and inpatient stays.

Phase I clinical trials

The primary purpose of a phase I clinical trial is to measure the safety and toxicity of different doses of a new substance in the human body. Some phase I studies may also assess tumor response, the amount of drug that accumulates in the body, and a substance's general behavior (pharmacokinetics) in the body.

Phase I trials are preceded by animal studies that measure toxicity, so an estimated safe human dose is already known. Rigorous controls are enforced to be sure that no patient suffers adverse effects. For example, blood or urine values of certain body substances may be measured several times a day to ensure that the liver and kidneys are not compromised. Doses that are found to be unacceptably toxic are lowered.

Phase I trials usually enroll just a few patients, perhaps ten to thirty. Often these patients have a variety of different cancers, for the activity of a new substance against different tumors can be studied. Sometimes one group of patients will receive only a low dose of the drug, and a different group will receive higher doses. But in other studies, the same patients who initially receive a low dose may be given a higher dose later if toxicity is not too profound.

The advantages of a phase I trial are:

- You may receive a treatment that may be better than anything else currently approved by the FDA years before it becomes available to the general public.

- If this drug is already in use for other illnesses, its toxic effects might not be completely unknown.

- Candidate substances for cancer treatment are not approved for phase I trials unless the substance has shown reasonably acceptable toxicity and activity against cancer in cultured tumor cell lines and in animal studies. Of every five thousand substances tested in animals, only five enter phase I trials.

- Doses found to cause unacceptable toxicity are lowered.

The disadvantages of a phase I trial are:

- For every one hundred drugs tested in phase I trials, only seventy will prove successful or safe enough to carry forward into phase II trials.

- Because phase I trials are chiefly concerned with discovering dose-limiting toxicity, they are brief compared to phase II and III trials. You may receive too few doses of the test substance to destroy all of your cancerous cells.

- Phase I trials usually test one substance alone, yet experience has shown that, at least for the chemotherapeutic agents commonly used today, combined drug regimens are more effective against most cancers than single-drug regimens.

- The substance, although it may be an approved drug for other illnesses or even for other cancers, most likely has never before been used in humans for your illness. Although it has been tested in cultured tumor cell lines and in animals implanted with tumors it may not be effective against your tumor, or it may be no better than existing treatments.

- The substance, although it may be an approved drug for other illnesses or even for other cancers, may be administered to you at a much higher, more toxic dose.

- The dosage will be varied among those enrolled, thus its effects on your tumor may not be directly comparable to the effects on the tumors of others enrolled in the trial...and patients do talk among themselves.

- The use of patients with different tumor types makes it difficult for you to compare your progress to that of other patients.

- Toxicity may cause substantial discomfort, illness, or permanent damage, in spite of the safeguards designed to prevent damage.

- Often phase I trials are run by one principal investigator at one institution. You may have to travel to participate in a phase I trial. (Phase I trials for pediatric NHL, however, are sometimes offered at multiple locations.)

Here are the titles of a few phase I trials for NHL selected from the NCI clinical trials database. These trials illustrate the broad variety of cancers being studied simultaneously in phase I trials. Note that the titles state the phase number, and at this phase make no reference to randomization or blinding. Don't be distracted by the overly technical verbiage in these titles. You'll become more familiar with the terminology as you read more about your illness:

- Phase I Study of Oral Penclomedine in Patients with Malignancies

- Phase I Study of Aminocamptothecin by Prolonged Infusion for Metastatic and Recurrent Solid Tumors

- Phase I Study of Irinotecan Administered as a Prolonged Infusion for Adult Solid Tumors

Phase II clinical trials

Phase II trials measure the effectiveness of new treatments against cancer. Some phase II trials also attempt to measure how best to deliver the drug to the tumor—orally, by infusion, and so on—and how often the dose should be given.

Phase II trials enroll many more patients than phase I trials, perhaps fifty to one hundred, so that the substance will receive a more thorough test and the statistics collected will be more meaningful.

Sometimes, but not always, phase II clinical trials are divided into arms, with one arm getting one version of the experimental treatment and a second arm getting another—perhaps the same experimental agent combined with an established, FDA-approved cancer-killing drug, or delivered by another route, or on a different dose schedule.

Owing to the results of phase I testing, a clearer idea exists regarding what cancers will benefit most from this treatment when it's used in a phase II trial. The kinds of cancers considered eligible for phase II trials of a substance, therefore, are usually more narrowly defined than for phase I trials.

Phase II trials take more time than phase I trials because, unlike phase I trials, more of the new agent is administered in an attempt to cause tumor regression.

The advantages of a phase II trial are:

- Candidate substances for cancer treatment are not approved for phase II trials unless phase I trials have shown that the substance has some activity against cancer in humans.

- You'll be receiving a treatment that may be better than anything else currently approved by the FDA several years before it becomes available to the general public.

- Only doses of acceptable toxicity, determined during phase I testing, are utilized.

- Randomizing and blinding usually are not used in phase II trials. Therefore, you are assured of receiving the experimental treatment.

The disadvantages of a phase II trial are:

- More than half of the drugs used in phase II trials will be found ineffective against cancer or too problematic for use. Of the original one hundred drugs that entered phase I trials, of which seventy survived to pass to phase II, only thirty-three will survive phase II testing.

- The substance, although it may be an approved drug for other illnesses or even for other cancers, may not prove to be better than existing treatments for your illness.

- Although its toxicity was determined in the phase I trial of this substance, the substance is still an evolving treatment with the potential for unexpected side effects.

- More of your time will be needed for a phase II trial than for a phase I trial.

- You may have to travel to participate in a phase II trial.

Here are a few examples of phase II trials for NHL selected from the NCI clinical trial database. Note the occasional use of randomization, and the trend toward fewer cancer types being eligible, as opposed to phase I trials:

- Randomized Phase II Study of Filgrastim and Stem Cell Factor in Priming of Bone Marrow for Autologous Transplantation in Patients with Relapsed or Refractory Hodgkin's Disease (HD) or Non-Hodgkin's Lymphoma (NHL)

- Phase I/II Study of Epstein-Barr Virus (EBV)-Immune T Lymphocytes from a Normal HLA-Compatible Donor to Treat EBV-Associated Lymphomas and Other Lymphoproliferative Diseases

- Phase II Study of Antibiotics and Gastric Acid Inhibition for Gastric MALT Lymphoma

Phase III clinical trials

Phase III clinical trials test a new substance's efficacy compared to existing standard treatments by using patients who are closely matched on several characteristics, such as stage of disease.

Phase III trials are usually much larger than phase II trials, and are sometimes multi-center trials—that is, trials run in many sites simultaneously. Often they run for months or years with long follow-up.

Phase III trials are usually randomized and sometimes, but not always, blinded or double-blinded.

The advantages of a phase III trial are:

- A substance that has survived the scrutiny of phases I and II is very likely to be better than current treatments: either more efficacious, or equally effective but less toxic.

- You'll be receiving a treatment that may be better than anything else currently approved by the FDA a year or two before it becomes available to the general public.

- If, during the trial, a new treatment shows itself to be profoundly superior to existing treatment, those receiving the existing treatment are switched to the arm of the study utilizing the new substance.

- If a new treatment shows itself to be clearly or dangerously inferior to existing treatment, those receiving the new treatment are switched to the standard treatment regimen.

The disadvantages of a phase III trial are:

- Of the thirty-three drugs that survived phase II testing, only about twenty-five will be found effective in phase III trials.

- Randomizing and blinding may not appeal to those who are determined to receive only the new treatment, not the contrasting current treatment.

- The new substance may prove to be just as effective as, but no better than, the existing treatment.

Here are a few examples of phase III trials for NHL selected from the NCI clinical trials database:

- Phase III Randomized Study of Cyclosporine and Methotrexate or Cyclosporine and T-Cell Depletion for Graft Versus Host Disease Prophylaxis During Peripheral Blood Stem Cell Transplantation in Patients with Advanced Malignancies Eligible for Allogeneic Transplantation from Matched Related Donors

- Phase II/III Study of Iodine I 131-Labeled Monoclonal Antibody Lym-1 in Patients with Intermediate or High Grade Recurrent or Refractory B-Cell Non-Hodgkin's Lymphoma

- Phase III Study of Liposomal Cytarabine (DepoFoam Encapsulated Cytarabine; DTC 101) Versus Standard Therapy for Neoplastic Meningitis in Patients with Leukemia, Lymphoma, or Solid Tumors

Which phase is best?

As you can imagine, phase II trials might appeal to patients who find phase I trials too risky and phase III trials too controlled. It would be a mistake, though, to assume, based only on the structure of the system, that phase II trials are the only good choice. A phase I trial of a drug with a long history of use for, say, an autoimmune illness such as rheumatoid arthritis might be a very safe choice for an NHL survivor if animal studies have shown the agent is active against NHL. A phase III trial using a new monoclonal antibody that just varies an ancillary feature of treatment, such as one antibiotic against another to control infection, might be as good a choice as a phase II trial of a less well-known, less promising substance.

Where are clinical trials run?

Clinical trials are found most often at the NCI-designated Comprehensive Cancer Centers and Clinical Cancer Centers, and at other university medical hospitals that receive federal funding and cooperate with the NCI on clinical trials. Your community oncologist may participate through association with the NCI's community clinical oncology programs. See Chapter 2, *Finding the Right Oncologist,* for more information on NCI-designated cancer care centers.

How can I find trials for NHL?

If you're an adult with NHL, you must take an active role in finding the best care for your disease. Adults with cancer are seldom asked to join a trial unless they are being treated in a regional cancer care center. The approach is different from that used for children with cancer, whose families are commonly approached regarding enrollment in clinical trials, and 75 percent of whom eventually are enrolled in clinical trials. The NCI estimates that less than 5 percent of those eligible for clinical trials enroll, and that minorities are under-represented in the clinical trial process.

You can use several methods to find clinical trials:

- You can ask your oncologist which trials would suit your medical circumstances. This has its advantages and disadvantages, one advantage being that you need do very little except trust. The disadvantages are described below in the section, "Why research trials on your own?"

- You can call the National Cancer Institute on 1-800-4-CANCER and ask about trials for your subtype of NHL, being sure to specify whether you're willing to travel—otherwise they'll send you local trials only—and asking for the full document, not the summary. Be warned that if you call often with this request, which is not an unreasonable thing to do, because new trials are added every month, eventually they may decline to send you any more listings. This has been the experience of some cancer survivors who've used this service, which is provided by various regional cancer care centers under the auspices of the NCI.

- You can research U.S. and international clinical trials on your own at the NCI's web site, listed at the end of this paragraph. This, in conjunction with learning to use Medline, is by far the most comprehensive way to check on new treatments being tested. This service alone may be worth the cost of a personal computer and the time spent learning to use it. Once available only to those who subscribed to the NCI's Information Associates' program for $100 per year, now the NCI provides this tool free of charge on the Internet. We strongly suggest that you examine all trials available for NHL, not just those in your area. At the time of this writing, the URL for the protocol search geared to physicians (another, less edifying tool is available for patients) is *http://cancernet.nci.nih.gov/ prot/protsrch.shtml*.

- You can use CenterWatch on the Internet (*http://www.centerwatch.com/*) to track new cancer treatment trials. CenterWatch has many good features, such as an email news notification service, but the titles and descriptions of clinical trials posted at this web site are so general they require you to do much more research. For example, they don't show what agent is being tested or where the trial is really held. Just the city is shown, which is inadequate if you're searching for trials at a top-notch cancer center in a large urban area. The listings are by state, forcing you to read the same over-generalized titles again and again for each state if you're willing to travel and want to be familiar with all trials available.

- You can use the services of commercial Internet service providers such as America Online (AOL) to receive email press releases from pharmaceutical companies concerning new products in development. Be aware, though, that press releases often will simply echo in less detail the medical information you may already have found elsewhere. Furthermore, press releases typically are written to attract or reassure investors, rather than impart information to cancer survivors.

- To find trials specifically for children, search the National Childhood Cancer Foundation site at *http://www.nccf.org/nccf/protocol.htm* in addition to the NCI site listed above.

Why research trials on your own?

Some people who have depended only on their oncologists for comprehensive and up-to-date information on clinical trials have been disappointed. In many cases, oncologists in clinical practice—and that means most oncologists—are aware only of the high-priority trials that receive emphasis in publications such as *Oncology Times*, or those that are offered nearby. Some still do not use a computer to search the NCI's database for all applicable trials. Perhaps they haven't the time to do so—remember that most oncologists in the trenches must track information on every cancer known, whereas you have the opportunity to focus intensely on your own cancer, subtype, and stage.

At the other end of the NHL oncologist spectrum is the hematologic oncologist associated with a university medical school or cancer research center. You can usually expect very good to excellent treatment from such a specialist, but often when consideration of clinical trials is appropriate, they are biased toward their own research or toward trials run by colleagues at their own institution.

The following story is an all too common example of our need to educate ourselves about clinical trials:

> Several months ago I had a phone call from a friend who now has NHL following treatment as a child for bone cancer. She thanked me for sending her information on the FDA's November 1997 approval of the naked monoclonal antibody, Rituxan.
>
> She was originally enrolled in an antiviral trial at a prestigious east coast cancer center, a trial targeting the Epstein-Barr virus, but the trial was halted following concerns about safety. When she showed her doctors the information on Rituxan, they immediately put her on it. "They had never heard of it," she said. Her first gallium scan since receiving Rituxan was clear, and her CT scan was improved. Today, ten months later, she continues in remission.

The ideal oncologist is one somewhere in the middle: educated about all trials and aware of what's a good fit for you, but not biased toward her own work or that of colleagues.

Life doesn't often approach the ideal, so it's a good idea to learn to search for clinical trials on your own, and to repeat your search every month, because new trials are constantly opening. At the time of this writing, there are one hundred forty-six trials for adults with NHL and fifty-three for children. Once you have found a trial for which you believe you qualify, you should bring it to your doctor's attention. What if you find several trials that seem to admit patients with your profile? How can you tell which trial would be best for you? Clearly this is one of the most important questions that will arise in your experience with cancer.

At this point, you need to acquire skills for searching Medline and reading the studies that result from your searches. The substances used in each clinical trial may have results published regarding their previous use in animals or in humans. These studies should be found, evaluated, and compared, by you and your doctor, to single out the substance most likely to benefit you. Detailed techniques for searching Medline are discussed in Chapter 24, *Researching Your Lymphoma*.

If your oncologist is unwilling to help you, is negative, or is at best ho-hum about your proactive attitude toward searching for trials, find a new doctor, because you'll need your doctor's recommendation to get admitted to a trial.

Getting admitted to a trial

Once you have found one or more clinical trials that you think you're eligible for, you must ask your oncologist to consult with and refer you to the treatment center running the trial for an evaluation to be admitted. If your doctor is unwilling to do so, seek a second opinion. You might try phoning the principal investigator listed in the trial description. Often they'll speak directly with patients about what's involved, but a few may insist on speaking first with your doctor.

You and your medical records will be scrutinized closely by your doctor, the doctors at the institution offering the trial, and perhaps your insurance company, to see if you're truly a candidate. Various physical parameters such as the condition of your heart and liver may be factors. The kind of tumor you have, how large it is, or whether your disease is progressing must be considered.

One of the chief considerations in evaluating patients for most clinical trials is how much previous treatment they've had, and what kind. Some trials want only those who have been heavily pretreated; others require patients who have not had any treatment resembling that proposed for the trial. Still others seek patients who have had no treatment at all.

You should read all of the entry criteria listed for the clinical trial and become very familiar with the results of your various tests so that you'll have a good idea whether you're eligible before you approach your doctor for a referral. Questions that many other cancer survivors feel overwhelmed by— questions such as how long the trial will run, where it is located, and what the side effects are—will not be a problem for you, because the description of the study will have answered many of these questions for you.

In order to be accepted, there may need to be a great deal of rapid cross-communication among you, your medical care providers, your insurance company, which will almost certainly insist on pre-approval, the oncology nurse in charge of administering the trial at the center you've targeted, the social worker, the housing assistant (if you must travel for this care), and the principal investigator, an M.D., running the trial. You may need to make one or more trips to the cancer center for an evaluation. You may be pleasantly surprised by how kindly you're treated—some doctors phone personally, for instance—or you may be dismayed by lost records, lack of communication, and red tape. Other patients experience heartache and anger when, after passing all the benchmarks, a reviewing M.D. employed by their insurance company denies payment for the treatment after finding some discrepancy. More on this topic is discussed below, under "About payment."

The evaluation process is the time to ask for your own copy of the full protocol. The protocol is the document that describes what will be done, when, and what action will be taken if certain undesirable effects occur. Do not sign a consent form until you have received and read a copy of the full protocol, and have considered all other clinical trials for which you might be eligible.

Many principal investigators are willing to speak directly with prospective patients about the details of the trial and the patient's medical history. The names and phone numbers of the principal investigator and participating doctors can be found at the end of the document that describes the clinical trial.

You can expect to feel conflicting emotions at this time. The excitement of finding a treatment that may be a cure, the fear that the treatment might have unknown effects, concerns about being away from home, nagging worries about financial considerations, and the thrill of empowerment on finding the best care may suddenly emerge as overwhelming feelings after months or even years of relatively calm feelings about coping with your illness.

No doubt the very detailed information that is part of the full protocol will answer many of your questions, and will spontaneously trigger many others. In addition, consider these less-than-obvious questions, which are adapted from Nancy Keene's book *Working with Your Doctor*:

- Who reviews this study, and how often?
- Who monitors patient safety?
- Why do the principal investigators believe that this treatment is better than standard treatment?
- What are all of the potential physical side effects of this treatment, both short- and long-term?

- Will participation in the study mean that I have to change oncologists?

- Must I be hospitalized to participate?

- What will be my costs, and what will my health insurance pay?

- Does the study follow patients for the long term?

- Who pays for any care I'll need if the treatment has unexpected negative effects?

Once you're in

Detailing exactly what to expect after you're enrolled in a clinical trial is not possible in this or any book because each trial is quite different, but in general, most people find they feel well cared for in a trial setting. It might be wise, however, to expect the unexpected. One cancer survivor, for example, traveled a great distance to take part in a clinical trial, only to be told upon arrival that the trial had been closed owing to safety concerns. Others meet delays because the paperwork necessary was never forwarded by those who promised to do so, especially insurance company pre-approvals for payment.

Once treatment is underway, some people are surprised that the extensive and detailed protocol outlining the treatment really is just a guideline. Although a great deal of homage is paid to adhering to the protocol for the sake of science, the truth is that the protocol can be changed if you're suffering adverse effects. Often a change in protocol will not adversely affect your chances of succeeding on the treatment. This is particularly true in a phase I trial that's measuring toxicity.

If at all possible, have a friend or relative with you during treatment to verify what medications are given, to provide emotional support, and to be an advocate if you need one. This is especially important if you have traveled some distance for care or are using morphine, for example, to control side effects.

Remember that you have the right to withdraw at any time from a clinical trial, to read your medical records, and to ask that deviations from the protocol be made if you're experiencing very bad side effects.

Marilyn is a survivor of small lymphocytic lymphoma who eagerly joined a clinical trial of a monoclonal antibody joined to a radioactive isotope. The following few paragraphs describe her experience over several months in this trial:

I found out today as I was being injected with the radioisotope Yttrium that I am the first subject (number 101) on Phase III of the IDEC Y2B8 clinical trial. The clinical trial is a random phase III trial of the monoclonal antibody Rituxan alone, versus Rituxan plus Yttrium; the sponsoring pharmaceutical company is IDEC. I got the hot version, that is, Rituxan with Yttrium. It's only two weeks of treatment. Week one, which was last week, consisted of getting Rituxan intravenously, then Indium, a mild gamma isotope, then scans the rest of the week to see how the liver and other organs uptake the indium and get rid of it. Then today I had Rituxan via IV again, and an injection of Yttrium, but no scan. I'm done except for blood draws weekly, and CT scans in three or four weeks. I feel weird, tired, and a bit nauseous, but this is absolutely nothing compared to chemotherapy. Something this easy can't work, right? I am a bit disheartened from reading that this treatment may work better on follicular NHL than on small lymphocytic lymphoma (SLL), which is my new diagnosis, but my oncologist said my tumor's CD20 cell surface markers were what's needed to qualify for this treatment. I'm looking forward to at least some months of remission—we'll see about a cure.

Eight weeks later, Marilyn reports:

My eight-week bone marrow biopsy flow cytometry results showed very low residual disease. However, my oncologist, who is Mr. Positive, said that eight weeks is purely arbitrary. He had a patient exactly like me (sure!) whose marrow showed complete remission not after eight weeks, but after twelve weeks. (Do you think he just loves to do bone marrow biopsies?) We are at a point that he says I should do a stem cell harvest in the meantime, in case I need a bone marrow transplant in the future. Okay. The good news is that there was a guy in the waiting room who did the Rituxan plus Yttrium thing a year and a half ago in the earlier phase I/II trial, and he's still in remission. Now if that will just rub off on me, I'll be a happy camper.

During one of my preliminary Indium scans before the real treatment started—during one of the sessions where I had to lie in an uncomfortable position for a half hour—the doctor, a physicist who calculates the effects of my scans, chatted with me and answered a lot of my questions. First of all, he said that in his opinion, chemotherapy as we know it today will be obsolete in five years, to be replaced by monoclonal antibody treatments. Secondly, he said that a lot of people are doing work on

lymphoma. He knows of many experiments on other monoclonal antibod-
ies which are in the very early stages. I asked him, "When I relapse, will I
be able to get more of the Yttrium?" He said, "Why do you think you'll
relapse? You should talk to your doctor, because we're thinking of this as a
cure." Of course I'm thinking he doesn't know what he's talking about, so I
pushed him further, and he said that I could get four doses of this much
Yttrium in my lifetime. So we'll see how long a remission this will give me
(times three), right? It does damage stem cells, but not enough to cause
concern. So I am so happy I can't stand it! I know that the oncology group
I am using is overly optimistic, but I'll take some good days. Why not
enjoy myself for a few days?

Experimental drugs outside clinical trials

There are several ways, other than clinical trials, to obtain drugs that are still in testing phases.

Investigational new drugs (IND)

Thanks to activism by AIDS patients, gaining early access to drugs still being tested is possible under the FDA's Treatment Investigational New Drug (IND) program, sometimes called the compassionate-use program. This access is reserved for those with life-threatening diseases that have no other satisfactory treatment. According to FDA statistics, more than 20,000 patients with cancer have received treatment under a treatment IND since 1987. For more information, contact your doctor, the drug manufacturer, and the FDA at (800) 532-4440.

Paralleling a trial

Once a drug is approved by the FDA for a given condition (commonly referred to as its indication), a doctor is free to prescribe this drug for any illness. This is called off-label use, and demonstrates the FDA's faith in the medical community's integrity and knowledge.

If a clinical trial is testing drugs that are already approved by the FDA, but in new combinations or at new dose levels, your doctor might be willing to administer these drugs to you as they would have been given within the trial. Contact your doctor for more information.

Importation of a foreign drug

If an illness has no cure using drugs currently approved by the FDA, drugs made in foreign countries might be imported. Only those drugs meeting strict FDA regulations, though, are permitted. Among other requirements, the manufacturer must file an investigational new drug application with the FDA, and a letter justifying importation must accompany the request. For more information, contact your doctor, and contact the FDA at:

CDER Executive Secretariat (HFD-8)
Center for Drug Evaluation and Research
5600 Fishers Lane
Rockville, MD 20857
(800) 532-4440

About payment

Many people have found that they have difficulty getting their insurance companies to approve payment for care administered under the auspices of a clinical trial or for an investigational new drug. One might surmise that, because cancer is a very expensive chronic disease, it would be to the financial benefit of insurance companies if better treatments were found. Nevertheless, individual companies often are unwilling to assume the costs of these studies. The trend, however, is that more companies are paying for trials than in the past, or can be convinced to make exceptions for those who need treatment in trials. The federal government has set a good example by ruling that federally insured employees will be covered for their treatment within NCI-sponsored clinical trials, and the state of Rhode Island has passed a law requiring insurance companies to pay for cancer clinical trials. The state of Maryland is assessing similar legislation that will require payment of fees for treatment given as part of a clinical trial for any illness, as long as the trial is approved by the National Institutes of Health.

Some cancer survivors have had success getting insurance payment approval by having their doctors supply evidence that previous tests of the new treatment showed some superiority over existing treatments, or by writing "letters of necessity" demonstrating that this experimental treatment is the only good choice available. Others have luck when their employers intervene. Still others use the news media to generate publicity that is embarrassing for the insurance company. Some cancer facilities offering clinical trials make provisions for those who want to participate but cannot pay. Compassionate-use programs may offer drugs at a reduced price.

Importation of foreign drugs for single-patient use under the FDA's strict guidelines will almost certainly be an expense you'll have to bear on your own, but do check with your health insurance company, as policies vary widely.

Listed below are several institutions that charge little or nothing for participating in clinical trials.

The National Cancer Institute in Bethesda, Maryland, offers free treatment for those who qualify for their trials. This is a top-notch scientific institution run by the federal government, having some of the best cancer researchers in the country. Those who have used their services sometimes say, though, that they were very aware that they were in a research setting, as opposed to a setting oriented toward patient care and comfort. Call (800) 4-CANCER.

Non-U.S. citizens are also admitted to trials at the NCI at the discretion of the principal investigator. Criteria that are weighed in making this decision include whether a U.S. citizen would be denied treatment if a non-U.S. citizen were enrolled, and whether treating this particular individual's illness would benefit medical progress.

For children being treated at the NCI, the Children's Inn at NCI provides free room and board for the children and their families. The Children's Inn accommodates both U.S. and non-U.S. citizens.

Shriners' Hospitals, twenty-two free children's hospitals across North America, are supported by the Shrine of North America, an international fraternity. These hospitals specialize in orthopedic and burn care. Children under age eighteen who suffer spinal cord injury from radiotherapy or who need joint replacements for avascular necrosis of bone that develops following steroid therapy for NHL might benefit from clinical trials offered at the Shriners' Hospitals. In the United States, call (800) 237-5055. In Canada, call (800) 361-7256.

The St. Jude Children's Research Hospital in Memphis, Tennessee, offers free treatment for children and is on the forefront of developing successful treatments for children's cancers. Highly successful treatment for childhood leukemia was developed at St. Jude's in conjunction with other pediatric cancer groups. Call (901) 495-3300.

Summary

The National Cancer Institute recommends that clinical trials, a means of testing new therapies in order to improve cancer treatment, can be a good choice for those with low-grade NHL, or intermediate- or high-grade NHL that has failed to respond to first-line therapy or has relapsed.

Clinical trials are organized into three phases that evaluate increasingly complex aspects of treatment success. Each phase has its advantages and disadvantages. A careful assessment of all clinical trials is necessary to choose the one that's best for your circumstances.

Patients' rights and safeguards are carefully observed in the clinical trial setting. You are free to withdraw at any time, and you cannot be denied care if you do so.

You can find information on clinical trials by asking your doctor, calling the National Cancer Institute at (800) 4-CANCER, or searching for trials on your own. See Chapter 24 for more information on searching for trials.

Being admitted to a trial may be preceded by a flurry of administrivia surrounding your evaluation that may thrill you with its cut-to-the-chase aspect, or may disappoint you with delays and miscommunications. The administrative offices of certain cancer care centers can be quite disorganized in spite of the institution's fine reputation for practicing excellent medicine.

Plan to have a friend or loved one act as an advocate for you during your treatment. Your emotional reactions might be surprising and conflicting, but overall you can probably expect to be confident that you've made a good choice.

CHAPTER 20

Transplantation

The art of healing comes from nature, not
from the physician. Therefore the physician
must start from nature, with an open mind.

—Paracelsus

Doctors have struggled for years against their inability to give some patients enough chemotherapy or radiation therapy to destroy all cancer cells. The barrier they face is that very large doses of radiation or chemotherapeutic drugs destroy other tissue along with cancerous cells, including the soft inner core of bone called bone marrow. Permanently destroying most or all marrow eventually results in death, because blood cells are made only within bone marrow. Bone marrow transplantation provides a solution to this problem.

Bone marrow transplantation was attempted in the 1930s and 1940s as a cure for aplastic anemia, but was abandoned after many failures later attributable to a lack of knowledge of tissue rejection factors. In the early 1950s, studies with mice revealed that bone marrow could regenerate itself following an ostensibly fatal dose of radiation if some of the marrow was saved before treatment and reinjected a few days after. By the late 1960s, some researchers, equipped with a somewhat better understanding of white blood cell compatibility and marrow regeneration, began once again to use marrow transplantation to treat some leukemias and lymphomas.

But suppose the marrow itself contains NHL cells, as is frequently the case for some subtypes? Reinserting one's own diseased marrow would seem risky—and it is. For these circumstances, either marrow purging or donor marrow is used.

At one time, transplantation was considered the last resort in treating cancers for which all other treatments had failed. This is no longer the case. Some highly reputable oncologists may recommend an immediate transplant at diagnosis for widely spread low-grade NHL, for patients with several bad-risk features, for lymphomas that are particularly aggressive, or at first relapse for other NHLs and many leukemias. Moreover, if the transplant fails, other options exist, such as boosting donor marrow to act against NHL or, if a transplant using your own marrow fails, retransplantation using donor marrow.

This chapter assumes you've made up your mind to proceed with transplantation after weighing the risks and benefits discussed in Chapter 6, *How the NHLs Are Treated*. We'll discuss what kinds of transplants are possible, who gets them, how they're performed, and where they're done. How to find a good transplant center and how you can prepare for your transplant are discussed as well. The responsibilities of a marrow donor are outlined. Even so, we're able only to touch on the main points of transplantation. For a more detailed discussion, see *Bone Marrow Transplants: a Book of Basics for Patients* by Susan Stewart.

Terminology

Terminology about transplants can be confusing. Even medical personnel tend to interchange terms such as marrow and stem cells, transplantation and marrow rescue. The following sections clarify the terms we'll use.

Transplant versus rescue

Although many people use the word "transplant" to describe any procedure involving reinfusion of blood precursors after marrow-suppressing (non-myeloablative) or marrow-destroying (myeloablative) treatment, a true transplant involves receiving marrow or blood products from a donor. When one's own blood products are used, the procedure is more correctly called a marrow or stem cell *rescue*. Nonetheless, many people, including many medical personnel, refer to both of these procedures as transplants.

Marrow versus peripheral stem cells

Stem cells are the young offspring of bone marrow, capable of becoming any kind of blood cell. They are found in the blood, but are found in greater abundance within bone marrow. They can be harvested from either, and when they are harvested from blood via a vein, a colony stimulating factor such as Neupogen, or certain chemotherapies such as cyclophosphamide and etoposide, or both in tandem, are sometimes used first to force more of them out of the marrow

Using peripheral stem cells in place of marrow appears to make no difference in the success rate of the transplant with respect to freedom from relapse. Accordingly, many transplant centers now use stem cells collected from the donor's or the patient's arm veins in place of bone marrow drawn from the hipbone. Stem cells from peripheral blood engraft more quickly than marrow upon reinfusion, and are less painful and less risky to harvest than marrow, because no anesthetic is required and the hipbone (iliac crest) does not need to be punctured.

In the discussion that follows, occasionally we will use the terms stem cell and marrow interchangeably.

Autologous transplants (rescues)

Autologous transplantation is performed using the patient's own stem cells or marrow. This procedure is also called marrow or stem cell rescue, autologous transplantation, or abbreviated as autologous transplant, ABMT, PSCT, or APSCT. It is done to allow extremely high, cancer-killing doses of anticancer therapies to be used—doses that also destroy most or all marrow—as opposed to a true transplantation from a donor, which aims to replace diseased marrow with healthy marrow.

As long as bone marrow appears unaffected by NHL, it's generally considered safe to reinfuse the patient's own marrow after high-dose chemotherapy and radiotherapy. Often, though, the marrow still is subjected to a purging process, either to kill cancer cells or to select healthy cells, even if no cancer cells are detected in it.

Donor transplants

There are several kinds of transplants performed using donor tissue, each having advantages and disadvantages. First, though, it's wise to have an understanding of how donors and recipients are matched to each other.

Matching haplotypes

Before a recipient's body can accept donor marrow or stem cells, testing must be done to ensure that the donor and recipient tissues can tolerate each other. This acceptance or rejection is mediated by proteins that extend from the surface of white blood cells. These sensors recognize and accept similar tissue, but trigger an attack against foreign tissue, including foreign white blood cells.

A sound knowledge of genetics, expensive equipment, and time are required to locate and analyze these white blood cell proteins in order to match donors and recipients properly. Engraftment failure, graft rejection by the host, or a very serious illness called graft-versus-host disease in which the donor's white blood cells attack the recipient's body organs may result from immune system mismatches. A closer match of white blood cell characteristics is required for marrow or stem cell transplantation than for other organ transplants, because it's the immune system itself that's being transplanted.

Currently, donors and recipients are matched on white blood cell characteristics, called haplotypes, that are controlled by certain genes on chromosome 6. Haplotypes HLA-A, HLA-B, and HLA-DR are always tested, with the DR locus being the most critical, but HLA-C is emerging as an important genetic site, or locus, on which to match as well. Nonetheless, currently only the first three are routinely tested for matching. Red blood cell type, commonly known as ABO typing, has no major effect on marrow compatibility.

Within these haplotypes are subtypes of almost inestimable variation. For this reason, the older serological testing method that uses intact white blood cells in a cross-reaction with others, called major histocompatibility (MHC) testing, is being replaced by direct testing of the genes extracted from the nucleus of the white blood cell—high-resolution DNA typing—for the more subtle differences in genetic makeup.

To make matters even more complex, each of us has two copies of each of these haplotypes, owing to our having inherited one copy of chromosome 6 from each parent. This means that the sites that must match actually are double the number discussed in the paragraphs above.

You'll hear matching success referred to as a 6 out of 6 match, or a 4 out of 6 match, and so on, abbreviated as 6/6 or 4/6. (As other genes are discovered to have a bearing on tissue rejection, eventually you'll hear the match described as a 7/8 or 8/8 match, an 8/10 or 10/10 match, and so on.) As newer direct DNA typing techniques become more common, you'll hear of matches on alleles—slightly different versions of the same gene—as well as the older term, haplotype matching. It's likely the two techniques will coexist for a time.

You inherit half of your genes from each parent. As a result, the odds of matching one parent's haplotypes are usually only three out of the currently used six genes, unless your parents are from a closely related ethnic community within which coupling outside of the tribe is discouraged.

Matching other family members is to some extent a roll of Mother Nature's dice. It's more likely that you will match a sibling, because genetic material of sibs is drawn from the same two sources, the parents. The odds of having a sibling match increase with the number of siblings you have. Fortunately, on some occasions a match can be found among first cousins.

Least likely of all is the chance that you will find a good match among those not related by blood. Nonetheless, in spite of these reduced odds, the National Marrow Donor Program now contains well over three million volunteers, among whom many matches for those needing transplants have indeed been found.

When a donor outside the family must be sought, problems may arise. African Americans and Asian Americans have white blood cell characteristics that are quite distinct, whereas Caucasian Americans, Latin Americans, and Native Americans have more white blood cell characteristics in common. This means that the full three million NMDP pool is not equally useful to all applicants. It's important to increase awareness of the need for marrow donors among ethnic groups. Friends and loved ones may join the NMDP by calling (800) MARROW-2. A blood sample only—not marrow—is required for donor testing.

Most transplant centers aim for a 6/6 match if an unrelated donor is used, and a 5/6 or 6/6 match if a related donor is used. A few centers specialize in transplantation using partially matched 3/6 or 4/6 related donors, and others are conducting clinical trials to improve partial-mismatch transplants. But many transplant centers still view partial mismatches as too risky within the constraints of technology that exist today.

More detailed discussions of inheritance and the calculation of odds of inheriting genes can be found in any textbook on genetics.

Allogeneic transplants

Allogeneic transplants are transplants using marrow or stem cells from someone who may or may not be a relative, but who is genetically *not identical* to the recipient. Allogeneic transplants are also known as allo-BMTs.

If an unrelated donor is used, very careful matching of white blood cell characteristics is done first, as described above under "Haplotypes," to reduce the chance of graft failure, graft rejection, or of very serious illness called graft-versus-host disease that may result from immune system mismatches.

If a related donor is used, careful matching of haplotypes is performed, but in general, fewer problems arise with a related donor, no doubt owing to the serendipitous matching of immune-related antigens of which we're not yet aware.

Preparation for an allogeneic transplant may differ from that used for an autologous transplant, because many transplant centers attempt to destroy the existing capacity of the patient's marrow to regenerate, regardless of the presence or absence of NHL in the marrow. It is thought that any remaining active marrow within the recipient may cause donor marrow to fail to engraft, or fail to replicate.

There are some studies underway, however, to test the effect of chimerism—a mixture of donor marrow and residual patient marrow—on NHL, and other studies are being performed to test the feasibility of converting the patient's marrow to donor marrow slowly, via repeated donor leukocyte infusions, without first destroying all of the patient's marrow.

Mary Butler describes her satisfaction with having had an allogeneic transplant:

> I had an allogeneic donor marrow transplant for (what my doctor now says was) intermediate-grade, mixed large- and small-cell, with sclerosis, follicular non-Hodgkin's lymphoma. I was in stage four by the time I was diagnosed, and also upon relapse after six rounds of CHOP.
>
> It's true my quality of life is diminished from what it was prior to diagnosis, but it beats being dead. I got to see my son graduate from high school and I also saw him set off for college. I share wonderful quality time with friends and family that I otherwise would not have experienced. I have had to adjust to chronic fatigue, but it is manageable and I can still do the things that matter most to me. I get to laugh, cry, see the

sunset, hug the people I love, see great movies, read good books, play on my computer, and so on.

I have come to accept that life is change. Everyone, whether there is a cancer diagnosis or not, has to adjust to some changes and to things that didn't go quite the way they had planned. I am a very happy person despite my limitations, and maybe in part because of them. It has taught me to let go, to stop wasting my time with things that don't really matter, because they are a waste of energy, and mostly to express my feelings and communicate with the people in my life.

I'm just delighted to be here, alive, still sucking in air. Without the transplant I would be dead. A choice between diminished and dead, for me, was clear.

Syngeneic transplants

Syngeneic transplants are transplants from an identical twin.

The earliest efforts at bone marrow transplantation for aplastic anemia in the 1930s succeeded most often when the donor was an identical twin. Until then, it was thought that the ABO red blood cell matching system was the important factor in successful transplantation. The likelihood that marrow donated by an identical twin would engraft where others failed gave a strong indication that other compatibility factors were at work.

With identical genes in marrow from both the donor and the recipient, no graft-versus-host problems are expected, but on rare occasions they do arise.

Transplants using an identical twin as a donor are slightly more likely to fail owing to relapse of NHL than transplants using matched related or matched unrelated donors. It appears that genetic makeup may play a role in the development of NHL; thus, receipt of marrow identical to one's own may provide a second hospitable environment for NHL. Another explanation might be that graft-versus-host disease, which usually arises following a transplant from a nonidentical donor but not from a twin, may also provide a graft-versus-lymphoma effect.

Umbilical cord blood transplants

Umbilical cord blood is rich in the precursor cells that develop into mature white cells, red cells, and platelets. More importantly, because the newborn child has had no opportunity to develop white blood cells that are trained to attack anything, including foreign tissue, the naive status of T-cells within umbilical cord blood makes it ideal for transplantation. While graft-versus-host disease may develop following an umbilical cord transplant from an unrelated donor, it's usually less pronounced than that which develops after using marrow from a mature donor.

In the last ten years, the public has been encouraged to donate or store umbilical cord blood, which is usually immediately discarded just after childbirth. Storage for one's own use or donation to a cord bank make these products available for future use by your family or others. To donate cord blood, call the National Cancer Institute at 1-800-4-CANCER or the International Cord Blood Foundation at (415) 635-1456.

At this time, cord blood from a single umbilical cord contains only enough material to transplant children or small adults. Research with combining cord blood from several donors to provide a larger volume is underway, as is research using technology to replicate cord blood stem cells.

Donor leukocyte infusion (buffy-coat infusion, adoptive immunotherapy)

Donor leukocyte infusion (DLI), also called adoptive immunotherapy or buffy-coat infusion, is usually done following an allogeneic transplant that has failed to engraft, following a relapse of NHL after allogeneic transplantation, or perhaps as part of a trial measuring the added success of following marrow infusion with leukocyte support. Mature white blood cells are collected from the donor in the same way stem cells or platelets are collected— several hours of apheresis, using two arm veins—and are infused into the NHL survivor.

Often, this boost of donor material will trigger engraftment or will cause an immune response to be mounted against the tumor. The price paid is an increase in the likelihood of graft-versus-host attacks against body organs, which can cause serious illness.

Who gets which transplant?

Several factors must enter into your decision to choose a transplant technique. Your general health, what kind of NHL you have, and whether any suitable marrow donors exist are a few of these factors.

Type of disease

The type of NHL you have can impact whether an autologous or allogeneic transplant is recommended.

Some researchers believe that certain NHLs are best treated with an allogeneic transplant, especially when NHL has invaded the marrow, but the different types of NHL vary widely in their response to high-dose treatment. This variation makes it impossible to say that all NHLs that involve bone marrow should be treated with an allogeneic transplant. In fact, Burkitt's lymphoma and the Burkitt-like lymphomas of adulthood respond well to brief-intensity, high-dose treatment *without* transplantation; in these instances, your marrow might be harvested and held in reserve for future autologous transplantation should you relapse.

Your doctor is your best source of information about how your specific subtype of NHL impacts the choice of allogeneic versus autologous transplants.

Age

In the past few years, the upper age limit for treatment with autologous transplantation techniques has climbed steadily from about age 40 in 1991 to age 60 and beyond.

Many transplant centers are reluctant to treat patients over age sixty with allogeneic techniques, however, owing to the severity of side effects following allogeneic transplant. There are isolated instances, though, of patients well beyond age sixty being transplanted with sibling marrow following high-dose therapy. Donor transplants are not yet commonly performed in this age group, however.

If you have Internet access, you can visit the National Cancer Institute's clinical trials database (*http://cancernet.nci.nih.gov/prot/protsrch.shtml*) and read the entry criteria for clinical trials of transplants. You'll see that some trials specify the upper limit of age as "physiological age 65," or a similar phrase. This means that a patient older than sixty-five might be accepted if he or she is judged to be otherwise as physically sound as most people aged sixty-five.

In short, your state of health may be more important than your age in determining what treatment you can withstand.

Other health factors

In general, other health problems that existed before your diagnosis with NHL may cause your doctor to consider an autologous transplant instead of an allogeneic transplant, because the side effects and long-term effects of an autologous transplant are less severe than with allogeneic transplantation.

Availability of donors

Even if your doctor believes that your subtype of NHL is best treated with an allogeneic transplant, the lack of a suitable and willing donor may leave autologous transplant as the only choice.

Which type of transplant is better?

In general, autologous transplants are physically easier to sustain, and have better survival statistics associated with the treatment itself, while allogeneic transplants may be more effective in protecting against NHL relapse, but entail a higher risk of death associated with treatment alone. As marrow purging techniques improve, the success rate of autologous transplants against NHL may approach those of allogeneic transplants.

The NHL patient usually has a much easier time recovering and far fewer long-term side effects from an autologous transplant than from an allogeneic transplant using donor marrow. On the other hand, transplants with marrow or blood products from a related or unrelated donor who is not genetically identical to the recipient appear to have an antilymphoma effect, called graft-versus-lymphoma (GVL), suggesting that either genetic differences or graft-versus-host interactions are meaningful in controlling lymphomas.

As of this writing, the mortality rate associated with high-dose transplant-related treatment procedures alone, as opposed to mortality from NHL, is about 3 percent for autologous transplantation and about 20 percent for allogeneic transplantation.

Finding a donor—quickly

When your health team determines that your subtype of NHL is best treated with an allogeneic transplant, the search for a donor must begin. In some cases, if the NHL is transforming to a higher, more aggressive type, the search must move quickly.

The best place to start the search is within your own family, owing to the increased likelihood of finding a very good match among close relatives, as described above under "Matching haplotypes." In many of today's smaller families, however, a good match might not be found. It may be necessary to search among unrelated donors for a good match.

Some donor centers typically test about ten donor blood samples per patient per day, but if they are made aware of the need for haste, they may be able to test up to one hundred samples per day. Some cancer survivors have found that this is an area in which their direct and personal communication efforts make a real difference.

If you're aware of your ethnic heritage, you might consider publicizing your need for donor testing in your community or in similar ethnic communities around the country. Ask ethnic associations to spread the word to other cities and states. You might also try asking local radio and TV stations for air coverage. Most have a consumer advocate or goodwill officer who will be glad to listen to you.

It would be a mistake, though, to rely only on your ethnic group(s) for help, because some ethnic groups share white blood cell characteristics with many others. Europeans—in spite of ethnic pride and ongoing squabbles in some parts of Europe—are almost indistinguishable from each other with respect to haplotype, with a few exceptions such as the closed communities of Gypsies, originally from India. This means that a donor drive targeted only to a U.S. Lithuanian community will miss many potential matches in Scandinavian, German, Polish, Russian, or French U.S. communities.

It's also wise to ask what your haplotypes are, and research which ethnic groups have the highest percentage of these haplotypes so that you can better target your recruiting efforts:

> After I volunteered to become a marrow donor, out of curiosity I asked the bone marrow coordinator at Johns Hopkins to read me my haplotypes. Using a few reference texts, I discovered that my haplotypes are not most often found in the ethnic groups my family lays claim to, but instead are much more common among Hispanics, American Indians, and Asians. One of my six haplotypes is found more often among Jewish people than among the groups our family claims as ancestors.

See the bibliography and Appendix A, *Resources,* for references you can use to verify which ethnic groups have the highest frequencies of your haplotypes. In particular, the 1996 text by Cavalli-Sforza is an excellent reference, and an abridged version now is available in paperback. The National Marrow Donor Program's recent research paper on the frequency of haplotypes in North America is available on the Web.

You should also make sure all donor registries are contacted. In addition to the NMDP, try:

- American Bone Marrow Donor Registry Search Coordinating Center, Patient Search Information: 1-800-7-A-MATCH (1-800-726-2824)
- International Bone Marrow Transplant Registry: (414) 456-8325

How transplants are done

The several steps of transplantation are described below: preparation for transplant, induction therapy to achieve a remission, harvest of marrow or stem cells, purging marrow or stem cells, consolidation (high-dose therapy), reinfusion of marrow, and isolation.

Preparation

Before you can undergo the high doses of chemotherapy and radiation therapy used in transplantation, you must be tested to determine if you're healthy enough to withstand this treatment, and to establish base lines against which organ function can be measured later. In an outpatient setting, your heart, lungs, kidneys, and liver will be assessed, and a dental examination will be done. If one or more of your body systems is weak, the drug regimen used for the transplant may be modified to spare that organ more damage.

A venous catheter will be inserted under your skin, most likely in your upper chest, to deliver chemotherapy directly into the large veins near your heart instead of using arm veins. Having a catheter in place will benefit you in these ways:

- Using a catheter for blood draws will spare you repeated punctures with IVs and needles.
- It can save your arm veins from damage, as the veins near the heart are of much wider diameter than arm veins, and so are less affected by drugs.

- The catheter's location near the heart will assure that drugs are pumped evenly and quickly to all parts of the body.

- Apheresis, the collection of various blood cells such as platelets and stem cells from blood, is easier and more comfortable when a catheter is used. When arms veins must be used, one vein in each arm must be used simultaneously: the first to withdraw blood, and the other to return the blood to your body.

- A central venous catheter might be used as access to the vein in which it resides to measure important body functions such as central venous pressure (CVP), which help your doctor determine the amount of IV fluids a patient needs.

- If mouth sores become severe and you cannot eat, parenteral nutrition will be necessary. Due to the thickness of these feeding solutions, they will cause arm veins to become terribly sore if infused into an arm vein. Having access to a larger vein via a catheter will be an asset.

Several kinds of catheters are available. See Chapter 5, *Tests and Procedures*, for a discussion of the advantages of different kinds of catheters.

An NHL survivor describes how having a catheter inserted turned out to be a much easier experience than she had imagined:

> *My doctor had planned to send me to a well-known cancer center for the stem cell harvest. I would not have had so much trouble with this had he not also told me I would need a Hickman catheter for that procedure, since it would involve higher pressure in the lines. I was weak, exhausted, and suffering from horrific headaches, which the doctor attributed to stress and I did not. I dreaded the thought of a five-minute, much less a two-hour car ride. Every movement or sound seemed torturous, and I had never had any history of migraines or similar ailments.*
>
> *More than that, I was viscerally repulsed by the thought of the surgery given my experience with the insertion of the Groshong catheter. I seriously considered not undergoing any apheresis. I don't know how I finally talked myself into going ahead with the catheter insertion, but I may have reacted to my husband's appeals to my sense of what was the right thing to do.*
>
> *My reward was to find that the surgery was a magical thing…both my husband and I told anyone who would listen what my fears were. It*

seemed to be a routine matter for the staff to respond. It is amazing what
a pinch of anesthesia will do—just enough to put you to sleep while the
local is administered, yet allow you to be awake for the rest of the proce-
dure.

In general, you'll feel best if your room is like home, and if you have your own comfortable clothing to wear. Transplant units sometimes limit the kinds of materials, including gifts, that can enter your room. Some allow only what can be autoclaved: cotton clothing, books, and so on. Their rules are geared to the period of time during which you'll have no functioning white blood cells and will be vulnerable to infection.

If your child is being transplanted, see Nancy Keene's book *Childhood Leukemia*, which contains an excellent chapter on transplantation for children. This book is particularly suitable if you have a child with NHL being treated on an ALL protocol.

Induction therapy

For lymphomas and leukemias, an induction phase may be used first to try to induce a remission before transplantation. Induction resembles standard chemotherapy, although the doses may be somewhat higher than you've had in the past, or the drugs used may differ. Because it's so much like first-line chemotherapy, the induction phase may be done in your hometown by your local oncologist, even if your transplant is to be done out of town.

Some people do not achieve remission in the induction phase before going ahead with the transplant. Often this is of some, but not of overwhelming concern to the medical team, because the high-dose treatment you'll receive soon after will destroy any remaining NHL. For some subtypes of NHL, being in remission first may improve your chances of survival, but keep in mind that prognoses and survival are very much a function of treatment, that new treatments are always being devised, and that the subtypes of NHL vary too widely to generalize.

Patient's harvest

If you're having an autologous transplant, the harvest will be done now, before high-dose treatments are started, and kept frozen (cryopreserved) until your high-dose treatment has ended.

Marrow

If stem cells from marrow will be used, you'll be given a general anesthetic for the procedure, and you may have an overnight stay in the hospital. Four to six very small cuts that do not require stitches are made in the skin over your hipbones, and many punctures through the bone, into the dozens, are made to withdraw about a quart of marrow. About twice as much marrow is withdrawn from a patient than from a donor to compensate for the possibility of damaged, unproductive, or cancerous marrow, and to freeze extra against the possibility that the first infusion does not engraft.

You may have a sore derriere for a few days to a week after this procedure. You may feel as if you slipped on ice and landed on your bottom. You may also feel tired and lightheaded for a day or two. Anesthesia alone can cause these feelings of fatigue.

Peripheral stem cells

Many transplant centers now use stem cells collected from your arm veins or your catheter (depending on type) in place of bone marrow drawn from the hipbone. The collecting of stem cells in this way is called apheresis. The blood is drawn from one arm vein or from one catheter lumen, passes through sterile equipment used one time only, and is returned to your body via the other arm vein or second catheter lumen after stem cells have been separated from your blood.

There are fewer stem cells in circulating blood than there are in marrow, but the number of circulating stem cells can be boosted if drugs known as colony stimulating factors, natural body products that can be replicated in the pharmaceutical lab, are first administered. Granulocyte colony stimulating factor (G-CSF) or granulocyte-macrophage colony stimulating factor (GM-CSF) is administered by injection under the skin several times in the week before harvesting. G-CSF or GM-CSF may make your bones and joints feel sore. Ice packs and Tylenol should relieve this pain. GM-CSF may also cause fever, lung or heart inflammation. Call your doctor if you have fever, chest pain, or difficulty breathing.

The apheresis session will probably last several hours. The nursing staff will have movies you can watch and blankets to warm you, because the blood that is returned to your body will have cooled and will make you feel chilled.

Very rarely, an allergic reaction to the anticlotting agent used in the apheresis equipment may occur. If you feel shortness of breath or hives, let the nurse know. Generally, they're at your side throughout the entire procedure.

The anticlotting agent may reduce the calcium supply in your blood. If you sense an unusual heartbeat, feel numbness around the mouth, tingling sensations, or weakness, tell the nursing staff immediately. Intravenous calcium will be given to you.

It's not unusual for an NHL survivor to have to undergo repeated hemaphereses, perhaps up to six times, until enough stem cells are collected, because NHL or its previous treatment sometimes compromises the marrow's ability to produce stem cells.

> *The calculation based on my body weight did not require a long series of attempts to harvest enough stem cells. It only took four days. The Hickman catheter presented a few problems in terms of balky access, but it was nursed along.*

Donor's harvest

The harvesting of marrow or stem cells from a donor is very much like that for the patient, described above in "Patient's harvest," with a few exceptions:

- The marrow is usually not frozen. Instead, it is collected and used immediately. If the donor is an unrelated donor found through the NMDP, the marrow is collected locally, then chilled and flown to the transplant center. It's no longer the case that the donor must be flown to the transplant center.

- Much less marrow—only about a pint or two—is taken because donor marrow is presumed to be healthy.

- If peripheral stem cells are used, usually fewer apheresis sessions are needed to collect an adequate supply from a healthy person.

- The donor's body will replace marrow and stem cells in three to four weeks.

- Side effects from either procedure and recovery time are likely to be less pronounced for the donor than for the patient whose own marrow is used.

Purging marrow or stem cells

Before the collected marrow or stem cells are put into your body, they are cleaned and sorted. Healthy blood precursor cells from marrow must be separated from pieces of bone, fat globules, red cells, mature white cells, platelets, and, most importantly, from cancerous cells. Stem cells that have been apheresed must be separated from mature white blood cells and from cancerous cells.

Although purging cancerous cells from marrow or stem cells is not always done, many researchers feel that it's wise to purge marrow, because small amounts of NHL may have lodged there. If your marrow was found to contain NHL, it's likely that marrow purging will be performed.

Marrow or stem cells that have been purged of all mature white blood cells may take longer to engraft. Some transplant centers prefer to leave certain types of some mature white blood cells in the mix to facilitate a good engraftment, but their presence may increase the chances of graft-versus-host disease (GVHD). Most transplant physicians strive for a balance of good engraftment versus GVHD.

Purging can be done using several techniques, but these techniques fall into two categories: destroying cancerous cells, or separating and saving healthy stem cells.

Much research is underway on selecting only healthy cells. Healthy stem cells, for instance, express a surface antigen identified as CD34 that cancerous cells do not express. CD34+ (CD34 positive) selection techniques also permit a one-step method to separate stem cells from mature white blood cells.

Consolidation (high-dose therapy, conditioning, mobilization)

For an autologous transplant, high-dose therapy follows the harvesting of marrow. If donor marrow is to be used, high-dose treatment of the patient may coincide with donor marrow harvesting. This high-dose therapy is called consolidation or consolidation of remission, and is also referred to as high-dose therapy, conditioning, or mobilization.

The purpose of high-dose conditioning is threefold: to kill all cancer cells; to vacate the marrow, leaving space for inbound stem cells to engraft and grow;

and to reduce the chance of a host-versus-graft attack that your body will mount against incoming donated stem cells.

Many different chemotherapeutic regimens are used for high-dose treatment of NHL, and new combinations are always being tried. Your oncologic team will choose a combination of drugs that will best preserve your organ function while optimizing the killing of all remaining cancer cells. Some drugs being used in various combinations as of this writing are cyclophosphamide, busulfan, etoposide, carmustine, cytarabine, melphalan, and cisplatin, but other drugs and new combinations are always being assessed for superiority. Usually, high-dose chemotherapy is administered over two or three days.

Radiotherapy may also be used, and in several ways. Irradiation of only the tumor may be done to reduce its bulk, either during the consolidation phase or at the original site of the tumor after the transplant. Total body irradiation (TBI), which if used in sufficiently high doses destroys all bone marrow, is used when marrow is diseased, when donor marrow is going to be used, or when the subtype of NHL is such that a relapse in the marrow is likely if TBI is not used as a preventive treatment.

When TBI is used as part of consolidation, the dosage is spread over several days. This spreading, called fractionating the dose, permits more radiation to be given than the body would be able to withstand were it given in one large dose.

Reinfusion of marrow

Reinfusion, which is done in your room using your catheter, takes thirty minutes to several hours. Marrow and stem cells are reinfused using an IV line, much like any IV drug. Although the marrow is warmed before it's given to you, you may still feel cold as it's being infused.

Some NHL survivors consider the reinfusion of marrow an anticlimax after high-dose treatment. Others have a celebration while it's being infused, especially if they searched long and hard for a donor.

Marrow or stem cells are not reinfused until one or two days after high-dose consolidation treatment has ended in order to allow chemotherapy and radiotherapy time to have maximum effect against cancer, and to allow these and other toxins to exit the body. Too lengthy a delay would endanger the patient, though, because reinfused marrow takes two to four weeks to engraft. During that time, the patient must be protected from all pathogens because he is incapable of mounting an immune response.

During reinfusion, you may experience fever, chills, hives, shortness of breath, or chest pains. If so, tell the nursing staff immediately. They'll give you antihistamines to curb the allergic reaction.

Isolation

Within five to ten days following your high-dose therapy, you will experience a profound drop in white blood cell counts as your marrow dies. At this point, you have no immune system to protect you from bacteria, fungi, or viral agents until the reinfused marrow engrafts and begins producing new white blood cells. This process takes from eighteen to thirty-six days, or, in rare instances, longer.

To avoid infection, you will be kept in isolation until your new marrow engrafts and becomes productive. Isolation requirements differ among transplant centers, with some having rigorous curtailment of visitors and confinement in laminar airflow rooms. Others simply require visitors to wear masks and wash hands upon entry. Check with your treatment center about visitors, and gifts that are considered sterile or sterilizable, before your transplant begins.

Some transplantation protocols require administration of colony stimulating factors after reinfusion to encourage the new marrow to produce white cells more quickly.

Common side effects

Most side effects of high-dose treatment begin to appear several days after treatment ends. This means you may have just a bit of time to enjoy your new marrow, and then you may feel poorly for a few days or weeks.

In general, those receiving an allogeneic transplant are likely to feel worse and to have a longer recovery period than those receiving an autologous transplant, especially if an acute case of graft-versus-host disease develops.

Many patients who receive their own marrow have no side effects or minimal side effects that are easily controlled with medication. One autologous transplant recipient reports the ease with which she dealt with the procedure:

I am feeling so, so great. I sailed through the transplant with no nausea, vomiting, or diarrhea. The only side effects I experienced were throat and anal pain due to sores from the chemotherapy, and the skin peeled off those areas. I am feeling just about back to my precancer self, except for being tired and still needing to lose the forty pounds that I gained. I have to return for tests in a few weeks, including CT scans and gallium scans. Then I will be restaged, although I think that I am in complete remission. After that I will be getting low-dose "mop-up" radiation followed by four rounds of chemotherapy (once every three months for one year).

Many of the side effects experienced during and after transplantation resemble those of standard-dose treatment, and can be found in Chapter 9, *Side Effects of Treatment*. Listed here are the side effects specific to transplant recipients, and how they're managed:

- **Fungal infection.** Although neutropenia and infection are discussed in the chapter on the side effects of treatment, fungal infection is of particular concern to transplant recipients because these infections can spread widely throughout the body and can be difficult to eradicate. If your transplant team suspects a fungal infection, cultures to confirm this will be done, and you may be placed on antifungal medication such as amphotericin.

- **Veno-occlusive disease.** (VOD) The high-dose treatment you're given may cause blood vessels in your liver to swell shut, a potentially fatal reaction. There is a higher risk of VOD if you first develop a fever, or are receiving an allogeneic transplant or a second transplant. If VOD develops, it's most likely to happen one to four weeks after the transplant. You may have pain in the upper right abdomen, swelling, jaundice, or fluid in the chest or abdomen. Supportive care is given for VOD, which usually goes away on its own. Cessation of drugs that stress the liver helps to ease the condition.

- **Viral hepatitis.** Many viruses that are latent in our bodies are able to take advantage of an immune-suppressed state, and can settle in the liver. There's no cure for a viral infection except time and good supportive care, although immunoglobulins and antiviral drugs can shorten the duration of some infections if they're given soon enough.

- **Acute graft-versus-host disease.** If you receive donor marrow, you may develop acute graft-versus-host disease (GVHD). Caused by white blood cells attacking liver, blood vessels, skin, the gastrointestinal tract, and other tissues, it can be controlled by immunosuppressive drugs. Earliest signs of GVHD appear as a rash or peeling on the skin of the hands and feet. At its most severe, GVHD can be fatal if it is not controlled.

- **Drowsiness, mental confusion.** Many transplant recipients report undesirable cognitive effects, particularly from TBI or cranial irradiation. This condition cannot be treated directly, but good nutrition, rest, and time may improve cognitive skills within a few weeks, although some transplant recipients report lingering effects years afterward.

- **Pneumonia, pneumonitis, adult respiratory distress syndrome (ARDS).** If you develop a dry cough or difficult, painful, rapid breathing within about two months after your transplant, you may have pneumonia, pneumonitis, or ARDS. Viruses such as cytomegalovirus (CMV) can cause pneumonia; radiation therapy can cause pneumonitis or pulmonary fibrosis; some chemotherapies can cause pneumonitis. Treatment depends on the diagnosis.

Engraftment

Everyone eagerly awaits engraftment. As time passes, many transplant recipients begin to worry a bit.

It takes about fourteen to twenty-eight days for marrow to engraft, but sometimes longer. Engraftment is presumed to have occurred when the patient's absolute neutrophil count or ANC—the number of mature white blood cells—begins to rise, as tracked by daily blood tests. Sometimes the rise is not steady. The counts may waver back and forth over several days, but the overall trend should be upward. It may be months or even years for the new marrow to produce enough cells to equal the amounts usually found among the general population, values called the normal range, although this is a somewhat arbitrary range that changes with age.

In general, stem cells will engraft more quickly than marrow. Those who have received an autologous transplant will engraft more quickly and produce adequate numbers of cells sooner than those who have received an allogeneic transplant.

Failure to engraft

Marrow sometimes fails to engraft well or at all. This can be detected in several ways:

- For an allogeneic transplant, genetic testing reveals that the marrow being produced is still the patient's marrow, not the donor's. This may pose a risk of relapse if the patient's marrow was found to contain NHL before the transplant.

- For an allogeneic transplant, the marrow is chimeric: a mixture of donor and patient marrow. This phenomenon is not well understood, but it is thought that a risk of relapse may be present if the patient's marrow was found to contain NHL before the transplant.

- For either an allogeneic or autologous transplant, the numbers of cells produced never reach normal levels. This is a poor engraftment rather than a failure to engraft.

A failure to engraft can be addressed with a second transplant, an infusion of additional donor white blood cells, a second infusion of more of the patient's own saved marrow or stem cells—or time, because sometimes very late engraftments occur. Failures to engraft are seen more often with marrow or stem cells purged of all mature lymphocytes than with unpurged products.

Outpatient follow-up

Many transplant centers are shifting their aftercare procedures to the outpatient setting. You may be released from the inpatient unit when your absolute neutrophil count in blood exceeds 500 on two consecutive days. If so, you will be expected to stay nearby for several weeks to facilitate care during possible medical emergencies, and for blood testing several times a week. Other tests will be performed from time to time, such as bone marrow biopsies to verify the productivity of marrow and the continued absence of NHL. You may be placed temporarily on antibiotic, antifungal, or antiviral medications as a precaution if your blood counts remain low.

The high-dose drugs used during a transplant can cause a form of depression known as chemical depression. Antidepressants are recommended, if needed.

It will take several months or more, perhaps up to a year, to recover from a transplant, although there is tremendous variability in individual recovery times. You may need to stay away from work for most or all of this time, depending on the health risks your job poses. Contact with small children or hard manual labor, for instance, might be considered large risks.

Pets after transplant

Transplant centers differ in their recommendations about being near family pets after transplantation. Some recommend complete avoidance; others recommend that the patient and the pets stay in separate parts of the house for the first few months; still others recommend avoiding handling the pet's bedding, smooching, and being licked or scratched. You should ask your discharge staff and your doctor what's best, but many post-transplant patients find that their veterinarians are better informed than human doctors about diseases that are contagious from animals, called zoonotic diseases.

In general, hand washing after handling pets is recommended, as well as delegating the task of cleaning waste from the kitty pan, the birdcage, and backyard dog droppings to someone else.

Toxoplasmosis frequently is mentioned as a special concern. Most cases of human toxoplasmosis are traced to eating undercooked meat, but there is a possible risk from contact with the feces of an infected cat. The risk of toxoplasmosis from cat feces is limited to those who come in direct contact with feces that are more than twenty-four hours old, as the eggs of *T. gondii* take twenty-four hours to hatch. Only those patients with cats that have an active case are at risk—usually those with kittens, as older cats have developed immunity long since. Outdoor cats, and indoor cats who catch mice, are potentially exposed to Toxoplasma gondii.

If you are told you must remove your pets from your home, you don't need to "get rid of them." You can find a temporary caretaker, a friend or relative, perhaps, or someone your veterinarian recommends. Your veterinarian may agree to board your pets at a reduced rate.

Long-term effects

Most long-term effects are discussed in Chapter 16, *Late Effects, Late Complications*; only those specific to transplantation are discussed here.

Chronic GVHD

If you have had an allogeneic transplant, there exists an ongoing risk of graft-versus-host disease.

(It is rare, but not impossible, to develop any form of GVHD, acute or chronic, after an autologous or syngeneic transplant. Researchers have experimented with deliberately creating GVHD in those who have had an autologous transplant for its graft-versus-lymphoma effect by administering and abruptly withdrawing immunosuppressive drugs.)

Unlike acute graft-versus-host disease, which appears soon after the transplant, chronic graft-versus-host disease (GVHD) appears three or more months afterward. It's less serious than acute GVHD, emerges less abruptly, can be controlled more easily, and is seldom fatal. Usually the skin is affected first, exhibiting itching, scaliness, or rash, although any organ can be affected, such as glands in the eyes or mouth. Often liver enzyme values in blood will become elevated, signaling the beginning of chronic GVHD. Graft-versus-host disease can affect connective tissue, tightening tendons and making movement painful.

Alexandre Azevedo, M.D., transplantation specialist, says:

> Chronic GVHD impairs the immune system, rendering the patient highly susceptible to recurrent bacterial infections. Most of these infections are caused by bacteria such as Haemophilus influenzae and Streptococcus pneumoniae. Most often, patients have recurrent upper respiratory infections of the sinuses and throat. These infections should always be regarded as potentially dangerous in patients with chronic GVHD, in whom the risk of disseminated infection (sepsis) is always a concern. Most often, these patients receive long (sometimes lifelong) courses of prophylactic antibiotics such as penicillin or erythromycin. Post-transplant immunization against common pathogens is not reliable in the presence of chronic GVHD because of the severe immunologic dysfunction that is associated with the disease, as well as with its treatment with immunosuppressants.

Some researchers believe that a small amount of GVHD is beneficial against NHL. For this reason, the immunosuppressive medications you will be given may be carefully titrated to allow some GVHD to develop, but not enough to cause serious health problems.

Chronic graft-versus-host disease may eventually burn itself out, but usually not for five or more years.

Complications of immunosuppressive medication

Immunosuppressive drugs given to control GVHD pose their own risks.

Chief among these is the increased risk of infection. Those taking immuno-suppressive drugs should take care to avoid breaking the skin, avoid crowds, thoroughly wash and cook all foods, postpone receipt of live vaccines, and avoid those who have had live vaccines. Check with your doctor about avoiding other risks, such as bacteria and fungi in soil that you may contact while gardening. Most transplant centers provide extensive information about such precautions.

Long-term use of immunosuppressive drugs such as cyclosporine may raise blood levels of lipids and cholesterol in some people, increasing the risk of blocked arteries. Different immunosuppressives can be substituted, cyclosporine levels can be adjusted, or cholesterol-lowering drugs can be prescribed.

Cyclosporine acts chiefly on T cells, disturbing the upward cascade of the immune response to threat by interfering with the action of interleukin 2 (IL-2). Certain cancers are known to be more likely among those whose T-cell function is suppressed, and many of these cancers are virally induced:

- NHL is about one hundred times more likely to develop among those with lowered levels of T cells than among the general population. It's usually a type of polyclonal NHL associated with Epstein-Barr virus (EBV) that usually regresses if T-cell function is restored by lowering the dosage of immunosuppressive drugs.

- Kaposi's sarcoma, a cancer induced by a human herpesvirus, may appear on the skin or in other organs, and is more prevalent among those whose T-cell function is suppressed.

- Melanomas are more likely among those with suppressed T-cell function.

Other late complications

Shingles, cataracts, peripheral neuropathy, kidney and liver function, infertility, weakness, fatigue, and cognitive and emotional problems as well as other problems may appear following a transplant. See Chapter 16 on late effects and Chapter 17, *Sexuality, Fertility and Pregnancy,* for discussions of these conditions.

Choosing a transplant center

Bone marrow transplantation is a lengthy, serious procedure. It demands state-of-the-art medical expertise and a good deal of experience to succeed.

Your medical insurance carrier may constrain your ability to pick a transplant center if they have contracted for this service with a particular group. It may be possible for you to convince them you should have it done elsewhere if you can prove that another center is better at handling your particular circumstances.

The American Society of Clinical Oncology and the American Society of Hematology have drafted a joint standard that specifies that a transplant center must do ten or more transplants per year in order to be certified. This guideline may be too broad for your circumstances, though. You may believe that the center that has done the most transplants for NHL, or a center that specializes in autologous or allogeneic transplants for NHL, is the best choice.

A transplant center's experience reflects to some degree the areas of expertise of the researchers involved and the kind of research for which they've succeeded in getting funds. Some transplant centers specialize in transplantation from unrelated donors; others prefer to transplant only patients who have a related donor. A few centers specialize in doing mismatched transplants. Still others specialize in treating children.

You also need to assess the center for more practical aspects such as any nearby housing they may provide, and psychological, emotional, and educational support for your family. A center with a lengthy waiting list, for instance, will not be a good choice if your NHL is converting to a more aggressive grade.

Here are resources you can use to choose a transplant center:

- Every two years, the Oncology Nursing Society publishes an extensive guide to transplant centers. You may call them at (412) 921-7373.

- The Blood and Marrow Transplant Newsletter contains useful information for choosing a center. Their phone number is (847) 831-1913, and you'll find their web site listed in Appendix A.

- The National Cancer Institute's Cancer Information Service (CIS) at (800) 4-CANCER can refer you to transplant centers that specialize in NHL.

- The National Marrow Donor Program has a booklet on transplantation using an unrelated donor. Call (800) 654-1247 or (800) 526-7809.

Getting insurance company approval

In 1998, the average cost of a transplant was $160,000, with prices ranging from $75,000 to $200,000. Costs for long-term follow-up care over the years can easily approach half a million dollars or more.

Owing to this extraordinary expense, some insurance companies scrutinize closely any medical plan that involves a marrow transplant. Staff with no medical training may use arbitrary means to deny approval, such as saying that transplantation for your disease is an experimental procedure, and thus not covered by your policy.

If your employer offers an open enrollment period annually—a period during which no previously existing medical conditions can be held against you—use this opportunity to upgrade your policy to the most liberal one offered.

Until legislation provides cancer survivors with fully reimbursed access to clinical trials, this battle is in your court. To overrule insurance company objections, you need to be familiar with state-of-the-art treatment for your subtype of NHL. See Chapter 24, *Researching Your Lymphoma*, for help in finding the latest and most reliable information about treatment of NHL.

If you're not satisfied with your insurance company's decision, do challenge it. Ask your oncologist for a "letter of necessity," and ask your employer to intervene, a tactic that is surprisingly successful, especially for those working for companies that are self-insured.

Self-insured companies often have their plans administered by an independent health insurance firm, but always pay the cost of your treatment from their own pocket. This means that, if you're working for a self-insured company, your employer, not the insurance company, is denying you payment. This is a sensitive situation you can turn to your benefit by arguing that it's in the company's best interest to keep you healthy or, more frankly, to avoid your embarrassing them.

Only a fraction of an insurance company's clients ever challenge the insurance company's decisions. The funds saved on the majority who are silent easily pay the costs of the few who do challenge these rulings. The Blood and Marrow Transplant Newsletter has a list of lawyers who specialize in transplant approval problems.

You might want to consider using a facility that has few or no charges. Free treatment is provided at the National Cancer Institute in Bethesda, Maryland, but within clinical trials only. Treatment for children is free at the St. Jude Research Hospital in Memphis, Tennessee. Some transplant centers will work out a financial repayment agreement with you if you are left with an unusually high bill after health insurance reimbursement. In some states, state-funded hospitals must provide you with care if you are unable to pay.

For more information on financing a transplant, see Chapter 14, *Insurance, Finances, Employment, Record-Keeping*.

Becoming a donor

Only 20 to 30 percent of patients needing allogeneic transplants are able to find a donor because there are too few donors in the marrow registries.

Family and friends of those with NHL should consider joining the National Marrow Donor Program. A blood sample only—not marrow—is used for testing.

Many who have donated marrow describe it as one of the most fulfilling experiences of their life, second only to becoming a parent. Most say they will do it again, eagerly and without hesitation, if called.

A decision to become a marrow or stem cell donor is a serious commitment. You must remain on call, be willing to undergo additional blood testing, and be willing to donate as soon as you're called, regardless of your other plans, including vacation plans or any minor illnesses. You will be responsible for saving a life. A donor should never back out of donating once treatment of the patient has begun, because often this treatment is intended to destroy all of the patient's marrow. Without donor marrow at this point, the patient will die. The process of harvesting marrow or stem cells is described above in the section called "Donor's harvest."

After you have donated, you may be asked to donate again later for the same patient if she relapses. Often the second donation is simply an apheresis of stem cells or mature white blood cells, even if marrow was used the first time.

Once you have donated for a patient, you will not be considered eligible to donate for a second patient for twelve months.

If you donated marrow or stem cells to an unrelated patient through the National Marrow Donor Program, you and the patient may contact each other after one year, if both agree.

You may join the NMDP by calling (800) MARROW-2.

Summary

Having a marrow or stem cell transplant is one of the riskiest and most intense forms of treatment for NHL. Being well-prepared makes the journey a much easier and less frightening one.

Much more can be said on the topics touched on in this chapter. For an in-depth description of transplantation from the patient's perspective, see Sue Stewart's 170-page *Bone Marrow Transplants: A Book of Basics for Patients*, or call the National Cancer Institute at (800) 4-CANCER and ask for their publication on transplantation, *Bone Marrow Transplantation and Peripheral Blood Stem Cell Transplantation*.

CHAPTER 21

Traveling for Care

I traveled among unknown men, in lands
beyond the sea . . .

—William Wordsworth

Robust research is underway on NHL at many prestigious national cancer centers. This means that there might be times when, after you have researched progress in treating your illness, you realize that the best care for your subtype of NHL is provided at a major treatment center away from home—perhaps very far from home.

This, of course, adds several layers of complexity to your treatment plans, not the least of which are financial considerations. Some health insurance policies cover airfare but not lodging; some pay a per diem to apply to food and lodging, but do not cover airfare; still others pay only so much per travel mile. Some policies pay nothing for travel and lodging.

This chapter doesn't have answers to all of these questions, but it will help you with the financial aspects of traveling for care. It is organized to address monetary needs, and focuses on free services. Canadian resources are reiterated in a separate section.

Assess needs and benefits

Your first step should be to verify what travel expenses your health policy will cover, because this coverage varies greatly.

Next, do some planning. If airfare isn't reimbursed by your health policy, driving might be an option. Driving may be out of the question, though, if the distance is great, if your car isn't in such good shape, or if you feel just plain awful. Lodging for family members who go with you is yet another expense. And who will remain behind? If children accompany you or a sick sibling, what about their schooling?

Air travel

In many instances, the only practical way to travel to the treatment center of your choice is by air. There are charitable groups that exist to fly you, free of charge, to distant treatment centers.

Some of these groups have requirements—for example, that the patient be able to embark and disembark the plane without airline assistance or that support equipment, if needed, be manageable without airline intervention.

Each service is described below, but the best starting point if you're pressed for time is Mercy Medical Airlift's National Patient Air Transport Helpline (NPATH), the only national toll-free number that can direct patients to the nearest and best air travel resource for their travel needs: (800) 296-1217.

Mercy Medical Airlift

Mercy Medical Airlift is the coordinating organization for three sectors of charitable air services in the U.S. They utilize fixed-wing (not helicopter) aircraft to help financially needy patients go to and from care centers for previously scheduled evaluation, diagnosis, treatment, and rehabilitation appointments. They do not provide emergency transport.

The three sectors of aviation involved in MMA are:

- The corporate aviation sector, consisting of 750 corporations who allow cancer and multiple sclerosis patients to use empty seats on regularly scheduled flights. The Corporate Angel Network is the focal point for this program. In 1997, 900 patients were transported. You do not need to demonstrate financial hardship to use CAN; there is no limit on the number of trips you can make. Cancer patients, their companion, or bone marrow donors are eligible. Children may be accompanied by two parents. Patients must be able walk up stairs to board the plane without assistance, and must be able to fly without any form of life support or medical assistance. Call (914) 328-1313 for other requirements.

- The private aviation sector, consisting of 4,500 pilots within thirty-two volunteer pilot organizations across the U.S. who use their own time and aircraft to fly patients free of charge to care centers. Organizationally, these groups cluster under Air Care Alliance. In 1997, more than 8,000 patients were transported. You may call ACA at (888) 662-6794 in the U.S.

- The commercial airline sector. Several commercial airlines offer, at times, special ticket prices or free tickets to those who need to travel for medical care, but cannot afford full ticket prices. These special offers vary by airline and are not necessarily ongoing offers.

In addition, Mercy Medical Airlift operates the Patient Assistance Center (PAC; (888) 675-1405), whose programs are:

- The National Patient Air Transport Helpline (NPATH) is, as mentioned earlier, the only national toll-free number that can direct patients to the nearest and best air travel resource for their travel needs. Call (800) 296-1217.

- Special-Lift and Child-Lift Programs to assist with transport of those needing care for pediatric or rare diseases at medical research centers.

- Programs to develop the charitable services of the private air sector, under the auspices of the Air Care Alliance.

- Programs to encourage and unify charitable ticket use programs among the commercial airlines.

The Red Cross

For military personnel only, the Red Cross can assist with emergency travel and communication. Call (202) 728-6400, or their 24-hour line at (202) 728-6401 to find the chapter nearest you or your destination.

Mission Air Transportation Network

This Canadian group uses corporate, government, or commercial aircraft to fly Canadians who cannot afford air transport but need medical care. Call (416) 222-6335.

Mission Aviation Fellowship

MAF supports air ambulance services and medical assistance in 57 countries. Call (909) 794-1151.

Land travel

Fewer organizations exist to help with land travel than for air travel.

American Cancer Society

The ACS regional offices in many cities have networks of volunteers who can provide transport by car to and from your treatment center. Call your local office or (800) ACS-2345.

The Leukemia Society of America

LSA can provide up to $750 in assistance per year for travel and other services, such as reimbursement for specific, approved drugs, blood transfusions, or x-rays. Only bills incurred *after* you have applied to LSA for aid are eligible for reimbursement. Call (800) 955-4LSA.

Traveler's Aid Society

Traveler's Aid provides emergency travel and lodging for those in dire financial need. Check local phone books for contact information. For the Traveler's Aid phone number at your destination, check your public library for phone books for other major cities.

Lodging

Having the means to pay for travel for care is part of the solution. However, finding affordable housing remains a barrier to travel for some NHL survivors. Several groups offer lodging for free or for a nominal fee.

Note that the cost of meals usually will be your responsibility. Facilities such as Hope Lodge, however, have kitchens you can use to reduce your expenses by avoiding the higher cost of restaurant meals.

American Cancer Society's Hope Lodge

The American Cancer Society sponsors free lodging in various cities for cancer patients being treated at nearby hospitals and their families. Their service is also offered to non-U.S. citizens traveling within the U.S. for medical care. Lodging is free and is provided on a first-come, first-served basis, so contact the ACS for the phone number of the Hope Lodge nearest the hospital you'll be using to verify that space is available. Each Hope Lodge has kitchen and laundry facilities. Call (800) ACS-2345.

National Association of Hospital Hospitality Houses

NAHHH offers a list of member hotels who provide reduced rates and special services to patients at nearby hospitals. Call (301) 961-3094, (317) 883-2226, or (800) 542-9730.

Ronald McDonald Houses

Ronald McDonald Houses, sponsored by the McDonald's Corporation, offer free lodging to children who must travel for medical care and their families. Pregnant women considered high-risk pregnancies are also eligible. Financial need may be a prerequisite for entry at some sites. A nominal fee of ten dollars a night may also be charged, but this may be waived if financial hardship is demonstrated. Call (312) 836-7100.

Children's Inn at the National Cancer Institute

The National Cancer Institute offers free meals and housing for children under age eighteen who are being treated at the NCI. Lodging might also be available for family members on a case-by-case basis. Both U.S. and non-U.S. citizens are accommodated. Call (800) 4-CANCER for more information, or contact:

Peggy Nelson
The Children's Inn
NCI, 7 West Drive,
Bethesda, MD 20814
Phone: (301) 496-5672.

For family members who cannot be lodged at the NCI, the American Cancer Society's Hope Lodge in Baltimore is an alternative, as are nearby hotels who have agreements with the NCI to offer reduced rates to the families of cancer patients treated at the NCI.

Adult care at the National Cancer Institute

Adult patients who have been treated at the NCI report that their spouses were allowed to stay overnight in the patient's room. You should verify this with the NCI and with the nurses on the floor.

Hospital-hotel agreements

Many hospitals have agreements with nearby hotels for reduced rates for patients and families. Contact the hospital's social worker or the admitting desk in advance of traveling for such information.

Hospital outpatient facilities

Some major cancer centers, such as Johns Hopkins in Baltimore, have outpatient lodging run by the institution for those requiring long-term follow-up care, such as that following bone marrow transplantation. Discuss these resources with the hospital admitting staff before you travel. The cost of you and your family staying in such hospital-run facilities may be covered by your insurance policy.

Travel insurance with medical features

Your health insurance might not cover out-of-state emergency medical care, so before you travel for pleasure, you should verify your health policy's coverage. If it's restrictive, consider getting travel insurance that covers emergency medical care. This ensures that if you take a vacation out of state and need, for instance, to get a transfusion or other emergency care while you're away, you'll have coverage to do so.

Here's a partial list of companies that offer such coverage, although this list does not imply recommendation or endorsement:

- Travel Assistance International: (800) 821-2828
- Medex: (888) MEDEX-00
- Travel Emergency Assistance (TEA): (281) 364-7726

Organizations that help with travel plans

Several groups can help you organize your travel plans for the least expense and worry.

The Leukemia Society of America

The Leukemia Society of America, described above in the section "Land travel" can help with travel arrangements. Call (800) 955-4LSA.

Candlelighters

The Candlelighter Childhood Cancer Foundation can offer much practical and instrumental help with travel and lodging plans. In the U.S., call (301) 657-8401 or (800) 366-CCCF. In Canada, call (800) 363-1062.

The National Children's Cancer Society, Inc.

This independent national organization can provide financial assistance for various needs. Call (800) 5-FAMILY.

Schooling

Some treatment centers, such as the Fred Hutchinson Cancer Center in Seattle, offer on-site schooling for sick children and their siblings. Contact the cancer center you're planning to use to see if they accommodate children who travel for care or who accompany others.

Your child's school, of course, might be willing to design a lesson plan that you can oversee to continue schooling your children who must travel.

Canadian assistance

This section describes Canadian services, some of which also are discussed elsewhere in this chapter.

- The British Columbia Medical Services Plan coordinates sharing travel expenses with commercial transportation firms such as airlines and ferries. Your doctor must fill out a Travel Assistance form. Call (800) 661-2668 or (250) 387-8277.

- The Mission Air Transportation Network uses corporate, government, or commercial aircraft to fly those who cannot afford air transport, but need medical care. Call (416) 222-6335.

- The Canadian Cancer Society offers various forms of assistance. Call (604) 872-4400 or (416) 961-7223.

- Canadian Cancer Society resource numbers by province:
  — Alberta: (403) 228-4487
  — Manitoba: (204) 774-7483
  — New Brunswick: (506) 634-6272
  — Newfoundland and Labrador: (709) 753-6520
  — Nova Scotia: (902) 423-6183
  — Ontario: (416) 488-5400
  — Prince Edward Island: (902) 566-4007
  — Quebec: (514) 255-5151
  — Saskatchewan: (306) 757-4260

Summary

The search for excellent care sometimes leads us far from home. The emotional issues regarding care away from home and the logistics of accommodating family members who must remain behind are difficult. Adding the expense of travel to these often seems overwhelming. This chapter offers ways to make traveling for care financially easier.

CHAPTER 22

If All Treatments Have Failed

Death, the refuge, the solace, the best and
kindliest and most prized friend…

    —Mark Twain
      Adam

The regrettable irony in almost anything written about death is that it is written by the living. We are sometimes privileged, though, to record the thoughts of the dying, who give us priceless insights regarding life's final phase.

This chapter assumes that one's treatment options have been exhausted, or are potentially too uncomfortable or damaging to continue. Please consider carefully whether reading this chapter will be bad for you emotionally if you still have options remaining.

Speaking to and for the patient is our chief goal, not for family and friends, as this chapter must attempt to communicate a great deal in limited space, and many books already exist for those who will grieve.

In its philosophical and religious aspects, preparing to die may differ little from living well, yet preparing to die becomes unique as we weaken permanently, or if we begin to experience profound and unrelenting physical discomfort. Thus we will offer information about dying as an incipient event rather than addressing the problems of living well with lymphoma. The physical and emotional aspects, but not the philosophical, religious, or financial aspects of approaching death will be discussed.

In the last twenty years, and especially in the last few years, many good books have become available on the topics of dying and dying well. Some, such as several by Elisabeth Kubler-Ross, tend to address those nearest the dying rather than speaking directly to the dying person. Others by Kubler-Ross, and such books as *How We Die* by Sherwin Nuland, *The Art of Dying* by

Patricia Weenolsen, *The Dying Time* by Furman and McNabb, and *A Graceful Exit* by Lofty Basta speak directly to the dying person. Please see Appendix A, *Resources*, for these and other books.

Marilyn's perspective

Marilyn Tyler, a survivor of low-grade NHL, describes the difference her disease has made in her outlook on life and her plans for her death:

> *I've told my children it'll take just one phone call when I go. All of my affairs are in pretty good order, with pertinent facts recorded in a loose-leaf notebook. A good tip: insurance agents, accountants' phone numbers, copies of trust and wills and deeds, with memos written on the face of them as to where safe deposit boxes are located with the original documents, and so on, can be recorded in this notebook. All of this makes for peace of mind. I not only don't want to be a burden in life, I sure as hell don't want to be a burden after I'm dead! I also don't want to spend my time imagining how my children will be able to enjoy my life savings after I'm gone. I'm giving it away now and am loving seeing how it makes their lives better.*
>
> *I'm frugal and have made my own money, but I'm generous. By early 1999, if I'm still here, I'll have succeeded in giving away about a quarter of a million dollars, so they won't have to pay estate taxes on it. I'll start $10,000 college accounts for each of the twins my daughter is expecting, and I'll double the accounts on January 2nd. I'm sending my niece to college, giving her the opportunity of two years in Madrid. It's been almost as much fun for me as doing it myself—and I think at age eighteen and nineteen she had a lot more fun than I would have at sixty-two and sixty-three, eh?*
>
> *My mother and I both prepaid for our cremations. For a slight additional fee and rider, one can arrange that cremation be taken care of no matter where in the country one dies. I think my siblings were most grateful for this prearrangement when my mother's time to die came. None of them had to deal with such choices as picking out caskets or spending big bucks on fancy funerals. We had a beautiful memorial service in the Lutheran church.*

I'm having the time of my life…every day is a peak experience, because I have no fear of death, and when you don't fear that, it's easy to wear the world like a loose garment.

I know I am not just my earthly manifestation. I'm through fighting anybody or anything (part of the philosophy I live by), and I just accept whatever comes along.

Preparing emotionally for death

There are probably as many emotions about dying as there are human beings, and there is no one correct way to die. Not surprisingly, if our death is expected and not too rapid, the emotions of loss that we experience are likely to mirror those we felt at first diagnosis of NHL. In fact, the evolving feelings associated with loss that were described in Chapter 1, *Symptoms and Diagnosis*, were first described by Elisabeth Kubler-Ross following her observations of the dying. They are common to many people in the time approaching death:

- Initially, *denial* that death is approaching

- *Anger* that you're being taken too soon or unfairly

- *Bargaining* with God or with others for more time, less pain, or comfort for our loved ones

- When bargaining fails, *depression and sadness* that death is inevitable

- Finally, *acceptance* that death will occur

Not everyone goes through all of these stages, nor do all people evolve through them in the same order, nor do we linger in these stages for the same amount of time. The person experiencing great pain, for instance, is likely to long for and accept death's approach quickly rather than being angry about its approach:

When my grandmother was in the advanced stages of cancer, she was in considerable pain because it had spread to her spine, and she was unable to keep food down. As a teen with little experience of death, I wasn't able to think of much to say to her, so I blurted out a cheerful remark about Christmas approaching. "I hope I'm dead by Christmas," she replied. It was years before I understood her willingness to let go, her longing for release from pain.

These stages are not necessarily sequential and discrete: you don't necessarily feel anger until it's spent, and only then move on to bargaining, for instance. The stages often are overlapping or concurrent.

Asking for honesty

We might not be able to prepare to die as we would like if those around us are not willing to admit it's imminent. At the very least, we should expect and ask for honesty from our doctors, even if family members continue to deny our approaching death in order to protect themselves a little longer.

If you have trouble getting honest answers from those around you, you might try pointing out how much it means to you to make sense of this final experience and to be ready for it. You might also attempt to tell them if you are convinced that death will occur soon, as often the patient is more aware than others, sometimes even more aware than medical personnel, that the end is quite near.

Difficult family issues

Unfortunately, at this very difficult time we often need to deal not only with our own feelings, but those of our loved ones, and this may be made even more difficult if their experiences with loss and grief are out of phase with our own. Our relatives' denial that we are dying is not the only issue that may sadden our final days. They may grieve earlier than we do, anticipating our death before we ourselves have accepted it—or indeed, perhaps before we're dying at all. They may lag behind us in the stages of acceptance, continuing to bargain with medical personnel for life-support measures when we're ready to let go. Or perhaps your family will express anger toward you for asking questions about dying, railing against any sign that you've given up.

You might be able to ease your family's acceptance of your death by reassuring them that they will be taken care of, by telling them that you love them, that you're weary of the battle and you welcome death, and by saying goodbye in loving ways, both overtly and symbolically.

What to say to children

Children need unique reassurances that they will be loved and well cared for after you're no longer available to love and help them. Of course, by now you've most likely done your best to arrange loving care for them, and they probably know of these arrangements.

Fortunately, there are many good books you can use to help your child understand death, in particular *I'm with You Now* by M. Catherine Ray (see Appendix A). In general, it's considered wise to give children as much honest and pointed information as possible, in terms that are appropriate for their age. For instance, it may be upsetting for your child to hear you say that you're in pain and are taking medicine for pain, but it's likely to be much more damaging if she sees you suffering and wasn't prepared to see this, and thinks your suffering cannot be mediated.

Make it clear to your children that your circumstances were not caused by anything they did. Children are egocentric, and must be reassured repeatedly that their thoughts and actions did not cause this illness.

Make it clear as well that your spouse and the child's siblings are not to blame. Expect that children will be openly or secretly angry with you for leaving them; spurts of this anger are natural and inevitable. At the same time, they may understand that it's not acceptable to blame you for dying. This doesn't leave the anger anywhere to go. Thus, the path that the young psyche may take—if they cannot blame you, and the burden of anger and self-blame is too great to carry alone—is to blame the surviving parent or a sibling. Make it as clear as possible that nobody is to blame, and that everybody is feeling sad and sorry about your dying.

Tell them over and over that you love them, and that you would not leave them if you had a choice.

There are specific points to be avoided, though, when talking to a child about dying. In her book *The Art of Dying*, Patricia Weenolsen suggests you avoid saying the following:

- Do not say you're simply going to sleep for a long time. Children may develop a fear of falling asleep if it's compared to dying, this phenomenon which is making all the grown-ups act so sad. They may even fear that they will never wake. If your faith includes a belief in an afterlife during which one awakes and is reunited with loved ones, try to explain using an analogy that does not parallel the child's normal daily actions.

- Likewise, don't tell them you're going on a long trip. They may never accept that you've died, and they may never again trust others to return.

Your death may raise enough issues with trust as it is; don't add to these issues by using allegorical detail with children who are too young to do other than take what you say literally.

- Be cautious about suggesting that your spiritual presence will remain nearby if your children believe in and act fearful of ghosts. They may become fearful of haunting after you've died.

Forgiveness and other emotional closures

Some religions emphasize that, before one dies, certain spiritual life tasks must be completed, such as forgiving those who have harmed you, forgiving yourself, and admitting your wrongdoings.

Only you need to be satisfied with the state of your inner being as you prepare to die. You may choose to adhere closely to religious beliefs, or you may decide they're bunk, that you wish to die peacefully without trying to contact everyone you've wronged, for example.

Detachment

Just as we may have withdrawn quite naturally from healthy, unaware friends after our diagnosis, cleaving instead to other cancer survivors, as death approaches we may find ourselves wanting and needing to withdraw from the living. This is a natural process, partly physical as we weaken and perhaps suffer physical pain, but partly it is a shift in the spiritual or emotional needs of the nonphysical self.

You may sense that people who have died are trying to communicate with you; you may dream about those who have died or about places distinctly not of Earth's confining dimensions. While it's beyond the scope of this book to speculate on the meaning or veracity of such events, we can share with you that others who are dying have reported such happenings, and appear to be much comforted by them. Often these dreams and perceptions occur in the last week or so of life.

An NHL survivor describes her conviction that experiencing a foreknowledge of death is possible:

> *About two weeks before my mom died, she dreamed that my father, who had died the year before, was calling her. When she told me, I was terribly upset—even angry with her—for being so superstitious.*

> *Recently, after my own NHL diagnosis, I also got a "call" from my Dad. He said he wanted to "come home." I interpreted that as meaning that somehow he knew I have NHL, and wants to help. (I hope he can.) I will no longer deny anyone's contact with the nonliving.*

The outside observer often is appalled by the sight of the family sitting in the dying person's room, talking among themselves as if the patient had already died. While ignoring the dying person's need to communicate does sometimes happen, at other times it's a reflection of the family's tacit understanding that the dying person is withdrawing from the living.

Permission to die: the last gift of love

Many reports of the experiences of the dying tell us that some people need permission from their loved ones to let go. If you are blessed with time, you might discuss this in advance with your family. Particularly if you are in pain, try to make it clear to them that they give you a great gift when they give you permission to die.

At times, even among those who have had this discussion, a final gesture of letting go by the family, verbal or tactile, appears to be necessary in one's final moments to allow death to occur.

An NHL survivor looks back with regret to her younger days when, during her father's final illness, she was unable to accept his willingness to die:

> *It was me who couldn't deal with events when my dad was dying. I am ashamed to say that I didn't visit him as much as I should have. My mother and brother did mostly everything. I was angry because he just accepted his cancer and wouldn't do anything to fight. Even when he died, I pretended it was someone else. Oh, if only I could relive those days. The guilt that I had to deal with for many years was awful. I'm older and wiser now, and can understand that my dad dealt with his illness the way he had to. I have now learned that people deal with illness in their own way. It's not that they don't care, they are just afraid of doing or saying the wrong thing...and especially afraid of losing a loved one.*

A parent's perspective

Janet, the parent of an eighteen-year-old with very aggressive high-grade lymphoma, has learned that no treatment options remain. Her writing reveals the terrible anguish of a parent, and her son's bravery as he faces death:

> How do I write these words? These are words that no parents can ever bear to think, let alone say out loud. My son is dying. Friday night came the doctor's words which I can't bear to repeat. This can't be true. This is not supposed to be happening. All this hard work. All Doug's pain, and strength, and fighting to beat this thing. Why did he have to go through all this? There is no fairness in the world. Children are not supposed to be sick and be told by their doctors they're going to die ... Last night at 5 P.M. Doug's doctors told him that the pneumonia wasn't really pneumonia: there's no infection in his lungs. They're filling with lymphoma, which is also now in his spleen and blood, and is going everywhere as fast as it can. My beautiful son was told he has from two days to two weeks to live. This morning we asked them to try anything, so they're trying three drugs never used together before to buy him just a little more time.

> Doug himself calmly asked, "I don't want to be morbid, but what is it going to be like?" They answered, "You won't have to suffer. You'll just have more and more trouble breathing." Then they told him, "Get your affairs in order, and if you want to call anyone or have anyone visit, call them now."

> They say, "Take no extraordinary measures, because there is no hope." How can they say that about my Doug? How can I give up my hope, with all his dreams and plans? How can I lose my son? This can't be happening. My son Glen is home, and lots of friends are coming to say good-bye to Doug. He's less than yesterday, but sleeping okay tonight. I was made to come home, and I hope there's no phone call in the middle of the night, and somehow, some way, that last-resort choice of drugs helps him. What am I supposed to do without hope? I can't do this.

Physical aspects of dying

Many NHL survivors and their families ask what dying will be like.

How will we die?

Dying from non-Hodgkin's lymphoma can occur in many ways, because the disease may appear in almost any part of the body. In general, life-threatening symptoms will be related to the failure of organs invaded by or near the tumor mass: lymphoma of the central nervous system may suppress the brain center that controls breathing or may cause seizures. Lymphoma spread to the liver or kidney may cause toxins to accumulate in the bloodstream that in turn causes coma. A large chest or liver tumor may cause the lungs or heart to fail. Because NHL can manifest in so many ways, your oncologist is the best person to prepare you for the physical symptoms you are most likely to face, and what level of pain, if any, you may need to counter with medication.

Leukemias and lymphomas are closely related, but, unlike death from many leukemias, death from NHL usually is not related to secondary infection or blood loss, although it can be if complications develop following marrow transplantation. Some, but not all, deaths from NHL are accompanied by pain, for which good relief can and should be provided by a hospice or a physician.

Even a death preceded by great pain and discomfort usually is, in its very last stage, peaceful and illuminated by a brief cognizance.

When will it occur?

No human knows the answer to this question: not for NHL, nor for any other form death may take. There are well-known physical signs associated with the very last stage of life, yet some people have revived after all signs of life are extinguished. Many people have rallied for months or years after feeling so ill they wished for and surrendered to death, or after their doctors had given up all hope for survival. We can know only that our death will occur in our lifetime.

The final moments of life

Most people at this stage of death seem not to be aware of what is happening to their body, or they seem to drift in and out of awareness. The perception of family members looking on at this stage is that the patient is in great discomfort, but those who have had near-death experiences do not report remembering great distress at this stage. The truth is unknown.

The visible physical signs seen most often just before death comprise the *agonal* stage, and may include muscle spasm, one or more large gasps for breath, breathing that starts and stops, heaving of chest or shoulders, a single deep exhalation, clear or unclear vocalizations, or noisy breathing. As will all muscles, bowel and bladder sphincter muscles relax. This might release no body waste, though, if no food was taken recently.

These signs may be visible for just an instant or may last for several minutes.

How medical staff define death

Currently, brain death is the criterion used to ascertain that death is irrefutable, because other classic signs of death, such as cessation of heartbeat, can be misleading or can be reversed using twentieth-century medical technology.

Signs of brain death include loss of all reflexes such as the blink reflex or the pupil's response to light, failure to respond physically or verbally to urgent or painful stimuli, and the absence of electrical activity within the brain as measured by an electroencephalogram (EEG).

Can we make dying easier?

Easing death can take several forms: receiving physical and emotional comfort, finalizing affairs, or perhaps forgiving one's self and others for old grudges and sins. Some of these topics are addressed in other chapters; spiritual comfort and philosophical adaptation are addressed in many fine books.

Pain control

The most pressing concern for many is the control of pain in the last stages of life. In the past, several studies have shown that dying cancer patients do not receive adequate medication to control pain, owing to misconceptions on the part of medical doctors about addiction or accidental overdose. In the time since these studies have been published, however, many physicians have become better informed about pain control for the dying cancer patient, and are doing a better job of providing palliative care. But patients and especially caregivers must remain vigilant about insisting on adequate pain medication.

It's wise to plan in advance on having a say in the comfort of your death. If you have the luxury of choices and the time to make them, draft a living will or advance directives, or both, and plan to die at home or in hospice care instead of within the hospital. Studies of care administered in hospitals show that advance directives expressing wishes against extraordinary life support measures often are ignored by doctors when care is administered in the hospital. Hospice care or care by loved ones is more likely to assure your comfort than life-saving hospital measures are.

Hospice and hospice home care

One of the most useful resources for the comfort of the dying person and his family is hospice care, a comfort-centered concept that emerged in Europe and migrated to the U.S. following many years' failure of medical technology to provide comfort for the dying. Hospice care is devoted only to making one comfortable and loved in her dying days, not to prolonging life. A peaceful and less expensive variation of hospice care is hospice home care, now quite common in the U.S.

Hospice nurses visit daily, or stay in the home, to administer pain medication and, in some cases, to help the caregivers with certain household chores. They are trained to recognize the signs of impending death, and can help the family with the arrangements that are necessary just after a death in the home has occurred. Their focus includes the physical and emotional comfort of the patient, and the well-being of the surviving family members after death.

Some hospice services charge little or nothing for those who cannot afford the service.

In some cases, a doctor's statement is necessary stating that the patient has less than six months to live in order for that patient to be eligible for hospice care.

Euthanasia

Unfortunately, there can be painful preludes to death for which no amount of medication is adequate. In some cases, the dying and their loved ones are willing, indeed almost compelled by horrific suffering, to end life earlier than the disease would end it.

Euthanasia, the hastening of the end of life by active intervention, has been much discussed in the U.S. recently. Groups such as the Hemlock Society and the American Medical Association have expressed divergent points of view. The American Medical Association states that doctor-assisted suicide violates their standards. The Hemlock Society publishes literature on dying and the right to die, including the book *Final Exit*.

In his book, *How We Die*, Dr. Sherwin Nuland, a surgeon, says,

> *In my medical practice, I have always assured my dying patients that I would do everything possible to give them an easy death, but I have too often seen even that hope dashed in spite of everything I try. At a hospice too, where the only goal is tranquil comfort, there are failures.*[1]

Some doctors will privately state that they have broken the law to ease a patient's going. One geriatric neurologist stated that, among her fellow medical doctors, about half will help a patient of their own to die when medicine and technology cannot relieve suffering.

> *My husband and I agree completely to help each other end life if one of us is suffering terribly with no recourse. We contacted the Hemlock Society to assess their point of view, and were amused to find that the literature we received included an application for lifetime membership! So, amidst our very serious planning, we were able to laugh.*

Planning your own memorial ceremony

It's an odd fact that many people who cannot bear to think of the dying process, who cannot even conceive of their mortality, are quite happy to plan their own memorial ceremony and burial. As death becomes a certainty, many people find comfort in planning how others will remember them and celebrate their life.

Some of the things you might want to consider are:

- Whether you would like to be buried or cremated, where and how you would like your remains to be preserved or honored

- What memories of your life you'd like retold at your funeral or memorial service

- If there are special poems or music you want read or played
- Whether the ceremony will be a religious one
- If your internment or the scattering of your ashes will be private

Janet's perspective

Janet, a survivor of mixed-cleaved-cell NHL, has reconciled to her death:

> Some years ago, I became interested in the subject of death and dying generally. I joined a group of academics and others who are sometimes called the 3D group (they have annual conferences on "Death, Dying, and Disposal"!). So I have ordered over time several books to add to my very interesting collection. It is surprising how helpful and enjoyable such books have been to me in their own way. There are often lighthearted things going on even at the time of illness and death, and certainly good funerals involve remembrance of the person including their humour and fun.

> There is also a movement in the U.K. to take the expense out of the last rites, so we have a supermarket where you can buy a coffin kit (among more traditional things)!

> I read recently of a lovely young lecturer who was terminally ill and used her coffin as a coffee table for several weeks; she had all her friends and relations write and paint remembrances all over it, so that eventually when she died she was carried into the funeral ceremony in something which represented a lifetime of love and friendship.

> There are interesting movements here in the United Kingdom. For example, the Woodland Burial movement enables people to be buried in a lovely piece of ground, to have a tiny named plaque flat on the ground and a tree planted in their memory by the plaque. The whole area is to be retained as a woodland park for people to enjoy. (At the moment available only in some areas, but developing quite quickly.)

> On an amusing note: when I tried to find out if there were one of these sites near where I live, I was told to contact someone who runs an animal farm, and discovered that he is thinking of adding to his horse (old nag!) cemetery to provide a woodland burial site for people. Although I was quite amused at the thought, I decided my relatives might not appreciate the joke.

I have instead been finding out about the way in which people can be used for medical research or organ transplants after their death and discovered that even with cancer they might find skin and corneas useful! Like the statement, "making a will won't kill you," I think there should be another one: "Planning a burial won't kill you!"

Summary

Dying cannot be described accurately by the living, much less by the well. Nonetheless, we have tried to listen to those preparing for death, to learn from what they say, from those nearest them, and to share these insights with you.

We are blessed to be living during a renaissance of interest in society about dying and death, and to benefit from cultural considerations of how to die well. You will find many books available to make the journey called dying as peaceful as possible.

CHAPTER 23

The Future of Therapy

Every great advance in science has issued
from a new audacity of imagination.

　—John Dewey

The spirit of cooperative academic endeavor, a coalescence of insights from multiple medical disciplines, governmental prioritization, a highly developed research infrastructure, and the uninterrupted scientific focus of nations at peace have positioned us well for the development of promising new cancer therapies in the years ahead.

This chapter will discuss peer-reviewed mainstream medical therapies for NHL. The first section is a brief overview of what causes cancer, followed by a section discussing broad trends in research. Next is an encyclopedic reference list of treatments now in trials, organized by mode of action. Finally, we discuss therapies we're likely to see in the more distant future, consisting of substances and approaches, such as tissue regeneration, that are not being tested against NHL at this time.

If you're pressed for time and want information on a single substance, check the index first to locate it within this chapter and elsewhere.

The sources of information for this chapter are the National Cancer Institute's clinical trials database and research papers accessible through the National Library of Medicine's Medline, a collection of more than nine million published medical papers.

Although the timing for testing and approving a typical cancer treatment is measured in years, cancer treatments are being improved constantly. This chapter represents merely a snapshot of new therapies at the time this book was written. Information presented here concerning how various anticancer substances work, for instance, reflects the knowledge currently available in the medical literature and is subject to change as research progresses.

You can gain access to new treatments that are still in clinical trials if you and your doctor decide it would be advantageous to do so. See Chapter 19, *Clinical Trials*, for more information.

None of the descriptions that follow should be construed as a recommendation for treatment. Any treatment you find here or elsewhere should be carefully evaluated by hematologic experts before your treatment decisions are made.

What causes cancer?

Many of the descriptions of newer treatments being developed today will be easier to understand if the known causes of cancer are understood. This topic is covered in detail in Chapter 3, *What Are the Non-Hodgkin's Lymphomas?*, but certain key points are reiterated here.

Many if not all instances of cancer are accompanied by changes in the tumor cell's DNA. At times, a gene is entirely missing, or has been half-spliced with another gene after DNA strands from two entirely different chromosomes accidentally overlap, break apart, and rejoin. In other cases, one chromosome will break, flip, and rejoin at the wrong ends. A third kind of damage involves deletion of one base pair of nucleic acids from an amino acid encoding sequence in a gene.

All of the body's work is accomplished using proteins built from genes. If the gene is damaged by chromosome breakage, for example, a protein built from it may be partly or completely nonfunctional, toxic, or even tumor-promoting.

A tumor may arise because such genes are:

- Incorrectly transcribed into aberrant proteins.
- Not transcribed at all, or are overexpressed.
- Expressed at the wrong time.
- Two erroneously spliced genes are being transcribed into a hybrid protein that is impotent or oncogenic.

Or the tumor may arise owing to a combination of any of these.

When these aberrant changes occur in or very near genes that regulate cell growth, trigger orderly cell death (apoptosis), or regulate maturation or cell division and reproduction, cancer may result.

An overview of research trends

Over the last twenty years, broad trends in cancer research in general, and in NHL research in particular, have taken several concurrent paths:

- A much more targeted approach to identifying and testing potentially useful anticancer substances, enabled by our much improved understanding of the genetic origin, development, and metabolic milieu of tumors within the body.

- An altered (and, to date, not entirely successful) effort in fighting cancer with substances our own bodies make, instead of using external plant-based or manmade substances.

- A willingness in some instances to halt, but not eliminate, a tumor's growth, changing a cancer from a fatal illness to a chronic, manageable, fairly symptom-free disease accompanied by a reasonably high quality of life and lengthy survival.

- An emphasis, at the request of many patients, to design drugs and procedures for supportive care—drugs that do not destroy cancer, but instead contribute significantly to survival by eliminating the secondary effects and illnesses related to treatment. The drugs that stimulate growth of new blood cells after chemotherapy, for example, fall into this category.

- An interest in preventing cancer and examining its causes.

Each of these is discussed below in general terms and reiterated in the specific categories of investigative drugs that follow this discussion.

Substance identification and testing

For many years, anticancer drugs were discovered by testing many natural and manmade substances wholesale—often in excess of 5,000 per year—against tumor samples that were kept alive in laboratories. Substances that worked in this setting were then tested in mice; those that worked in mice were tested in humans. Those that worked better in humans than existing drugs became part of standard treatment—all without understanding the drug's mode of action until afterward, if ever.

While this approach is still often used, a trend toward understanding a drug's mode of action *before* its use has emerged, owing to great advances in biochemistry, genetics, molecular biology, and many related fields of science such as engineering and computer science. You'll see this trend reflected in almost every drug category discussed later in this chapter—indeed, that they can be categorized at all reflects this new understanding.

For instance, a problem that often emerges in cancer therapy is the inability to deliver a high dose of toxin directly to the tumor, either because it's encapsulated within or entwined with healthy tissue, is many cell layers thick, or has high internal pressure that makes penetration difficult. Many of the newer approaches to cancer therapy target specific barriers such as these, rather than just a wholesale killing of the tumor by unknown mechanisms.

This refined testing relies on our much improved understanding of the genetic causes and biologic pathways of cancer. Using this understanding, a researcher might be able to identify the portion of a molecule that's responsible for the specific anticancer activity the researcher is hoping to accomplish. Often this design and simulation is computerized, atom by atom, including animation showing how the molecule will interact with the binding site of the tumor or other bodily substance that aids cancer growth. This isolation of design is followed by a computerized search of a database of millions of substances, retrieving all that match this characteristic. Sometimes among the substances that match will be a tried and true drug for another illness; sometimes it will be a drug tried for other purposes, but abandoned, such as thalidomide. Sometimes it will be a new plant-based biological compound found during a pharmaceutical company's last foray into the rainforest or ocean to collect samples of all flora.

Some researchers take this understanding several steps farther and attempt to build from scratch custom-made drugs that have a lock-and-key fit to the tumor cell type or to some biological mechanism that supports tumor growth. This approach is called rational drug design.

Biological anticancer substances

Almost any anticancer substance could by definition be called biological in that it has an effect on the body, but in this book the term includes only those substances made by the body to fight enemy substances. These substances have accumulated a tremendous following among many patients and some researchers as potential cures for cancer. As a distinct class of drugs, they are appealing for many reasons. One fairly overt reason is the popular contemporary cachet of "natural substances" and their alleged low toxicity. Another less obvious reason is the sense of balance provided by the theory that cancer is an internal process run amok, and that a corresponding internal substance may correct it. The third and best reason is that they may work, as interleukin-2 and interferon-alfa have against some kidney cancers and melanomas.

Unfortunately, none of this enthusiasm for cure has held up to scrutiny as these substances are used today against the NHLs. Substances such as naked monoclonal antibodies and interferon alfa-2B, for instance, have not succeeded in totally destroying non-Hodgkin's lymphomas. Although they can in some cases arrest or shrink tumor growth, the effect appears to be temporary; the tumor regrows when administration of the substance is stopped. Moreover, some of these substances cause considerably uncomfortable side effects, giving the lie to the notion that "natural" equals "harmless."

Two biological anticancer drugs, Rituxan and interferon alfa-2B, are FDA-approved and in use against NHL at the time of this writing. Rituxan targets cell surface antigen CD20, and appears to temporarily halt tumor growth or shrink the tumor. It appears that Rituxan can be given again after several months with no toxic effect, and perhaps with continued and repeated effectiveness—but not enough treatment time has elapsed to know this for certain.

Interferon alfa has been approved by the FDA to treat chronic myelogenous leukemia (CML), but is sometimes used for low-grade NHL as an off-label use or in clinical trials. Interferon appears to be effective against NHL only as long as it continues to be taken, and can produce flu-like side effects.

Much work remains to be done in the area of biological substances, because the concept is very promising and has hardly been tapped. Combining monoclonal antibodies with toxic substances that permit targeting only of the tumor instead of healthy tissue is being pursued hotly. Combining the interferons with some of the interleukins, notably interleukin-2, may yield better results than interferons alone have yielded. Combining these natural substances with traditional chemotherapies is the target of many clinical trials now being run. Creating a version of one or more of these molecules that's slightly different from those found in nature may make them more potent than those produced by our bodies.

It's useful to keep in mind that many of the substances that have long been used against the NHLs and other cancers, including three of the four drugs in CHOP, also are "natural":

- Adriamycin (doxorubicin) is a strong antibiotic derived from a fungus.
- Vincristine (Oncovin) is an alkaloid extracted from a member of the Vinca plant species.
- Prednisone is a manmade copy of our body's hormone prednisilone.

In other words, natural substances are not always harmless and magically effective, just as steroids—including such substances as estrogen, vitamin D, and cholesterol—are not necessarily rage-producing, dangerous, and illegal.

A subcategory of drugs that is sometimes considered biological therapy are the biological response modifiers, another somewhat ambiguous name, as any substance that modifies a bodily response might in theory fit this category. In this instance, though, we include only substances made by the body and replicated in the lab, such as the growth factors for red and white blood cells and platelets. These substances are discussed below under "Supportive care."

Tumor stabilization (stasis)

Over the years, there has been a shift from thinking of conquering cancer to controlling its presence in the body. This shift has come about not by design, but serendipitously, following the realization that some anticancer drugs can control cancer but not destroy it, and that, in some of these cases, the tumor does not become resistant to the drug.

Americans sometime seem to have difficulty accepting the concept of control over cure, perhaps because thirty years' effort following President Nixon's "War on Cancer" has formed the channeled, absolute goal of cure; perhaps because cancer still is thought of as an invader rather than a dangerously wayward part of the self; or perhaps because the social stigma of cancer and the resulting isolation remain so pronounced.

Regardless of the reasoning, it remains that some of us who are comfortable with the notion of controlling other potentially fatal health conditions such as high blood pressure, diabetes, or seizure disorders are still reluctant to choose gentle, repeatable, likely cancer control over a one-time, high-risk cancer cure.

Examples of drugs that can control but not always eliminate cancer are tamoxifen, which can halt the growth of some breast carcinomas, and interferon-alfa2B, which can stabilize some lymphomas.

Supportive care

Progress in this category is responsible for the success of certain cancer therapies, such as marrow transplantation, that depend more on ancillary care for success than on the procedure itself. Although this chapter does not discuss many investigative drugs used for supportive care simply because our space is limited, they should not be underestimated. Many of the gains made in lengthening life or curing cancer have come about because these drugs, such as Zofran for controlling nausea, permit the individual to retain nutrients, reestablish adequate levels of infection-fighting white blood cells, or overcome previously fatal fungal infections. A great deal of wisdom about supportive care has accumulated owing to the experiences the medical community has had caring for the immune-suppressed, including those with AIDS.

Cancer prevention

Years ago, cancer epidemiology consisted of asking those already diagnosed with cancer to recall incidents and lifestyle habits from many years ago. Their answers were examined for patterns that might correlate to the incidence of cancer in a population.

Today, we're seeing different kinds of detection and prevention trials, such as those designed to examine lifestyle, diet, and environmental factors as they're occurring, and to tally and track all cases of cancer in these groups as they develop. This is a more accurate way of assessing risk and correlation than asking patients in a highly stressful setting to recall, for example, dietary habits from thirty years ago.

Other trials include asking participants to adhere to a specific diet for a number of years, and then recording the incidence of cancers in this group as opposed to the incidence among those who had no dietary restrictions.

Still others may involve participants who are taking vitamin supplements, exercising to a schedule, or losing weight. These groups are followed for many years and any cases of cancer that occur are recorded and followed.

Current trials

Currently, there are more than two hundred clinical trials of treatment for all types of NHL. Some are trials of treatments already approved by the FDA, but with restructured timing or dosage for better results; some are of entirely new substances, techniques, or devices.

We will cover only those substances, techniques, and devices never before used against NHL. We will not cover the tactic of recombining already approved drugs in new ways, although these are unmistakably valuable, as optimizing timing, dose, and multi-agent therapy have been pivotal in the success of cancer therapy.

Novel substances are discussed first. New techniques and devices are discussed in the next section, "Novel techniques and devices."

Novel substances by mode of action

Novel substances being used in trials for NHL are listed below, grouped alphabetically by modes of action. You'll note that some substances, such as phenylbutyrate and bryostatin 1, fit more than one category.

Alkylating agents

DNA strands are held together by a variety of forces, one being electrical bonds. Alkylating agents form new electrochemical bonds within the DNA strand. This disrupts many normal functions of DNA, including its ability to divide. Alkylating agents are able to affect a cancer cell's DNA even when the DNA is not uncoiled and separated—in other words, they are not cell-cycle specific—which may explain their relatively high activity against many cancers. Many alkylating agents are already being used against NHL.

New alkylating agents being tested are mitomycin, carzelesin, tallimustine, diaziquone (AZQ), temozolomide, and penclomedine.

Antiangiogenesis therapy

Most tumors trigger growth of many new blood vessels to support the increased metabolic needs of the tumor. This growth of new blood vessels is called angiogenesis. Antiangiogenic agents interrupt the ability of the body to grow new blood vessels, causing tumors to shrink.

Some of the substances being studied now to reduce the blood supply to starve tumors, an approach called antiangiogenesis, cause concern because they also are likely to reduce the blood supply to normal tissues. The normal tissues of concern are found near wound healing and, for example, in the uterus of a menstruating woman. Refined methods of curtailing a tumor's blood supply are being examined, such as triggering clots only in tumor blood vessels by preferentially binding clotting substances to proteins found only on tumor cells.

Now in clinical trials for the NHLs are thalidomide, COL-3, carboxyamidotriazole, matrix metalloprotease inhibitors, tecogalan sodium, and TNP-470 (also called AGM-1470).

Antibody therapy

Antibodies are substances secreted by white blood cells called B-cells. They attach to foreign material and pathogens so that the invaders can be destroyed by T-cells and macrophages.

Antibodies engineered in the lab to attach to only one cell surface receptor—monoclonal antibodies—have long been used in research and cancer diagnosis to tag cancer cells for visibility and quantification. Now they're beginning to be used to treat cancers.

Some antibodies listed below are intended to attack tumors; others are being used to purge marrow before transplantation. Others, such as anti-CD3 antibody BC3, can be used to fight graft-versus-host disease after allogeneic (donor) transplantation by saturating the surface receptors of T cells that would otherwise attack foreign marrow.

Antibodies being tested are:

- Di-dgA-RFB4 targeted to antigen CD22
- CHOP combined with Rituximab (Rituxan targets antigen CD20)
- 131I-Labeled LL2 IgG (Lymphocide)
- MePRDL/MOAB BC3
- 131I-Labeled LL2 (Lymphocide) IgG with transplantation
- Yttrium Y 90 Anti-Tac (CD30) and pentetic acid calcium
- Rituximab consolidation following Rituximab induction

- Iodine 131 anti-B1 antibody radioimmunotherapy

- Immunotoxin LMB-2 targeted to Tac-expressing (CD30-positive) tumors

---

Anticytokine therapy

This is a broad category of anticancer drugs that contains some agents also in other categories.

By definition, cytokines are proteins our bodies manufacture to trigger activity in other cells, cyto- meaning cell, and -kine meaning activity. Using this definition, almost any protein or enzyme is a cytokine, but for cancer and for the lymphomas, special cytokines are in play. Lymphokines, for example, are cytokines secreted by lymphocytes. All of the interleukins and interferons are cytokines, as is tumor necrosis factor and the colony stimulating factors.

Some cytokines appear to cause cancer growth under certain circumstances, such as interleukin-6 (IL-6) in myeloma studies. Some cytokines work in opposition to each other, such as G-CSF and antihematopoietic cytokines.

The substances being tested as anticytokines are COL-3, carboxyamidotriazole, suramin (SUR), TNP-470, lisofylline, certain immunosuppressive drugs, and DAB389-IL2, a fusion protein (on which more is said below) targeting interleukin-2 receptors.

Antimetabolite therapy

As the word antimetabolite implies, these substances in some way impede the cell's metabolism, its building up and breaking down of cell parts. Each of the antimetabolites used for NHL works a bit differently from the others, and some may fit into other categories described in this chapter, such as the antifolates.

- Gemcitabine (difluorodeoxycytidine) is an antimetabolite being examined for use against NHL. Gemcitabine substitutes for an enzyme in the process that constructs DNA from RNA, causing the process to fail.

- Azacytidine is an antimetabolite that is similar to cytosine arabinoside, substituting for a component that is key in DNA replication.

- PEG-L-asparaginase (pegaspargase, polyethylene glycol-L-asparaginase) is a form of L-asparaginase bound to a carbonated molecule that seems to produce fewer side effects than L-asparaginase alone.

- 506U78, an ARA-G nucleotide, is a substance being tested whose exact mode of action is unclear, but it appears to interfere with nucleic acid synthesis. Without nucleic acids, DNA cannot be constructed, and cell division and replication are not possible.

- CGP-48664, a growth inhibitor, exerts its effects against NHL by inhibiting the enzyme S-adenosylmethionine decarboxylase, an enzyme necessary for building DNA. When DNA cannot be built, the cell cannot multiply.

Apoptosis induction therapy

Normal cells die in an orderly, shrinking way, melting their outer coat slowly into pieces called blebs, fragmenting their nucleus and its DNA. Eventually they are absorbed by neighboring cells. In contrast, infected cells die by swelling and bursting, called lytic death. Most untreated cancer cells don't die at all, and those that do are greatly outnumbered by new cancer cells.

Some studies have shown that certain substances can induce orderly cell death—apoptosis—in cancer cells, but the methods by which apoptosis drugs work still are being delineated. Some may act by reactivating death genes the cancer cell had succeeded in suppressing. Other substances seem to have unique properties, such as desferoxamine, which deprives the tumor of iron needed for life processes. Many drugs described in other sections of this chapter ultimately result in apoptosis, regardless of their modes of action.

Apoptosis-inducing drugs being tested for NHL are desferoxamine and perillyl alcohol.

Chemoprotectants

These agents are used to offset dangerous effects of chemotherapy by shielding healthy cells from damage or by promoting their regrowth.

Substances being tested for these purposes are:

- Amifostine (Ethyol) to protect marrow, central nervous system, and kidneys

- Dexrazoxane (Zinecard) to protect the heart

- Keratinocyte growth factor (KGF) to hasten regeneration of cells in the lining of the mouth and GI tract

- Pentetic acid calcium to combine with and remove excess Yttrium-90 during radioimmunotherapy

Chemosensitization/potentiation

Research has shown that some drugs, while having no direct ability to kill cancer cells, appear to heighten the cancer cell's vulnerability to other drugs. Other studies have shown that some drugs can both kill cancer cells and improve the ability of other drugs to do so.

Substances being tested for these purposes are novobiocin, bryostatin 1, P-Glycoprotein Antagonist PSC 833, and O6-Benzylguanine.

See also "Drug modulation" and "Radiosensitization."

Cyclin-dependent kinase inhibitor therapy

Cyclins are proteins that govern the progression of the cell from one stage of cell division to the next. The cyclin-dependent kinases are enzymes that join with cyclins, forming several unique cyclin/cdk complexes, to mediate this progression. Substances that can inhibit these enzymes inhibit tumor growth.

Flavopiridol is being tested for this purpose.

Cytokine therapy

Cytokines, as discussed above under anticytokine therapies, are proteins our bodies manufacture to trigger activity in other cells, such as the release of prostaglandins at the site of injury or the growth of new white blood cells. All of the interleukins and interferons are cytokines, as is tumor necrosis factor and the colony stimulating factors.

Manmade cytokines being tested for use against NHL include interferon-alfa, interleukin-2 (IL-2), and interleukin-12 (IL-12).

Demethylating agents

Genes that are coated with a carbon substance—methylated—cannot be translated into the proteins that carry out the work of genes. There are about nine known tumor-suppressor genes, of which p53 is the best known, and among which p53 appears to be the master gene. Tumor-suppressor genes are sensitive to the activity of the dividing cell. They signal when to demethylate and transcribe growth genes, when to arrest growth, and when to initiate cell death if irreparable errors are found in the cell's DNA.

Demethylating substances are being tested to uncover methylated tumor-suppressor genes in cancer cells: genes that normally control cell death and other normal cell functions. By uncovering and activating these normal genes, it is thought that cancerous cells can be forced to mature, rest, divide, and die as normal cells do.

Deoxycytidine is one agent being tested as a demethylator.

Differentiation therapy

Cell differentiation into distinct functional types is part of the normal cell's maturation process. When cancer cells are continually dividing, however, they are not maturing and differentiating into the adult, functioning form of the tissue in which they arose. The result is a large group of cells that not only fail to carry out the function the organ was designed to do, but that also crowd out other cells and commandeer a disproportionate share of the body's resources.

Some cancer cells are so young and so undifferentiated that it's not possible to tell what organ gave rise to the tumor, and the diagnosis is by default carcinoma of unknown primary origin (CUP).

Some substances can force cancer cells to mature as normal cells do, stopping the cycle of uncontrollable cell division that characterizes cancer cells. All-trans retinoic acid, for instance, is the best known example to date. ATRA is the missing product of a damaged gene, the hallmark of acute myeloid leukemia subtype M3 (acute promyelocytic leukemia). When manmade ATRA is supplied, the white blood cells mature, differentiate, cease their rapid multiplying, and resemble normal cells.

Bryostatin 1, phenylbutyrate, targretin, and all-trans retinoic acid are possible differentiators being tested for the NHLs.

Drug modulation

Certain anticancer drugs seem to make other drugs more effective in killing cancer cells for reasons that vary. 5-fluorouracil (5-FU), for example, works more effectively in the presence of methotrexate, trimetrexate, interferon-alpha, leucovorin, or N-(phosphonacetyl)-L-asparte acid (PALA).

Leucovorin, a reduced form of the B vitamin folic acid, is being tested with 5-fluorouracil and topotecan for use against NHL.

See also "Chemosensitization."

Drug resistance inhibition

Cancerous cells frequently are able to mutate to forms that are no longer killed by chemotherapy or radiotherapy. Efforts are being directed at resensitizing cancerous cells to cytotoxic drugs.

Drugs being tested for this purpose are novobiocin, cyclosporine, phenobarbital, and the P-Glycoprotein antagonist PSC 833.

Folate antagonist therapy

Folate, a form of iron, is needed to make the building blocks of DNA, purines, and thymidylates. In the absence of these, new copies of DNA cannot be made. Because cancer cells divide more rapidly than most normal cells, and because they commandeer major supplies of the body's nutrients, treatments such as folate antagonists are expected to affect cancer cells more strongly than most healthy cells.

Phenylbutyrate and ICI D1694 (also called ZD1694) are classified as antifolates.

Fusion protein therapy

Similar to monoclonal antibody therapy in its intent, fusion protein therapy consists of a toxin attached to a protein that can in turn attach to or be transported into a tumor cell, thus damaging or killing the tumor cell while leaving healthy cells undamaged.

DAB389-IL2 is a compound consisting of two proteins fused together: interleukin-2 bound to diphtheria toxin fragments A and B. This compound attaches to T-cell lymphocytes expressing the interleukin-2 receptor, whereupon the diphtheria toxins damage the lymphocytes. This therapy can be used against cancerous T cells or against normal donor T cells to control graft-versus-host disease.

Growth factor antagonist therapy

This approach is similar to antiangiogenesis therapy, which aims to stop growth of blood vessels supplying tumors with nutrients. Growth factor inhibition aims at depriving the tumor of other substances and structures needed for growth. Some of the drugs listed in this group also are classified as antiangiogens.

Substances being tested are oral COL-3, carboxyamidotriazole, suramin (SUR), and TNP-470.

Hormone therapy

Some tumors respond to various hormones, perhaps the two best known being breast and prostate cancers responding to some androgens and estrogens.

Many tumors, including some NHLs, have receptors on their surface for a brain hormone, somatostatin. By supplying the tumor with a substance closely resembling somatostatin (an analog), the reaction of the tumor resembles orderly, programmed cell death called apoptosis.

Octreotide, one analog for the hypothalamic hormone somatostatin, is being tested in this way.

Idiotype vaccines

See "Tumor cell derivative vaccines."

Immunosuppressant therapy

Glucocorticoids such as dexamethasone, prednisone, and methylprednisolone are manmade copies of the human corticosteroid hydrocortisone normally produced by the adrenal glands. They're used against hematologic cancers to suppress the rampant growth of cancerous white blood cells.

Tacrolimus (FK506) is being tested for use as an immunosuppressant in NHL therapy. Peldesine (BCX-34) suppresses certain T cells only, and may be used as either an immunosuppressant or as an active agent against T-cell malignancies.

Liposomal encapsulation

Some drugs appear to work better, to be less toxic to the liver or the kidneys, and to be effective when taken orally if they are first encased in a layer of lipids.

Drugs being used in this way are cytarabine and doxorubicin.

Leukocyte therapy

This approach uses white blood cells to challenge a tumor. Often these are from a donor, but they may be the patient's, which have been extracted from a vein, resensitized to the tumor, and reinserted. Trials that appear in this category may also fit others, such as bone marrow or stem cell transplantation.

The following trials are underway using leukocyte therapy:

- Phase I Pilot Study to Evaluate the Toxic Effects of Allogeneic Epstein-Barr Virus (EBV)–Specific Cytotoxic T Lymphocytes for EBV Associated Lymphoproliferative Diseases in Organ Transplant Recipients

- Phase I/II Study of Epstein-Barr Virus (EBV)-Immune T Lymphocytes from a Normal HLA-Compatible Donor to Treat EBV-Associated Lymphomas and Other Lymphoproliferative Diseases

- Phase I/II Pilot Study of G-CSF-Stimulated Donor Peripheral Blood Mononuclear Cells for Post-Transplant Relapse of Hematologic Malignancies

- Phase I Study of Cellular Adoptive Immunotherapy with Epstein-Barr Virus (EBV)–Specific Cytotoxic T-Cells Following Chemotherapy for Refractory or Recurrent EBV-Expressing, HIV-Associated, Intermediate- or High-Grade B-Cell Non-Hodgkin's Lymphoma

- Phase I Study of Cytotoxic T-Cell Infusion with PBSC Transplantation for Acute Leukemia, Hodgkin's Disease, Non-Hodgkin's Lymphoma, and Multiple Myeloma

Lymphokine-activated killer cell therapy

Lymphokine-activated killer (LAK) cells are white blood cells that have been conditioned by cytokines to attack tumors.

The following trials are underway using LAK therapy:

- Phase I Study of Cellular Adoptive Immunotherapy with Epstein-Barr Virus (EBV)–Specific Cytotoxic T-Cells Following Chemotherapy for Refractory or Recurrent EBV-Expressing, HIV-Associated, Intermediate- or High-Grade B-Cell Non-Hodgkin's Lymphoma.

- Phase I Study of Cytotoxic T-Cell Infusion with PBSC Transplantation for Acute Leukemia, Hodgkin's Disease, non-Hodgkin's Lymphoma, and Multiple Myeloma

Monoclonal antibodies

See "Antibody therapy."

Nonspecific immune-modulator therapy

Nonspecific immune modulators are substances that aid in redirecting, suppressing, or boosting the immune system in ways that are either somewhat general or perhaps poorly understood.

Vaccine adjuvants may contain aluminum or small pieces of protein, for instance, that are not related to the vaccine material, but are known to elicit a stronger immune response.

The vaccine adjuvant QS-21, like vaccine adjuvants in general, has been shown to heighten the immune response, and thus the effectiveness of a vaccine created from tumor cells. (See "Tumor cell derivative vaccines" later in this chapter.)

Peripheral blood lymphocyte therapy

See "Leukocyte therapy."

Protein kinase C inhibition

In a normal cell, DNA is surveyed for damage after it is copied in the early steps of cell replication. A substance called protein kinase C interacts with other substances to ensure a rest phase during which damaged DNA is repaired before the next step of cell division is begun. If damage cannot be repaired, the cell is marked for destruction by the p53 gene, a key player in overseeing the orderliness of our DNA and its replication. This is how the DNA, the genome, is kept pure and error-free.

In a cancerous cell, these checkpoints may be missing or out of control; the p53 gene and other key genes may be absent or damaged.

Substances that interfere with protein kinase C can stop the cancer cell from resting between the stages of division. This quickening of the cell cycle leaves no time for the cell to repair its damaged DNA, and thus these substances can be used to boost the DNA-damaging capabilities of other drugs. When the tumor's DNA is damaged and cannot be repaired, the tumor is less likely to reproduce successfully.

A substance in this category being tested is UCN-01.

Radioimmunotherapy

These substances are compounds consisting of manmade monoclonal antibodies (see "Antibody therapy" above) and a radioactive isotope. The antibody attaches preferentially to tumor cells; the isotope decays within, upon, or very near the tumor, damaging or killing the cell with radiation.

Monoclonal antibodies conjugated to radioisotopes include:

- Iodine-131 labeled LL2 immunoglobulin G (Lymphocide)
- Yttrium-90 labeled humanized Anti-Tac (CD30-positive)
- Iodine-131 labeled anti-CD20 (Bexxar)
- Yttrium-90 labeled anti-CD20 (IDEC-Y2B8)

Radiosensitization

Certain drugs can make tumors more sensitive to damage by radiotherapy.

Topotecan and broxuridine (BUDR) are being tested for this effect.

Topoisomerase inhibitor therapy

Topoisomerases are enzymes that our cells use to break DNA bonds before copying and to repair the breaks after copying. Topoisomerase inhibitors interfere with DNA repair, causing the cancer cell to die, because damaged DNA cannot be translated into proteins, such as transport and digestive proteins, that each cell needs to breathe or eat.

New topoisomerase inhibitors being tested against NHL include aminocamptothecin (9-AC), rebeccamycin, and irinotecan.

Pyrazoloacridine's effects resemble those of a topoisomerase inhibitor, but its exact mode of action still is unknown.

Tubulin inhibitor therapy

When a cell has made a copy of all of its chromosomes and is ready to divide, spindles made of tubulin form to pull the two copies of each chromosome apart into two identical clusters of forty-eight chromosomes apiece. Tubulin inhibitors stop spindles from forming, thus stopping the tumor cell from dividing.

A novel tubulin inhibitor being tested is rhizoxin.

Tumor cell derivative vaccines

Vaccines made from tumor cells that have been removed from the body and cultured in the lab can cause our bodies to become resensitized to tumors, resulting in renewed attacks against the tumor by our immune systems. This trial examines that technique:

- Phase I Adjuvant Study of Tumor-Derived Immunoglobulin Idiotype Combined with QS-21 for Follicular Lymphomas

(See "Nonspecific immune modulator therapy," for QS-21.)

Novel techniques and devices

Not only new substances are tested for efficacy against NHL, but new techniques and devices as well. Below are novel methods and devices currently being funded by NCI.

Bone marrow or stem cell transplantation

Transplantation has been used successfully for more than ten years to combat lymphomas and leukemias, but new and better ways to use this procedure are being examined.

Some of the new strategies and tactics include:

- Tandem or multiple successive transplants that attempt to eradicate all cancer cells.

- Transplants using umbilical cord blood or placental blood. Umbilical cord and placental blood is less likely to cause a severe graft-versus-host reaction in the patient because the blood surrounding the newborn has not had time to develop white blood cells against external challenges.

- Improved chemotherapeutic regimens, utilizing higher doses of drugs with fewer side effects.

- Boosting the engraftment of marrow transplanted from donors via subsequent repeated infusions of donor stem cells. This has been shown to gradually convert marrow, especially a poor engraftment or mixed patient/donor marrow, to production of donor marrow only.

- Use of marrow containing graft-facilitating cells, a kind of cell found intermingled in marrow, to ensure a rapid and strong engraftment.

- Use of interleukin-2 to stimulate stem cells in new marrow, hastening the recovery of marrow following transplantation.

- Non–marrow-destroying transplants that leave patient marrow mixed with donor marrow, attempting to establish host-versus-graft tolerance for donor cells so that graft-versus-lymphoma effects are possible.

- Colony stimulating factor therapy to harvest stem cells before transplantation and to support marrow recovery after transplantation.

CD34+ cell separation devices

One such device is on the market, and at least one other is pending FDA approval, for selecting from marrow stem cells that express cell surface antigen CD34. This is a means of reverse-purging of marrow, because cancerous stem cells seldom express the CD34 cell surface antigen.

Marrow purging

Often the marrow of NHL survivors is infiltrated by cancerous cells. When an autologous transplant is being performed, marrow purging is a means to ensure that no cancerous cells remain in marrow to be reintroduced to the body. The following tactics are now beginning use:

- Purging of marrow with various monoclonal antibodies having different properties, such as anti-T12 or anti-B3 antibodies

- Reverse-purging via selection of CD34-positive stem cells from marrow, a means of selecting healthy immature white blood cells

- Purging with Campath-1 for deletion of both B and T lymphocytes, as a means to reduce transplant-related Epstein-Barr malignancies that may be reintroduced via B cells if only T cells are depleted

- Purging of T-cells capable of forming E-rosettes when exposed to sheep blood cells, to leave behind marrow able to form new T cells

Whole-body hyperthermia

WBH is a treatment that attempts to exploit the observation that some chemotherapy drugs work better when body temperature is raised and held steady for a period of time. WBH sometimes involves using equipment resembling a warm bath or a tanning bed.

Future trials

The strategies detailed below are being discussed with great vigor among scientists, and some are being tested against other cancers, but they are not yet ready for human trials against NHL. Some may prove suitable for treating NHL; others may not.

Antisense molecules (antisense oligonucleotides)

DNA wants to exist in paired strands, except when a cell is dividing. Because cancer cells are known to have one or more faulty genes somewhere along the length of their DNA, some researchers are experimenting with delivering to the tumor short pieces of DNA or RNA that will match the faulty genes and couple with single strands of the cancer cell's DNA. In theory, these short pieces of DNA or RNA might interfere with a cancer cell's division and replication in a variety of ways.

Autologous graft-versus-lymphoma responses

Some studies have found that withdrawal of immunosuppressives following autologous transplantation results in a graft-versus-host response similar to that seen following allogeneic transplantation. This phenomenon might be exploited to increase the efficacy of autologous transplants by generating a graft-versus-lymphoma effect.

Chemoprevention

Trials of substances such as tamoxifen, vitamin E, and beta-carotene have shown some success in preventing cancers in certain groups of people. More such trials are likely to be held, perhaps testing substances found in vegetables, such as limonene from orange peel, lycopene from tomatoes, and resveratrol from grapes, or perhaps testing manmade substances that mimic products found in nature.

Cellular matrix exploitation

The cellular matrix is a medium somewhat like cement along which cells propel themselves, and in which cells eventually become anchored in order to thrive.

For either normal or cancerous cell growth to occur, the cellular matrix has to provide a foothold for new cells migrating to their home. Studies of the behavior of cellular matrix proteins such as laminin and some collagens, and the enzymes that interact with them such as the matrix metalloproteases, may shed light on cancer pathways that are amenable to normalization.

Some molecules involved with growth of new blood vessels—angiogenesis—appear also to be involved with activities of the cellular matrix.

Death receptors

Normal cells, cells being transformed into cancerous cells, and fully cancerous cells have on their surface certain proteins that act as binding regions for a protein, TRAIL (also called Apo2L), that triggers orderly cell death. Cells being transformed into cancerous cells can be destroyed by TRAIL, but normal cells protect themselves from this destruction using "decoy" receptors: they bind TRAIL, but do not transport it inside the cell, thus seeming to render it ineffective. Cancerous cells also appear to have many ways to avoid cell death. Future cancer therapies will examine these differences in behavior among normal, cancerous, and soon-to-be-cancerous cells.

Gene therapy

In its broadest sense, gene therapy is a name applied to several kinds of cancer treatment that involve modifying genes, such as triggering the body's white cells to attack tumors, but in the strict sense, gene therapy is the modification of the tumor's genes to cause it to self-destruct or to behave as a normal cell does.

Modification of white blood cells to attack a tumor can occur if a weakened virus is modified genetically to contain a piece of the tumor's DNA. When this weakened virus is unleashed in the body, our white blood cells recognize it as "enemy" and destroy it. Because the virus also is expressing part of the tumor's DNA, white blood cells become sensitized to this protein as well, and attack it wherever they find it, that is, either on the virus coat or on the tumor.

This has been done with some (but not total) success against melanoma. This application of the technology, referred to in this instance as a melanoma vaccine, now is being reviewed by the FDA for approval.

Conforming to the strictest definition of gene therapy are experiments to reinsert genes into cancer cells lacking properly functioning copies of these genes, or inserting a manmade suicide gene into the tumor cell that will make the cell more susceptible to the toxic effects of certain drugs.

Currently, there are thirty-one clinical trials classified as gene therapy for many different cancers in NCI's database, testing such possibilities as:

- Inserting a working copy of the p53 tumor suppressor and apoptosis gene into bladder and liver tumors via one of the common cold viruses.

- Inserting a functioning version of the herpesvirus thymidine kinase gene into brain and ovarian tumors via one of the common cold viruses. The thymidine kinase gene will cause the tumor to react to gancyclovir, an antiviral medication, as if the tumor were a virus.

- Inserting a copy of the cytosine deaminase gene into colon cancer tumors using one of the common cold viruses. The cytosine deaminase gene will cause the otherwise impervious cell to react to the harmless prodrug Flucytosine (5-fluorocytosine) and convert it to a drug that can kill the tumor.

In vitro sensitivity-directed chemotherapy

This approach requires a sample of one's tumor, against which a variety of anticancer compounds are tested to see which works best. In practice, there are problems with this approach, because tumor cells that respond well in a test tube may be inaccessible to the apparently useful drug when the same scenario is attempted within the body.

In other words, this technique may be useful to rule out agents to which the tumor fails to respond, but cannot be used with complete accuracy to determine agents to which the tumor will respond.

Some clinicians offer this service now, but its use is not widespread.

Mitochondrial DNA

Science and medicine have focused primarily on the activity of genes within the cell's nuclcus, but DNA also exists within the mitochondria of each cell.

Mitochondria are small organs (organelles) within each cell that burn oxygen to accomplish cellular tasks. It's thought that mitochondria are bacteria that were enslaved by the cells of larger species many millions of years ago, because each mitochondrium contains its own DNA and resembles a bacterium in certain other ways. Many of the cells of most higher species contain mitochondria; cells requiring higher levels of oxygen consumption, such as muscle cells, contain more mitochondria than do others.

Mitochondrial DNA can only be inherited from the female. Ova—being fully functioning cells—contain mitochondria, but spermatozoa do not.

These facts are meaningful for cancer research for at least three reasons:

- For diseases that are linked to NHL and found in both males and females, but found consistently only on the mother's side of the family, mitochondrial DNA may play a role.

- Mitochondrial DNA sometimes exhibits damage that is known to cause cancer, as does the much more closely studied nuclear DNA.

- Mitochondria appear to respond to chemotherapy and radiation therapy, and mitochondrial DNA can be modified to improve cancer treatment.

Molecular oncology

A tumor may arise because a gene is being incorrectly transcribed into an aberrant protein, is not transcribed at all, is over-expressed, or expressed at the wrong time, because two erroneously spliced genes are being transcribed into a hybrid protein that is impotent or oncogenic, or owing to a combination of any of these.

Molecular oncology attempts to substitute the correct or missing gene product for a faulty or missing gene. For example, all-trans-retinoic acid (ATRA) treatment for acute promyelocytic leukemia, APL, replaces a missing protein. APL develops owing to the fusion of two genes on chromosomes 15 and 17 that, separately, would work in equilibrium producing ATRA to control a metabolic process, but together cause it to continue unabated. ATRA treatment of these leukemias temporarily corrects this out-of-control condition, but usually does not cure it, as the leukemia can become resistant to treatment.

Proto-oncogenes, oncogenes, and tumor suppressor genes

As with many areas of cancer research, this is a well-studied but not yet fully understood area of genetics.

DNA in normal cells contains oncogenes and precursor genes called proto-oncogenes. Both can trigger growth, but these genes normally are tightly regulated, sometimes kept quite literally under wraps with methylation, so that they cannot be transcribed into proteins that would trigger growth until it's time for the cell to divide.

In contrast, and for biological balance, there are about nine known tumor-suppressor genes (of which p53 is the best known) that are sensitive to the activity of the dividing cell, that signal when to demethylate and transcribe growth genes, when to arrest growth, and when to initiate cell death if irreparable errors are found in the cell's DNA.

Errors in or near any of these genes can cause a cell to become cancerous.

Some studies are examining ways to regain control of oncogenes that have run amok or to substitute for the products of tumor suppressor genes that have been damaged.

Recombinant viral vaccines

Viruses engineered to target only cancer cells are being considered as one way to damage tumors and spare healthy tissue. The virus itself could attack and kill the tumor, or it could insert its DNA or RNA into the tumor—DNA that has been modified in the lab to contain a killer sequence, or to weaken the tumor's defenses or ability to replicate.

Telomerase inhibitors

At the end of each chromosome is a long string of repeating, nontranslated genetic material called a telomere. Not too long ago, it was discovered that, as a normal cell ages, the telomere, or tail, shortens. When it is entirely gone, the cell dies in an orderly, shrinking, dissolving way (apoptosis).

The telomeres of many cancer cells, however, never shorten.

Some researchers believe that an enzyme called telomerase is faulty in certain cancer cells, and that by manipulating this enzyme, the cancer cell might be forced to age normally and eventually die.

Tissue engineering

Currently, tissue engineering is in limited use to regrow skin damaged by burns and to repair damaged cartilage within joints. Artificial kidneys that are half human tissue, half mechanical device are being tested in animals. Although tissue engineering is not used yet following cancer therapy, it's conceivable that someday, new vocal cords, or intestinal, breast, or other tissue might be regrown in the laboratory and implanted into a cancer survivor weeks or months after laryngectomy, mastectomy, or colectomy.

The obstacles to this approach are several, the first being that usually a small piece of the patient's own tissue is required to grow the much larger quantity on a base consisting of anchor material and nutrients. For cancer survivors, the risk exists that microscopic cancer growths that might be included in this sample would survive, thrive, and subsequently be reimplanted. The second problem is that even seemingly simple tissues can be quite complex. Cartilage, for instance, is composed of several layers, each having a separate function. Results of cartilage implantation are too new to be certain that the tissue functions as it should for many years after. Although multilayered skin has been regrown and used successfully in burn therapy and is FDA-approved, it's not known whether all tissues, in all their complexities, can be regrown. A third obstacle is expense. One square inch of nutrient matrix for regrowing skin costs several thousand dollars. Tissue engineering for a very complex organ might be beyond reach, simply owing to expense.

Triplex molecules

In some cases, the antisense molecules described in an earlier section that bind to single strands of dividing DNA or RNA also can bind with double-strand DNA that is not in the process of dividing. When antisense molecules do bind to double strands, they form a triplex molecule. Some researchers are pursuing this strategy as a means of crossbinding DNA so that it cannot even begin replication, thus causing the cancer cell to become static or to die.

Tumor infiltrating lymphocyte therapy

In several cancer types, including both the Hodgkin's and non-Hodgkin's lymphomas, it has been noted that some white blood cells are able to infiltrate tumors and appear to be on the attack.

Boosting lymphocytes' tendency to infiltrate tumors may heighten or universalize this response against more tumor types at all locations in the body.

Summary

Many new concepts and treatment are evolving for cancer in general and the NHLs in particular. This chapter has addressed the treatments now in clinical trials, and those still in the planning stages.

It's wise to keep in touch with new treatments being developed for NHL by consulting your doctor, by browsing the NCI clinical trials database, or by calling NCI at (800) 4-CANCER and asking for a list of trials for your subtype of NHL. Chapter 24, *Researching Your Lymphoma*, contains information regarding evaluating clinical trials.

Researching Your Lymphoma

Chance favors the prepared mind.

—Louis Pasteur

Non-Hodgkin's lymphoma survivors and their loved ones choose to search for information for many reasons. Many of us feel a compelling need to learn all we can as quickly as possible about what we'll be facing, or we feel that we must do something to contribute to our recovery. Some of us just like to verify that our doctors are relaying accurate and up-to-date information, even when the care we've received has been very good. Others are faced with having to assume a greater responsibility for their health care, owing to living in areas with few doctors, or perhaps owing to having had a bad experience with a doctor's lack of knowledge. HMO policies that are based on cost control and that may deny us the best care in order to keep expenses down are a driving force for too many of us. Those with a rare subtype of NHL might have a doctor with little experience treating this subtype who may appreciate any information found. Loved ones of cancer survivors sometimes need to feel they're doing something to help, and finding information may satisfy that need.

The decision to research your illness is the beginning of an empowerment that will do more than just serve you in good stead for making decisions. Research on stress and cancer hints that a proactive attitude may contribute to long survival. The more you learn, the more control you have over how events unfold, not only because you'll be making better health and treatment choices, but because you can take back some of the control that is lost in the clutter of automation that now accompanies cancer diagnosis and treatment.

In general, the more you learn, the more confident and relaxed you'll ultimately be when dealing with NHL.

This chapter will offer you basic ways to find information about your illness, outside of simply relying on your doctor. First a few generalities about one's approach to learning are covered, then we discuss using medical libraries and research journals, as well as the National Cancer Institute's Internet, phone, fax, and clinical trials services, and hiring a search firm to do the legwork for you. Methods for checking drug side effects, verifying your chemotherapy dosage, finding support groups, interpreting test results, and evaluating unproven remedies are offered.

For each type of information, ways to access the source with and without a computer are outlined when it is possible to do so. For instance, the Merck Manual section on laboratory results is available both on paper and on the Internet. Certain unique resources, however, are found only on the Internet.

Prerequisites and perspectives

Before you start, you need to know a few specific facts about your diagnosis to make searching more fruitful. You also will benefit by knowing what to avoid, and what to insulate yourself against.

Prerequisites

You'll need four things before you start: the exact name of your NHL subtype, its stage, the classification system(s) used for diagnosis, and a medical dictionary.

If you don't know your precise diagnosis, you'll waste a lot of time and precious energy reading the wrong material. You may even frighten yourself unnecessarily by finding distressing but wrong information, not realizing that it doesn't pertain to you.

Your doctor's staff can read you the exact name of your NHL subtype and its grade from your pathology report. Better yet, ask them to send you a photocopy of this, and of all your medical records. Cross-check this information against Appendix D, *Classification Systems*, to see what your subtype is called in other systems. This way, if you find your subtype of NHL referred to in research papers by an unfamiliar term, you'll be better equipped to assess what you're reading.

Purchase a medical dictionary to help you with the terminology you will encounter, which becomes increasingly easy to understand with greater exposure. Several reasonably priced medical dictionaries are listed in Appendix A, *Resources*. One of the most useful is *The Cancer Dictionary*, by Altman and Sarg.

Perspectives

The following perspectives are helpful to keep in mind while researching your condition.

- Persistence. Please don't feel intimidated by the volume of information on NHL or its seeming complexity. As with any other task of assimilation, small steps ultimately will yield great gains. If you're wary of trying to search for information because medicine seems like an alien frontier to you, it might be helpful to know a few interesting facts:

  — Academic success does not account for all that much of success in life. Success also is a result of being flexible, adaptable, developing social skills, having luck, being persistent, patient, and so forth.

  — If one person can understand something, generally so can another person, and if the second person doesn't understand, it might be because the first person isn't explaining it very well.

  — Contrary to popular mythology about kids being computer whizzes and older people not, the fastest growing group of Internet users is over age 65.

  In short, if you're persistent in asking about, searching for, and trying to absorb medical information, in turning away from doctors who are condescending, seeking instead those who respect you, you'll succeed. You won't need a degree in medicine or an abnormally high IQ to understand what you find, just a medical dictionary and the motivation to acquire new skills. It might take you twenty minutes longer to understand a certain medical concept than it takes an M.D., but it's worthwhile if that twenty minutes makes the difference of a lifetime.

- Clarity. When asking for help, be specific about what you need. Educate yourself as to what options are available. We suggest you ask for full information, rather than edited versions that may exist. For example, when communicating with the National Cancer Institute (NCI), consider requesting the information for physicians, not for patients, if you already are somewhat familiar with NHL. (The patient information statement is quite basic, and, while it may be useful to you initially, soon it will seem less than edifying. If you find that this is the case, it's time to request the physicians' version of PDQ information.)

If you're looking for clinical trials, always tell the NCI staff whether you're willing to travel. If you don't specify a national search, they'll tell you only of trials in your own area. Always ask for the full information on clinical trails, not the summaries. If you ask friends for help or hire a search firm to do a medical search the same considerations about clarity and intent apply.

- **Humility.** Don't forget that you should always verify what you find with your oncologist. It's imperative that you focus on correct, current information, and that you understand what it means regarding your specific circumstances. At times people simply are not equipped to evaluate what they've found, but it's almost a certainty that your doctor has a good frame of reference for doing this evaluation.

- **Courtesy.** Good manners dictate that you make an appointment to discuss lengthy topics with your doctor or other health professional, or that you offer to pay for a telephone consultation. See Nancy Keene's book *Working with Your Doctor* for a good discussion of improving patient/doctor relationships.

- **Diplomacy.** Some doctors react badly to the idea that their patients are doing their own research or bring in information from the Internet, where information ranges from abysmal to superb. Share your research and questions with your doctor, asking for his advice. If you use the Internet to research, cite the original sources on which your Internet findings are based, such as the PDQ database of the National Cancer Institute or a specific medical journal.

- **Self-respect.** If your doctor is not interested in what you find, or seems threatened by your efforts, consider discussing this attitude with him or consider changing doctors.

- **Serenity.** When you have started researching your illness, you may find some information that's upsetting, such as survival statistics. Keep in mind that statistics always describe composite results of studies involving numbers of people, and cannot be applied to the progress and circumstances of a single individual. For example, when a researcher averages the survival times of eighty patients treated with drug XYZ whose survival ranges from 2 months to 212 months, he may calculate that the average survival following treatment is thirteen months. Nobody has an idea where to place themselves on this continuum, however, unless they know intimately the health factors of all eighty people and can match themselves to at least one of them. For the researcher, the average will tell her whether the treatment is worth further development, but for the individual, statistical averages are just data, not information.

A survivor of low-grade disease describes how her own search for information made a distinct difference in her decision about treatment:

> When I was first diagnosed, I was shocked, especially because I felt so well and had no symptoms of any disease. I just had a swollen lymph node in my groin. The tests were complete, and the diagnosis was a low-grade, follicular, cleaved cell, B-type. I went immediately onto the Internet and used several search engines to read about this particular type. There was lots of information. The most useful information I found at that point were the studies indicating there was absolutely no difference in long-term survival of people who had early, aggressive treatment with chemotherapy and those who had no treatment until they experienced symptoms of the disease.
>
> From this I knew that I had some time to think about my options, and to have a second, and even third, opinion from different doctors as to recommended courses of action. If I had not found that information, I would more than likely have rushed into treatment with a doctor who would not have been the best choice for me.
>
> Among the many complaints I hear from cancer patients is that they felt rushed into decisions and wound up with the wrong doctor, treatment, or facility. They wished they had done even a minimal amount of research before they made their decision. I know the Internet information made a real difference in my life.

Ways to find information

Here's a summary of ways that you can obtain information about non-Hodgkin's lymphoma. The sections that follow describe these methods in detail.

- If you have computer access, you can find an almost limitless amount written about NHL on the Internet, some of which is highly accurate, some of which is of lesser quality. The highly reliable information at the

National Cancer Institute's site should be your starting point, and the latest medical research papers an ongoing source of information.

- If you have siblings, children, or grandchildren with computer access, and you don't feel like starting from scratch using a computer amidst your worries about cancer—and who would blame you?—ask them to do Internet searches for you. Make sure you tell them the specifics of your diagnosis, and what you're looking for: treatment options, complementary therapies, stories of other patients, clinical trials, and so on.

- If you're friends with a doctor, nurse, or librarian, ask them to do searches of various resources, such as the National Library of Medicine's Medline database and the NCI's Physician's Data Query (PDQ).

- Pay a commercial firm that specializes in this activity to do a search for you.

- Visit an academic or medical library to research the medical journals in the periodicals section and their medical texts.

- Ask your doctor for help getting copies of research papers from medical journals, but offer to pay for any photocopying that's needed.

- Contact the Cure for Lymphoma Foundation, the Leukemia Society of America, the Lymphoma Research Society, or the American Cancer Society, and ask for information that can be mailed to you.

- Call the National Cancer Institute at (800) 4-CANCER and ask for information, or ask for help using their CancerFax service.

How to obtain NCI's information

The information on cancer amassed and maintained by the National Cancer Institute, a division of NIH, is the granddaddy of all cancer databases, and should be your starting point for learning the basics about NHL. It's accurate and current. You can access this information in several ways.

By phone

You can call NCI at (800) 4-CANCER and request that information on NHL be sent to you by mail free of charge. Remember that the information geared to physicians is much more useful and detailed than that written for patients. If you feel uncomfortable asking for physician information, you can give some justification or even make some up. For example, you could say that your doctor asked you to request this information. One patient said that he was writing a newspaper article that required in-depth material. You might want to ask as well for literature that describes all of the NCI publications that one might order, such as tracts that describe dealing with fatigue or depression.

By fax

The information available by phone request is also available by fax. Call (800) 4-CANCER and ask for instructions for faxing.

By personal computer

If you have computer access, you can read the National Cancer Institute's state-of-the-art NHL treatment statement for physicians, as well as an immense collection of other literature about NHL, at their web site (*http:// cancernet.nci.nih.gov*). Follow the path for health professionals to PDQ information and the word "treatment."

You may retrieve the NCI physician's statement on NHL via email by keying the encoded identifier *cn-100066* into the message area, with no other information, such as your signature, included in the message area. Send this email to *cnet@icicc.nci.nih.gov*.

If you'd like a list of all NCI information that's retrievable by email, send the single word *help* to the same email address, *cnet@icicc.nci.nih.gov*.

How to obtain medical research papers

Reviewing the research papers published in medical journals is the best way for an NHL survivor to get the most current information. Textbooks are out of date almost as soon as they're printed owing to the time delays of production. NCI PDQ information is a good foundation, but doesn't reflect every emerging trend still in the test phase—just state-of-the-art standards for care.

Medical journals that tend to have many articles on NHL are *Blood; Transplantation; Leukemia and Lymphoma; Journal of Clinical Oncology; The British Journal of Haematology; The American Journal of Hematology; Bone Marrow Transplantation; The European Journal of Haematology; Seminars in Haematology; Haematologica; The Annals of Hematology; Leukemia Research; Current*

Opinions in Hematology; Leukemia; Cytokines and Molecular Therapy; Hematology and Oncology Clinics of North America, and *The Journal of the National Cancer Institute.*

If you like to read about basic cancer research that's years away from becoming treatment, the journals *Science, Cell,* and *Nature Biotechnology* are good choices.

Many medical journals are now on the Web, including *Blood; Bone Marrow Transplantation; Science; The Journal of the American Medical Association; The American Journal of Hematology;* and *The Journal of the National Cancer Institute.* Some of these cannot be viewed online unless you're a subscriber to the standard paper edition.

Reading medical research papers is arguably the most difficult part of learning about progress against NHL, as well as the best way to keep abreast of progress. A medical dictionary will serve you well in this effort, and you should ask your doctor about parts that are not clear. Usually the abstract (summary) of a paper will suffice, as abstracts of cancer research studies normally contain conclusions, but at times obtaining the full text of the paper will be necessary.

If you use the full text of a paper, don't try to understand the whole thing at first. Just read the introduction, the conclusions, and the discussion. The middle sections deal with scientific methodology that's important in verifying that the research was performed to strict scientific standards, but this part has been peer-reviewed by other scientists and the editors of the journal. This material is usually, but not always, less important to a patient trying to find good prospects for care. As you become better acquainted with research papers and their terminology, occasionally you may want to read the remaining sections as well.

By subscription

Subscription costs for some of the journals such as these usually start at about one hundred dollars per year, and can go much higher. The disadvantage of subscribing to individual journals, besides the accumulation of hard-to-index paper copy, is that good research articles on NHL will be spread among all of these, and subscribing to several becomes prohibitively expensive.

By using Medline

An absolutely indispensable resource—some say the most important resource—that you can use is Medline, maintained by the U.S. National Library of Medicine (NLM). Various Medline search engines, such as NLM's, which at the time of this writing is free, are available on the Internet, giving you access to the nine million medical research papers in the National Library of Medicine.

If you don't have computer access, ask a friend or relative who does to do a search for you. Alternately, a nurse or someone affiliated with a hospital or library may have Medline access. The National Library of Medicine's Medline web address is *http://www.ncbi.nlm.nih.gov/PubMed/*

If you're using a computer, at most Medline sites you'll generally find a search engine that accepts keywords and returns summaries of the medical research publications that match your keywords. For example, if you key in the terms:

NHL, treatment, CHOP

and click on the search button, you'll receive in return the titles of the many studies regarding treating NHL with CHOP. Clicking the mouse on each title will cause the summary (abstract) of the study's results to display on your screen. You'll note that the latest studies are displayed first. After you've read a number of these studies, the terminology will become familiar, and you can repeat the search often in the following days or months, using new keywords.

Almost all of the Web-based Medline search engines use an organizational hierarchy called MEdical Subject Headings (MESH). MESH terms group references by category so that you'll get more research papers returned for your searching efforts, even if you're not familiar with the right medical terms or if you misspell a word slightly. Some Medline search tools invoke MESH terms behind the scenes when you enter a keyword; others, like PaperChase, will prompt you to pick a MESH term from a list that they produce that is associated with the keyword you entered. Still others have advanced searches you can invoke using MESH terms explicitly.

Here is a partial list of MESH terms that might be used behind the scenes or offered to you as a choice when the word "lymphocyte" is the keyword used in a Medline search:

- LYMPHOCYTE COOPERATION
- LYMPHOCYTE COUNT
- LYMPHOCYTE COUNT, CD4
- LYMPHOCYTE CULTURE TEST, MIXED
- LYMPHOCYTE DEPLETION
- LYMPHOCYTE DIFFERENTIATION ANTIGENS, B
- LYMPHOCYTE DIFFERENTIATION ANTIGENS, T
- LYMPHOCYTE EPITOPES, B

A good way to get background information on any medical topic is to seek out the review articles in Medline. Enter various search terms, like:

- immune, lymphoma, review
- leukocytes, immune, review
- dendritic, immune, review

This will retrieve the abstracts of review articles that are geared to physicians who might not be specialists—articles appearing in more generalized publications such as *Family Practitioner* or *Nature*—which contain more explanatory material and make fewer assumptions.

If you need help with searching, you can call the National Library of Medicine at (800) 272-4787 or (301) 496-6308.

If the Medline summaries (abstracts) you read are more tantalizing than edifying, you can order the full text of any research paper from companies that specialize in this service. Some of these companies, such as InfoTrieve, are Web-based; others can be found by calling a medical school library and getting recommendations from a librarian. Unfortunately, at the time of this writing, the National Library of Medicine's service does not offer full text retrieval to those not associated with an academic library. Those who are, however, can use the Loansome Doc service to order full text of papers.

On the Internet, the Medline service providers HealthGate, Medscape, Helix, PhyNet, PDRnet.Com, SilverPlatter, Ovid On Call, Infotrieve, PaperChase and others offer full-text services for a fee.

By using medical libraries

Another way to find articles in medical journals is to visit a medical or university library and examine their journals and recent texts, borrowing or photocopying what you find most useful. Copyright law permits photocopying one copy of a journal article if it's for your own immediate use. Avoid relying solely on textbooks that are older than two years, as the time it takes to bring a text to print makes the source material used to prepare a text quickly out of date.

Note that some university and medical libraries restrict entry to those affiliated with the institution is some way. You can find the nearest medical library open to the public by calling the National Network of Libraries of Medicine at (800) 338-7657.

Your local hospitals also may have medical libraries.

To find articles in medical journals, ask the main information desk where periodicals are stored and how to search them by subject. There's some variety in how different libraries store, search, and retrieve journal articles. Some academic libraries have all periodicals stored on CD-ROM, for example, but others are still stored as paper copy in the stacks. Regardless of these differences, there's always a way to search by subject, and this should be your starting point. The library you visit may also have access to Medline or Index Medicus.

Often the periodicals section of a medical or academic library will have staff devoted to helping you. All should have material you can read at your leisure describing how to search their collection. Don't be shy about asking for help. Most librarians are proud of their ability to root out obscure references and are in that career because they want to connect people to information.

Arrive prepared to pay for photocopy fees and with coins for photocopy machines.

By hiring a search firm

Before hiring a commercial firm to do a search of the medical literature, you might want to call the National Library of Medicine's Management Desk at 1-800-638-8480 and ask for whatever help they can provide.

You might choose to pay a search fee to one of a number of companies who provide this service. Tell them what topic you're interested in, but keep in mind that the more specific you can be, the better: treatments for ALL for preschoolers, rather than childhood leukemia, for instance, will yield more useful material on this topic. The search firm will locate copies of articles from medical journals and mail them to you.

Here's a partial list of such companies. Their being included here does not imply an endorsement of their service:

- The Health Resource, Inc.: (501) 329-5272

- Can Help: (360) 437-2291

- Schine On-Line Services: (800) FIND-CURE

How to obtain medical textbooks

Texts on cancer, immunology, hematology, and NHL can provide you with the foundation for understanding more timely sources such as the papers published in medical journals. In general, the more recent the text, the better.

A source of background information might be an immunology text aimed at pre-med college students or first-year medical students. The terminology might be a notch higher than many people are comfortable with, but not nearly as difficult as that found in medical journals, and definitely geared to providing broad, fundamental information. They'll probably range in price from $40 to $200, but it's fairly easy to get used copies at college and university bookstores.

Using the list of books in Appendix A as a guide to reliable texts, visit your local public or academic library or a medical bookstore.

Medical bookstores usually are found near medical schools. Some of the largest well-known bookstore chains also carry hard-to-find textbooks such as Magrath's 1997 text on NHL, or they can order them for you. Several bookstores have web sites that greatly facilitate ordering books, especially if you're not feeling well enough to drive, park, browse, and lug heavy texts home.

Because of the high cost of textbooks, borrowing texts is an attractive alternative for most people.

If you haven't used a public library lately to search for holdings, you might be pleasantly surprised to find that, in many cases, the old card catalogs are gone, replaced by fast and easy-to-use computer workstations. Their databases can tell you within a few minutes how many copies of a book are in their system, which branches of the library own the book, whether another borrower has charged it, and when it's due back.

If your public library is in a large urban area, the materials you need may be readily accessible, but if not, your library system may be able to borrow the materials you need even if it's not in their holdings. As with searching for medical research papers, it pays to ask for help. You may have to wait longer for an interlibrary loan, but it can save you the cost of an expensive text.

One book, *The Wisdom of the Body*, has a chapter on blood and the immune system. It might not be as complete as some would like, but it's readily available in many public libraries.

How to find clinical trials

New and possibly better treatments are available to NHL patients in carefully controlled settings called clinical trials, which are described in depth in Chapter 19, *Clinical Trials*. You should become familiar with the trials that are available before you need one, for frequently trials are needed when events have reached crisis level and time is running low.

In order to choose the best from among several clinical trials, it's necessary to be familiar with the track record, if any, of the chemotherapeutic agents being used in each trial. Each of the drug names appearing in a trial's title can be used as a keyword to search medical journals (as described earlier in the section "How to obtain medical research papers") for any previous research studies published. This is a daunting task; do not expect to finish it in one sitting or even in a few days. Once it's done, though, you only need to search for new drugs as they first appear in the clinical trials database or among your other sources of information.

You can use several methods to find clinical trials. These are discussed in the following sections.

Ask your oncologist

Ask your oncologist which trials would suit your medical circumstances. This has its advantages and disadvantages, one advantage being that you need do very little except trust.

Call the National Cancer Institute

Call the NCI at (800) 4-CANCER and ask about trials for your subtype of NHL. Specify whether you're willing to travel—otherwise they'll send you local trials only—and be sure to ask for the full document, not the summary.

Hire a search firm

Commercial firms exist that can do a medical literature search for you. A partial list of such companies appears earlier in the chapter.

Personal computer

You can use a computer to research U.S. and international clinical trials at the NCI's web site (*http://cancernet.nci.nih.gov/prot/protsrch.shtml*). This, in conjunction with learning to use Medline, is by far the most comprehensive way to check on new treatments being tested. Once available only to those who subscribed to the NCI's Information Associates' program for $100 per year, this tool is now provided free of charge by the NCI on the Internet. We strongly suggest that you examine all trials available for NHL, not just those in your area.

When you visit this site, you'll be presented with a menu of choices for finding trials by cancer type, location of trial, kind of trial, and so on. Use the down arrow next to Diagnosis to expand the list of cancers, then scroll down and click on one of these two:

- lymphoma, non-Hodgkin's, adult
- lymphoma, non-Hodgkin's, childhood

If you're using this search engine for the first time, it's a good idea to view all NHL trials available for adults or children. Use the down arrow next to Trial Type to select the word "treatment," then click the search button. The result will be a large list of all trials for NHL that focus on treatment.

You can repeat the search using the City and State fields to see trials only in your own area, or with the phase field to see only phase I, phase II, or phase III trials, which are explained in Chapter 19.

If you're interested in a particular kind of drug or method, you can use the Modality field to select only trials using this technology, such as monoclonal antibodies, which are categorized as such and also as antibody therapy.

Other means of finding clinical trials include:

- CenterWatch's site on the Internet to track new cancer treatment trials. Find them at *http://www.centerwatch.com/*.

- Commercial Internet service providers such as America Online (AOL) to receive email press releases from pharmaceutical companies concerning new products in development.

- The National Childhood Cancer Foundation site to find trials specifically for children. Find them on the Web at *http://www.nccf.org/nccf/ protocol* or call (800) 458-6223.

How to find support groups

Local hospitals, a local branch of the national Wellness Community, the American Cancer Society, and the Internet offer solid information and access to others who have been through it, too. Their help is beyond estimation. The American Cancer Society can be reached at (800) ACS-2345; ask for their I Can Cope program. The Wellness Community in your area is listed in the phone book.

If you have Internet access, the Association of Cancer Online Resources (ACOR) has pointers to all of the Internet hematologic cancer email discussion groups. Highly recommended are the NHL list, run by Robert Scott Pallack, for emotional support and medical information, and the NHL-LOW list for medical information only—no emotional support—about low-grade NHL. HEM-ONC, run by GrannyBarb Lackritz, is for discussion of all hematologic cancers; PED-ALL for children with NHL being treated on ALL protocols; and BMT-TALK for those planning a bone marrow transplant. A new Mantle-cell NHL Internet discussion group has just been formed. For these and other Internet discussion groups, ACOR (*http://www.acor.org/*) offers a handy automatic subscription feature.

For kids with NHL and a personal computer, Sickkids (*http://tile.net/listserv/ sickkids.html*) is a discussion group just for children, but supervised by adults.

Several of the groups listed in the following section, "How to find groups for curing lymphoma," also offer one-on-one phone support for those with lymphoma or those planning a bone marrow transplant.

How to find groups for curing lymphoma

These three nonprofit groups specialize in helping those with lymphoma and in supporting research:

- The Lymphoma Research Foundation of America. This group has an impressive record of funding lymphoma research. Call (310) 704-2040, or visit their web site at *http://www.lymphoma.org/*.

- The Cure for Lymphoma Foundation. Call (212) 213-9595, or visit their web site at *http://www.cfl.org/*.

- The Leukemia Society of America. Call (212) 573-8484, or visit their web site at *http://www.leukemia.org/*.

How to find information on transplants

The Blood and Marrow Transplant Newsletter is an excellent resource for all kinds of transplant information, and especially for finding a lawyer if you're having insurance payment problems. Call (847) 831-1913, or visit their web site at *http://www.bmtnews.org/*.

The American Cancer Society. Call (800) ACS-2345, or visit their web site at *http://www.cancer.org/*.

The National Marrow Donor Program can be reached on (800) 4-MARROW, or visit their web site at *http://www.marrow.org/*.

How to verify drug information

Pharmaceutical information tools are useful for finding drug side effects, mode of action, and marketing names. Your pharmacist, your library or bookstore, your computer, and the FDA can be sources of information.

You can call your pharmacist for information about drugs, or ask for the foldout paper of small print that comes from the drug manufacturer but is seldom included with your prescription unless you ask for it.

The Physician's Desk Reference (PDR), a compendium of information about drugs, is now reprinted in versions that are easier for the general public to understand, but you might appreciate the learning experience gained from reading the original PDR. In addition to the PDR, many other drug encyclopedias are available as well for the general public.

The Food and Drug Administration is a good means for verifying drug information. Call (888) 332-4543, (800) 532-4440, or visit their web site at *http://www.fda.gov/*.

You can report adverse effects of drugs to the FDA, too, or use their MedWatch web site: *http://www.fda.gov/medwatch/how.htm*.

The following sites have search engines requiring only the drug name:

- RXMed: *http://www.rxmed.com/*
- Clinical Pharmacology Online: *http://www.cponline.gsm.com/*
- PharmInfoNet: *http://pharminfo.com/drg_mnu.html*
- DrugInfoNet: *http://www.druginfonet.com/*
- HealthTouch: *http://www.healthtouch.com/level1/p_dri.htm*

How to verify your chemotherapy dose

You can use the general formula for calculating dosages of your chemotherapy drugs and can compare it to the amount that is recommended for you in your medical records. Keep in mind, though, that your doctor may be using a different dose for very good reasons.

Glaxo's DoseCalc site deserves special mention as a user-friendly research site because it's a great way to verify your chemotherapy dosage. Go to the URL, *http://www.meds.com/DChome.html*. Enter your height, weight, and a drug name. Behind the scenes, it calculates your square feet per meter (yes, square, not cubic, feet per meter—the basis for most chemotherapy dosages) and gives you the standard dose administered for a person your size.

You can also do this calculation using your body surface area and the standard recommended dose for your body surface area. Appendix C, *Body Surface Area in Square Meters,* is a chart of heights, weights, and body surface areas. If your height or weight falls outside the ranges of this chart, you can use one of the following web sites to calculate your body surface area:

Cornell University: *http://www-users.med.cornell.edu/~spon/picu/bsacalc.htm*

Medical College of Wisconsin: *http://www.intmed.mcw.edu/clincalc/body.html*

Martindale's HS Guide: *http://www-sci.lib.uci.edu/HSG/Pharmacy.html*

Or try a Web search on the phrase "body surface area." Note that some of these sites use slightly different fomulae, and so the results will differ slightly.

For the truly dedicated, calculation of body surface area can be done by hand. You will need a scientific calculator (there may be an application on your personal computer for scientific calculation). One formula for calculating your body's surface area in square meters is the DuBois & DuBois formula:

$(kg^{.425}) \times (cm^{.725}) \times 0.007184$

or

(your weight in kilograms raised to power 0.425) times (your height in centimeters raised to power 0.725) times 0.007184

First convert your weight to kilograms and your height to centimeters. (One pound equals 0.45 kilogram; one inch equals 2.54 centimeters):

If your weight is 140 pounds, multiply 140 by 0.45 to get 63 kg.

If your height is 5'6" multiply 66 by 2.54 to get 167.64 cm.

To raise a number to a power in Windows 95, click Start, Program, Accessories, Calculator. Click View, then Scientific. Using our example above, enter 63, then click the X^Y key and enter .425; finally, click equal. Do the same for height:

63 kg to the power 0.425 = 5.817

167.64 cm to the power 0.725 = 40.9896

Then multiply 5.817 X 40.9896 X 0.007184= 1.713

Thus, 1.71 rounded is your body surface in square meters if you're 5'6" tall and weigh 140 pounds.

Once you've calculated your body surface area, you need to know the recommended dose per square meter for each of the drugs you're getting. You can ask your doctor's staff for this information or use Glaxo's site, discussed above. If you notice a substantial difference between the calculated and actual dose given, ask your doctor why.

How to interpret test results

Here are a few ways to find the normal values of tests that you can compare to your own test results. Please note that a value outside of the normal range does not always indicate a problem. Your doctor is generally the best person to tell you how to interpret test results, but there are several references available for comparing your test results to normal values. Appendix B, *Blood and Marrow Test Values*, lists the normal adult values for a variety of blood tests.

The Merck Manual, either the paper version or at their web site, has a section devoted to laboratory pathology. Many public libraries have a copy of the Merck Manual in their noncirculating reference section. At Merck's Internet web site, just enter the test name and click on the search button. *http://www.merck.com/* is the home page from which you can find the search facility.

Each of the following web sites has a search engine for finding the normal values of various test results:

- The University of Michigan Pathology Laboratories Handbook (*http://po.path.med.umich.edu/handbook/*). Enter the test name and click Search.
- The Lupus Lab Tests web site (*http://www.mtio.com/mclfa/lfalt1.htm*) has tests commonly done for lupus, but many of these are also done for hematologic cancers such as NHL.

How to assess unproven remedies

If your treatment isn't giving you good results, you may become vulnerable to claims for a quick cure made by certain practitioners. While some of these treatments may have merit, others are simply the means by which charlatans realize financial gain. How can you separate treatments that may have unrecognized medical potential from those that have been tried and discarded by reputable researchers, and those that are, or were, the focus of legal action?

QuackWatch on the Internet gives the medical scientist's evaluation of those unusual remedies you've been hearing about: *http://www.quackwatch.com/*.

The National Cancer Institute publishes a great deal of information on untested remedies. Call (800) 4-CANCER.

The American Cancer Society has a list of questions you should ask before becoming involved with unusual remedies. Call (800) ACS-2345, or visit their web site at *http://www.cancer.org/*.

The Consumer Health Information Research Institute provides an integrity index and a credibility of publication index, including one that rates cancer books. Visit them on the Web at *http://www.reutershealth.com/* or call (816) 228-4595.

Unique web resources

If you don't have a personal computer yet, or if the kids won't let you near it, this section may convince you how easily and quickly you can get the answers you've been looking for.

Please note that web sites may be inaccessible on occasional days owing to data reorganization or maintenance, and that web site addresses can change.

- The Atlas of Hematology offers photographs of microscopic slides of normal and diseased blood, with accompanying text: *http://www.med.nagoya-u.ac.jp/pathy/Pictures/atlas.html*.

- The American Medical Association has a doctor locator and other useful features: *http://www.ama-assn.org/*.

- Steve Dunn's CancerGuide is an excellent source of information on clinical trials and researching your illness: *http://cancerguide.org/*.

- Oncolink, sponsored by the University of Pennsylvania, is a highly reliable source of cancer information: *http://www.oncolink.upenn.edu/*.

- The Merck Manual online is an indispensable source of medical information: *http://www.merck.com/*.

- Cancer News has links to several sites containing press releases: *http://www.cancernews.com/*.

- Mid-South Therapeutics, Inc. hosts a web site with information for patients about tests and procedures: *http://www.msit.com/patients.htm/*.

- HealthAnswers offers a web site with a search engine that can supply information about how to prepare for tests, and so on; it can be found at: *http://www.healthanswers.com/*.

- The Thrive Health Library is a good general site for questions and answers: *http://www.thriveonline.com/*.

What next?

Think of researching your condition as a cyclical activity. Although you can accumulate and absorb the basic facts about NHL in a burst of initial activity, certain parts of the literature search process should be repeated about once a month in order to stay in touch with improvements in care. Three areas in particular should be revisited on a regular schedule:

- The National Cancer Institute updates the physician's state-of-the-art treatment statement as new standards of care are chosen. If the treatise on NHL is modified, the NCI can notify you via email, or you can call the NCI at (800) 4-CANCER each month and ask them to check the date of last update on the NHL physician's statement. The NCI classifies changes to these documents as either substantial or editorial. Editorial changes might include replacing one citation with a better one.

- Every month, new research papers on NHL are published in many medical journals, and their summaries (abstracts) are collected in Medline and in Cancerlit, which is a subset of Medline consisting of cancer literature only.

- New clinical trials for treatment are added to the NCI database every month.

Summary

This chapter describes three critical techniques: tapping National Cancer Institute information repositories, accessing medical research papers, and locating clinical trials. Supplementary resources such as finding medical textbooks, verifying test results, locating information on drug side effects, and locating support groups, are also discussed.

Your approach to learning can make a difference, and the learning experience is a continuous one. It's best to keep an open mind and to repeat your search efforts from time to time.

You have a right to your doctor's respect for your efforts. If the response you receive from your doctor when you share what you've learned is cavalier or condescending, it may be necessary to discuss this attitude with him or to find a new doctor.

Resources

The lists that follow reiterate the various groups, publications, services, and web tools discussed throughout this book, and include additional resources that also may serve your needs. All entries in each category are listed in alphabetical order, not by importance.

Key NHL resources

This first category includes resources you're likely to use most often, those that are the richest sources of NHL-specific information.

NHL organizations

Cure for Lymphoma
215 Lexington Avenue
New York, NY 10016
(212) 213-9595

Offers support and information, and funds research to fight lymphoma.

Leukemia Society of America
600 3rd Avenue
4th Floor
New York, NY 10016
(800) 955-4572

Offers assistance to lymphoma and leukemia survivors.

Lymphoma Research Foundation of America
2318 Prosser Avenue
Los Angeles, CA 90064
(310) 470-4912

Offers support and information, and funds research to fight lymphoma.

National Lymphedema Network
2211 Post Street, Suite 404
San Francisco, CA 94115
(800) 541-3259

Provides information on swollen limbs, which may occur soon or many years after treatment.

NHL Internet support groups

A list of NHL-related Internet support groups follows. Because the Internet is a dynamic resource, this list may not be comprehensive. The number of subscribers given was approximate at the time of writing and will vary over time. The Association of Cancer Online Resources (ACOR) has pointers to all of the hematologic cancer email discussion groups. ACOR offers a handy automatic subscription feature for these and other discussion mailing lists, at *http://www.acor.org/*.

- NHL. Run by Robert Scott Pallack, offering medical discussion and emotional support for all non-Hodgkin's lymphoma survivors. NHL has about 300 subscribers.

- NHL-LOW. Discussion of medical treatment for those with low-grade NHL. About 170 subscribers.

- HEM-ONC. Run by GrannyBarb Lackritz, offering medical discussion and emotional support for the hematologic malignancies, including NHL. Several oncologists are subscribed to this list. About 800 subscribers.

- BMT-TALK. Medical discussion and emotional support for those who will be having or who have had bone marrow transplantation for any cancer. Several oncologists are subscribed to this list. About 500 subscribers.

- PED-ALL. Medical discussion for pediatric acute lymphocytic leukemia, which resembles some NHLs. This list was formed in early 1998.

- CLL. Medical discussion and emotional support for chronic lymphocytic leukemia, which can convert into one form of NHL, called small-cell lymphocytic leukemia (SLL). About 300 subscribers.

- SICKKIDS. A discussion group just for children, but supervised by adults, at *http://tile.net/listserv/sickkids.html*.

- YAP. A discussion group for young adults age 18 to 25 dealing with their own illness or that of a loved one. This list was formed in late 1998.

NHL reading and reference material

The Cancer Dictionary, by Robert Altman and Michael Sarg, is a good medical dictionary specifically for cancer survivors.

The Non-Hodgkin's Lymphomas, Second Edition, edited by Ian Magrath. New York: Arnold and Oxford University Press, 1997. As of this writing, this is the most current and comprehensive textbook available that is specifically devoted to NHL. You might be able to find a copy in your doctor's office, a hospital library, or a university library. It can be purchased through any bookstore, including web-based bookstores, by ordering it from the publisher.

The National Library of Medicine's MEDLINE database
http://www4.ncbi.nlm.nih.gov/PubMed/

The best place to find the published results of studies on cancer treatment and care. It houses more than nine million research papers. If you need help with searching, you can call the National Library of Medicine at (800) 272-4787 or (301) 496-6308.

The U.S. National Cancer Institute (NCI)
Bethesda, MD 20892
(800) 4-CANCER
http://cancernet.nci.nih.gov/

A division of the National Institutes of Health, the NCI has a hotline to help cancer survivors with a variety of issues such as physician referrals, an enormous web site, and numerous tracts, statements, booklets, and books about cancer treatment and care. Many of the statements about cancer come in two versions, patient's and physician's. You might prefer to start with the patient's version, but it's likely that, as you learn more, the physician's statements will provide better, more detailed answers to your questions. The physicians' information is often part of PDQ (Physicians' Data Query).

Document retrieval services can fax or mail you the full text of any published research paper. On the Internet, the Medline service providers Health-Gate, Medscape, Helix, PhyNet, PDRnet.Com, SilverPlatter, Ovid On Call, Infotrieve, PaperChase, and others offer full-text services for a fee. Do a web search for any of these names.

Companies that will do medical information searches for you for a fee:

The Health Resource, Inc.
(501) 329-5272

Can Help
(360) 437-2291

Schine On-Line Services
(800) FIND-CURE

General cancer resources

The following resources, while not specific for NHL, are varied and numerous, and are likely to offer you aid and services suited to your needs.

Cancer organizations

Agency for Health Care Policy and Research
P.O. Box 8547
Silver Spring, MD 20907-8547
(800) 358-9295

American Cancer Society (ACS) National Office
1599 Clifton Road NE
Atlanta, GA 30329-4251
(800) ACS-2345
http://www.cancer.org/

The American Cancer Society has many national and local programs to help cancer survivors with problems such as travel, lodging, and emotional support. ACS publishes an excellent book, *Informed Decisions—The Complete Book of Cancer Diagnosis, Treatment and Recovery*. This hefty book is a comprehensive guide to care and treatment for all aspects of all cancers. They also offer a 24-hour support line for both English- and Spanish-speaking cancer survivors. Check your local phone directory for the office nearest you or contact:

American Red Cross
430 17th Street NW
Washington, DC 20006
(202) 737-8300

The American Self-Help Clearinghouse
25 Pocono Road
Denville, NJ 07834
(973) 625-7101

Publishes a national directory of self-help groups.

Burger King Cancer Caring Center
4117 Liberty Avenue
Pittsburgh, PA 15224
(412) 622-1212

Provides counseling and a hotline service for those with cancer.

Cancer Care Counseling (National Cancer Care Foundation)
1180 Avenue of the Americas
New York, NY 10036
(212) 382-2078 or (800) 813-HOPE

Provides information and support for those affected by cancer.

Cancer Family Care
7162 Reading Road, Suite 1050
Cincinnati, OH 45237
(513) 731-3346

Offers counseling to families affected by cancer.

Cancer Research Institute
681 Fifth Avenue
New York, NY 10022
(800) 99-CANCER

Offers services such as PDQ searches for clinical trials and free literature on cancer.

Cancervive
6500 Wilshire Boulevard, Suite 500
Los Angeles, CA 90048
(213) 655-3758

Offers many services to cancer survivors.

Center for Medical Consumers
237 Thompson Street
New York, NY 10012
(212) 674-7105

Provides information referrals to other organizations and maintains a medical consumer's library.

Consumer Health Information Research Institute
300 East Pink Hill Road
Independence, MO 64057
(816) 228-4595
http://www.reutershealth.com/

Provides an integrity index and a credibility of publication index, including one that rates cancer books.

Hereditary Cancer Institute
2500 California Plaza
Omaha, NE 68178
(402) 280-1746 or (402) 280-2942

Evaluates families for risk and furnishes educational material to families with hereditary cancers.

Make Today Count
1235 East Cherokee
Springfield, MO 65804
(800) 432-2273

Offers peer support via local chapters for those with life-threatening illnesses.

Mautamar Project for Lesbians with Cancer
1707 L Street NW, Suite 1060
Washington, DC 20036
(202) 332-5536

Offers support to lesbians and their families.

National AIDS Hotline
(800) 342-2437

Furnishes assistance to those with AIDS, including AIDS-related NHL.

National Coalition for Cancer Research
426 C Street NE
Washington, DC 20002
(202) 544-1880

An activist group that monitors government spending on cancer.

National Coalition for Cancer Survivorship
1010 Wayne Avenue, 5th Floor
Silver Spring, MD 20910
(301) 650-8868

Formed by cancer survivors to offer support and to effect change in progress against cancer through legislative efforts. They have published the *Cancer Survivor's Almanac*, a good reference for any cancer survivor.

National Family Caregivers Association
9621 East Bexhill Drive
Kensington, MD 20895
(800) 896-3650

Provides a variety of services to caregivers.

People Living Through Cancer, Inc.
323 Eighth Street, SW
Albuquerque, NM 87102
(505) 242-3263
Email: *cancerhope@aol.com*

Offers many services to cancer survivors.

PWA Coalition Hotline
50 West 17th Street, 8th Floor
New York, NY 10011
(800) 828-3280

Furnishes assistance to those with AIDS, including AIDS-related NHL. A really nice group of people.

R. A. Bloch Cancer Foundation
4410 Main Street
Kansas City, MO 64111
(816) 932-8453

Offers a variety of services to cancer patients and survivors, such as telephone-based second medical opinions and one-on-one phone contact between cancer survivors.

Well Spouse Foundation
610 Lexington Avenue, Suite 814
New York, NY 10022
(800) 838-0879

Offers support to those whose spouses are chronically ill.

Wellness Community
2716 Ocean Park Boulevard, Suite 1040
Santa Monica, CA 90405
(310) 314-2555

Has branches throughout the U.S. Check your local phone book for the chapter nearest you.

Children's cancer resources

Included below are organizations and reading material specifically for children.

Organizations that help children with cancer

Association for the Care of Children's Health
7910 Woodmont Avenue, Suite 300
Bethesda, MD 20814
(800) 808-ACCH
(609) 224-1742

Provides information for making informed decisions about care.

Candlelighters Foundation
7910 Woodmont Avenue, Suite 460
Bethesda, MD 20814
(800) 366-2223

Provides information and support for parents of children with cancer.

Chai Lifeline/Camp Simcha
48 West 25th Street
New York, NY 10010
(800) 343-2527

Provides a free kosher camp for children of any religion with cancer, including transportation from anywhere in the world.

Children's Hospice International
1850 M Street NW, Suite 900
Washington, DC 20036
(800) 242-4453

Provides many types of assistance to children with cancer and their families.

Federation for Children with Special Needs
95 Berkeley Street, Suite 104
Boston, MA 02116
(617) 482-2915

Provides support for parents regarding educational and healthcare rights.

Hole in the Wall Gang Camp
565 Ashford Center Road
Ashford, CT 06278
(860) 429-3444
http://www.holeinthewallgang.org/

A free 10-day summer camp for children ages 7 through 15 with cancer.

Make-A-Wish Foundation of America
100 W. Clarendon, Suite 2200
Phoenix, AZ 85013
(602) 279-9474
http://www.wish.org/

Offers sick children ages 2 through 18 an opportunity for an adventure.

Sibling Information Network
University of Connecticut
249 Glenbrook Road, Box U64
Storrs, CT 06269
(860) 486-4985

Publishes a newsletter of interest to those who have children with developmental disabilities.

Special Love, Inc. (Camp Fantastic)
117 Youth Development Court
Winchester, VA 22602
(540) 667-3774

Offers recreational programs for children with cancer and their families.

Starlight Foundation International
12424 Wilshire Boulevard, Suite 1050
Los Angeles, CA 90025
(800) 274-7827

Provides entertainment for sick children between ages 4 and 18.

Sunshine Foundation
P.O. Box 255
Loughman, FL 33858
(800) 767-1976

Grants wishes to sick children.

Sunshine Kids
2902 Ferndale Place
Houston, TX 77098
(800) 594-5756

Offers sports, cultural events, and group activities for children being treated for cancer.

Vital Options
(818) 508-5657

A group dedicated to providing support to young adults with cancer and other serious illnesses.

Books about cancer for children

Clifford, Christine. *Our Family Has Cancer, Too!* Pfeifer-Hamilton Publishing, 1997.

Fromer, Margot Joan. *Surviving Childhood Cancer: A Guide for Families.* American Psychiatric Press, 1995. Written for children.

Harpham, Wendy Schlessel. *Becky and the Worry Cup: A Children's Book About a Parent's Cancer.* HarperCollins, 1997.

Kohlenberg, Sherry. *Sammy's Mommy Has Cancer.* New York: Magination, 1993. For preschoolers.

Martin, Ann M. *Jessi's Wish* (Baby-Sitters Club No. 48). Apple, 1991. Through Danielle, who has cancer, Jessi learns new things about herself.

Trillin, Alice. *Dear Bruno.* New Press, 1996. A cartoon book about adjusting to cancer, primarily but not exclusively for children.

Books about dying for children

Buscaglia, Leo. *The Fall of Freddie the Leaf.* New York: C. B. Slack, 1982.

Hitchcock, R. *Tim's Dad: A Story About a Boy Whose Father Dies.* Human Services, Springfield, Illinois, 1998.

Holden, L. D. *Gran-Gran's Best Trick: A Story for Children Who Have Lost Someone They Love.* New York: Magination, 1989.

Krementz, Jill. *How It Feels When a Parent Dies.* New York: Alfred A. Knopf, 1981.

LeShan, Ed. *Learning to Say Good-by: When a Parent Dies.* New York: Macmillan, 1976.

O'Toole Donna. *Aarvy Aardvark Finds Hope.* Burnsville, North Carolina: Celo Press, 1988.

Vigna, J. *Saying Good-bye to Daddy.* Morton Grove, Illinois: Albert Whitman, 1991.

White, E. B. *Charlotte's Web.* New York: Harper & Row, 1952.

General cancer reading

The Alpha Book on Cancer and Living. Alameda, California: The Alpha Institute, 1993.

Brenner, David J., and Eric Hall. *Making the Radiation Therapy Decision.* RGA Publishing Group, 1996.

Cancer Rates and Risks, 1996. The National Cancer Institute, (800) 4-CANCER.

Crane, Judy B. *How to Survive Your Hospital Stay.* Westlake Village, California: The Center Press, 1997.

Cukier, Daniel, and Virginia McCullough. *Coping with Radiation Therapy: A Ray of Hope.* Los Angeles: Lowell House, 1996.

Dollinger, M., E. Rosenbaum, and G. Cable, editors. *Everyone's Guide to Cancer Therapy.* Andrews & McMeel, 1998.

Drum, D. *Making the Chemotherapy Decision.* Lowell House, 1997.

Dunn, Steve. *CancerGuide.* Read this online at *http://www.cancerguide.org/sdunn_story.html.*

Friedman, A., T. Klein, and H. Friedman. *Psychoneuroimmunology, Stress, and Infection,* New York: CRC Press, 1996.

Glaser, Ronald, and Janice Kiecolt-Glaser. *Handbook of Human Stress and Immunity*. New York: Academic Press, 1994.

Harpham, Wendy Schlessel. *After Cancer: A Guide to Your New Life*. New York: W. W. Norton, 1994.

Harpham, Wendy Schlessel. *Diagnosis: Cancer*. New York: W. W. Norton, 1998.

Harpham, Wendy Schlessel. *When a Parent Has Cancer: A Guide to Caring for Your Children*. HarperCollins, 1997.

Hoffman, Barbara, ed., The National Coalition for Cancer Survivorship. *A Cancer Survivor's Almanac*. Minneapolis: Chronimed, 1996.

Inlander, Charles B., ed. *People's Medical Society Health Desk Reference: Information Your Doctor Can't or Won't Tell You*. New York: Hyperion, 1996.

Johnson, J., and L. Klein. *I Can Cope: Staying Healthy with Cancer*. Minneapolis: Chronimed, 1994.

Keene, Nancy. *Childhood Leukemia: A Guide for Family, Friends, and Caregivers*. Sebastopol, California: O'Reilly & Associates, 1997. A good reference for the parents of a child with NHL, some forms of which can resemble one form of childhood leukemia.

Keene, Nancy. *Working with Your Doctor: Getting the Healthcare You Deserve*. Sebastopol, California: O'Reilly & Associates, 1998.

Keene, Nancy. *Your Child in the Hospital: A Practical Guide for Parents*. Sebastopol, California: O'Reilly & Associates, 1997.

Lerner, Michael. *Choices in Healing: Integrating the Best of Conventional and Complementary Approaches to Cancer*. Cambridge: MIT Press, 1996.

McKay, J., N. Hirano, and M. Lampenfeld. *The Chemotherapy and Radiation Therapy Survival Guide*. New Harbinger Publications, 1998.

The Merck Manual, available in either the paper version or at their web site (*http://www.merck.com*), is a vast resource. Many public libraries have a copy of the Merck Manual in their noncirculating reference section. The new 17th edition will be published in early 1999.

Murphy, G., L. Morris, and D. Lange, editors. *Informed Decisions—The Complete Book of Cancer Diagnosis, Treatment and Recovery*. The American Cancer Society. New York: Viking Press, 1997.

The National Cancer Institute's *PDQ State-of-the-Art Treatment Statements for Physicians* on: Adult Non-Hodgkin's Lymphoma; Childhood Non-Hodgkin's Lymphoma; Breast Cancer and Pregnancy; Non-Hodgkin's Lymphoma During Pregnancy; AIDS-Related Lymphomas; Cutaneous T-Cell Lymphoma; Primary Central Nervous System Lymphoma, and others.

Olson, Kaye, RN. *Surgery and Recovery: How to Reduce Anxiety and Promote Healthy Healing.* Traverse City, Michigan: Rhodes and Easton, 1998.

Radiation Therapy and You, a fifty-page booklet, is available from the U.S. National Cancer Institute by calling (800) 4-CANCER.

Schover, L. *Sexuality and Fertility After Cancer.* New York: John Wiley & Sons, 1997.

Spiegel, David. *Living Beyond Limits: New Hope and Health for Facing Life-Threatening Illness.* New York: Fawcett Columbine, 1994.

Youngson, Robert, with the Diagram Group. *The Surgery Book.* New York: St. Martin's Press, 1993.

Zakarian, Beverly. *The Activist Cancer Patient.* New York: John Wiley & Sons, 1996.

Zukerman, Eugenia, and Julie Ingelfinger. *Coping with Prednisone (and other cortisone-related medicines).* New York: St. Martin's Press, 1997.

Cancer magazines

Cancer Communication
Published by PAACT
Patient Advocates for Advanced Cancer Treatments
1143 Parmelee Northwest
Grand Rapids, MI 49504
(616) 453-1477

Coping
P.O. Box 682268
Franklin, TN 37068
(615) 790-2400

Living Through Cancer
323 Eighth Street, SW
Albuquerque, NM 87102
(505) 242-3263

Medical resources

Medical information targeted to special topics is available through the resources listed in these categories.

Bone marrow transplantation

This expensive and lengthy treatment procedure is addressed by the publications and support groups listed below.

Reading material for transplantation

Bone Marrow Transplantation and Peripheral Blood Stem Cell Transplantation. The National Cancer Institute offers this treatise on marrow or stem cell transplantation. On the Web at *http://cancernet.nci.nih.gov/* or call (800) 4-CANCER.

Martin, Paul, M.D. (Member, Fred Hutchinson Cancer Research Center, Professor of Medicine, University of Washington.) *A Short Primer on HLA and Bone Marrow Transplantation.* On the Web at *http://www.giftoflife.com.*

Stewart, Susan L. *Bone Marrow Transplants: A Book of Basics for Patients.* Highland Park, Illinois: BMT Newsletter, 1992.

Transplant Center Access Directory. National Marrow Donor Program. Call (800) 526-7809; or on the Web at *http://www.marrow.org* and *http://www.bmtinfo.org/.*

Reading material for finding a donor

Tissue Typing for Beginners: *http://www.umds.ac.uk/tissue/what1.html*

HLA Gene and Haplotype Frequencies in the North American Population: The National Marrow Donor Program Donor Registry: *http://www.swmed.edu/home_pages/ASHI/prepr/Motomi.htm*

Haplotype searching: *http://www.swmed.edu/home_pages/ASHI/prepr/mori_abd.htm*

Histocompatibility: Interpretation and Correlation of HLA Typing for Bone Marrow Transplantation: *http://www.bmtinfo.org/bmt/topics/htm/type_b.htm*

HLA Class I and II Sequence Alignments: *http://www.anthonynolan.com/HIG/data.html*

Transplant advocacy and support groups

Blood and Marrow Transplant Newsletter
1985 Spruce Avenue
Highland Park, IL 60035
(847) 831-1913

Offers support, publications, and guidance to legal aid for those getting transplants.

Bone Marrow Transplant Family Support Network
P.O. Box 845
Avon, CT 06001
(800) 826-9376

Offers counseling and support for those going through a transplant.

Living Bank
4545 Post Oak Place, Suite 315
Houston, TX 77027
(800) 528-2971

Motivates and facilitates organ donor commitment.

National Bone Marrow Transplant Link
29209 Northwestern Highway, No. 624
Southfield, MI 48034
(800) LINK-BMT

Offers peer support and a variety of services for those being transplanted.

National Marrow Donor Program
3433 Broadway Street, NE, Suite 400
Minneapolis, MN 55413
(800) MARROW-2

Coordinates national and international testing and matching of marrow donors and recipients.

Organ Transplant Fund
1027 South Yates
Memphis, TN 38119
(800) 489-3863

Provides a variety of services, including financial services, to those receiving transplants.

Verifying doctor and hospital credentials

The American College of Surgeons
633 North Saint Clair Street
Chicago, IL 60611
(312) 202-5000

Can verify whether your surgeon is board certified in a surgical specialty.

American Medical Association Directory of Physicians in the U.S., published by the American Medical Association, provides a means to verify your doctor's credentials. The AMA's *Physician Select* web site, found at *http:// www.ama-assn.org/aps/amahg.html*, is an excellent means to check your doctor's education and board certification.

The American Society of Pediatric Hematology/Oncology (ASPH/O) established standard requirements for programs treating children with cancer and blood disorders.

Center for Medical Consumers
237 Thompson Street
New York, NY 10012
(212) 674-7105

Provides information referrals to other organizations and maintains a medical consumer's library.

College of American Pathologists
325 Waukegan Road
Northfield, IL 60093-2750
(800) 323-4040

The Consumer Health Information Research Institute
(816) 228-4595
http://www.reutershealth.com/

Provides an integrity index and a credibility of publication index.

The Joint Commission on Accreditation of Health Care Organizations (JCAHO)
1 Renaissance Boulevard
Oakbrook Terrace IL 60181
(630) 792-5800

National Council Against Health Fraud
P.O. Box 1276
Loma Linda, CA 92354
(909) 824-4690

The Official ABMS Directory of Board Certified Medical Specialists 1998. 30th Edition. 1997 Marquis Who's Who. This is a directory of board-certified physicians who have chosen to specialize in a particular area of medicine.

QuackWatch (*http://www.quackwatch.com/*) gives the medical scientist's evaluation of those unusual remedies you've been hearing about.

U.S. News and World Report's annual "Best Hospitals" edition. Write to 2400 N Street N.W. Washington, DC 20037-1196, or call (202) 955-2000.

Drug and dosage information

The Physician's Desk Reference (PDR), a compendium of information about drugs, is now reprinted in versions that are easier for the general public to understand, but you might appreciate the learning experience gained from reading the original PDR. In addition to PDR, many other drug encyclopedias are available for the general public.

U.S. Food and Drug Administration (FDA)
5600 Fishers Lane
Rockville, MD 20857
(301) 827-4420
(888) 332-4543
(800) 532-4440
http://www.fda.gov/

You can report adverse effects of drugs to the FDA, too, or use their Med-Watch web site: *http://www.fda.gov/medwatch/how.htm*.

Clinical Pharmacology Online
http://www.cponline.gsm.com/

DrugInfoNet
http://www.druginfonet.com/

Glaxo's DoseCalc
http://www.meds.com/DChome.html

HealthTouch
http://www.healthtouch.com/level1/p_dri.htm

PharmInfoNet
http://pharminfo.com/

RxMed
http://www.rxmed.com/

Calculating body surface area

Cornell University
http://www-users.med.cornell.edu/~spon/picu/bsacalc.htm

Martindale's HS Guide
http://www-sci.lib.uci.edu/HSG/Pharmacy.html

Medical College of Wisconsin
http://www.intmed.mcw.edu/clincalc/body.html

Tests and procedures

These resources can help you learn how tests are done, and what the results mean.

Information on how tests are done

Andrews, Maraca, and Michael Shaw. *Everything You Need to Know About Medical Tests*. Springhouse, 1996. An excellent, comprehensive (691 pages) reference written for the patient in a readable and respectful style.

Barry, L., ed., with Peter Zaret, and Lee D. Jatlow. *The Patient's Guide to Medical Tests*. Houghton Mifflin Co. (Trade), 1997.

The Biology Project. University of Arizona: *http://www.biology.arizona.edu/*.

Brodin, Michael B. *The Encyclopedia of Medical Tests*. Pocket Books, 1997. A 1982 book with the same title written by Pinckney and Pinckney should be passed over in favor of this newer book. 592 pages.

Department of Pathology, University of Washington, Seattle: *http://www.pathology.washington.edu/*.

The Family Internet site at *http://familyinternet.com/*.

HealthGate at *http://www.healthgate.com/*.

Keene, Nancy. *Childhood Leukemia: A Guide for Friends, Families, and Caregivers*. Sebastopol, California: O'Reilly and Associates, 1997. An excellent reference for those who have a child with leukemia or lymphoma, especially for the form of NHL related to and treated like childhood acute lymphocytic leukemia.

Keene, Nancy. *Your Child in the Hospital: A Practical Guide for Parents, Second Edition*. Sebastopol, California: O'Reilly and Associates, 1999. Covers all aspects of the child's experiences with hospitalization, from tests and treatment to emotional issues such as sibling reactions.

Magrath, Ian, editor. *The Non-Hodgkin's Lymphomas, Second Edition*. London: Arnold and Oxford University Press, 1997.

Mid-South Imaging & Therapeutics, P.A. at *http://www.msit.com/*.

Mosby Consumer Health Series at *http://www.mosbych1.com/mhc/top/003833.htm*.

Pagana, Kathleen, and Timothy Pagana, editors. *Mosby's Diagnostic and Laboratory Test Reference*. Mosby, 1992.

Shtasel, Philip. *Medical Tests and Diagnostic Procedures—A Patient's Guide to Just What the Doctor Ordered*. Harper and Row, 1990.

Stauffer, Joseph, and Joseph C. Segen. *The Patient's Guide to Medical Tests: Everything You Need to Know About the Tests Your Doctor Prescribes, Fourth Edition*. Facts on File, 1997.

ThriveOnline: http://www.thriveonline.com/.

University of California at Los Angeles: *http://anima.crump.ucla.edu/*.

Normal values of tests

The Lupus Lab Tests web site (*http://www.mtio.com/mclfa/lfalt1.htm*) has tests commonly done for lupus, but many of these are also done for hematologic cancers such as NHL.

The University of California Division of General Internal Medicine. Enter the test name and click Search: *http://www.oncolink.upenn.edu/*.

The University of Michigan Pathology Laboratories Handbook. Enter the test name and click Search: *http://po.path.med.umich.edu/handbook/*.

Clinical trials and investigational new substances

The Food and Drug Administration (*http:///www.fda.gov/*) contains regulations for investigational new drugs and for importing foreign drugs for single-patient use. Call (800) 532-4440.

The book *Intuitive Biostatistics,* by Harvey Motulsky, can help you understand published results of clinical trials, and can help you assess trial design if you're planning to enroll in a trial.

The National Cancer Institute Clinical Trials web site (*http://cancernet.nci.nih.gov/prot/protsrch.shtml*) is the most comprehensive way to locate trials of new substances and treatments.

QuackWatch (*http://www.quackwatch.com/*) gives the medical scientist's evaluation of those unusual remedies you've been hearing about.

Steve Dunn's Cancerguide is an excellent resource for learning how to assess clinical trials and how to research your illness. Email *dunns@h2net.net* or on the web at *http://www.cancerguide.org/sdunn_story.html*.

Resources for pain and other side effects

The American Cancer Society has many programs to help cancer survivors with problems such as pain. Call (800) ACS-2345 or check your local phone directory for the office nearest you.

American Society of Anesthesiologists
515 Busse Highway
Park Ridge, IL 60068
(847) 825-5586

American Society of Clinical Hypnosis
2200 East Vine Avenue, Suite 291
Des Plaines, IL 60018
(847) 297-3317

National Lymphedema Network
2211 Post Street, Suite 404
San Francisco, CA 94115
(800) 541-3259

Provides information on swollen limbs, which may occur soon or many years after treatment.

Legal, financial, employment, and insurance resources

Beyond the physical aspects of cancer lie its effects on our careers and finances. The resources listed below can offer guidance and aid.

Organizations that help with legal and financial issues

The Blood and Marrow Transplant Newsletter
1985 Spruce Avenue
Highland Park, IL 60035
(847) 831-1913

Offers guidance to legal aid for those getting transplants.

The Center for Medical Consumers
237 Thompson Street
New York, NY 10012
(212) 674-7105

Provides information referrals to other organizations and maintains a medical consumer's library.

Consumer Credit Counseling
(800) 388-2227

Can provide help getting expenses under control.

The Federal Trade Commission
(202) 326-3650

Can provide information about the federal Consumer Credit Protection Act, a landmark series of laws passed in 1968 to protect debtors.

Health Care Cost Hotline
(900) 225-2500

Can furnish the median fee and range of fees charged by doctors for various services and procedures. The call is $2.00 to $4.00 per minute.

Health Insurance Association of America (HIAA)
555 13th Street NW
Washington, D.C. 20004
(202) 824-1600
http://www.hiaa.org/index.html

Has more than 250 members consisting of insurers and managed care companies. HIAA can supply booklets on disability income, health insurance, long-term care, medical savings accounts, and general insurance information, including a directory of state insurance departments.

Lexis Law Publishing
(800) 542-0957

This group can send you a copy of any law.

The Medical Information Bureau (MIB)
P.O. Box 105, Essex Station
Boston, MA 02112
(617) 424-3660

Records all entries made by insurance companies about your health, and will send a copy of this information to your physician if you request it. If you find an error in these files, you can contact the bureau for the procedures necessary to correct errors.

The Organ Transplant Fund
1027 South Yates
Memphis, TN 38119
(800) 489-3863

Provides help with fundraising to those receiving transplants.

Magazines for legal and financial issues

Health Pages reports on ranges and norms of doctor's fees. Call (212) 929-6131.

Medical Economics reports on ranges and norms of doctor's fees. Call (201) 945-9058.

Social Security Administration bulletins

The chief resource in this category is the 1997 Social Security Handbook, 13th edition. On the Web at *http://www.ssa.gov/OP_Home/handbook/ ssahbk.htm.*

Other, more specific SSA bulletins include:

Social Security: What You Need To Know When You Get Disability Benefits (6/96; Pub. No. 05-10153)

Social Security Disability Programs (5/96; Pub. No. 05-10057)

Social Security: If You Are Blind, How We Can Help (6/96; Pub. No. 05-10052)

A Guide to Social Security and SSI Disability Benefits for People with HIV Infection (6/95; Pub. No. 05-10020)

How We Decide If You Are Still Disabled (4/96; Pub. No. 05-10053)

How Social Security Can Help with Vocational Rehabilitation (9/94; Pub. No. 05-10050)

Working While Disabled…How We Can Help (1/96; Pub. No. 05-10095)

Red Book on Work Incentives for People with Disabilities (8/95; Pub. No. 64-030)

Free treatment resources

The National Cancer Institute
Bethesda, MD
(800) 4-CANCER

The Shrine of North America
Shriner's Hospitals
In the United States, call (800) 237-5055
In Canada, call (800) 361-7256

The St. Jude Children's Research Hospital
(901) 495-3300

Free travel and lodging for care

See Chapter 21, *Traveling for Care*, which consists of many more resources than we can duplicate here.

Air Care Alliance helps cancer patients travel to distant health centers for care. You may call ACA at (888) 662-6794 tollfree in the U.S. Direct number (757) 318-9145, or visit their web site at *http://www.angelflightfla.org/air-careall.org/acahome.html.*

The American Cancer Society (ACS) sponsors Hope Lodges, which provide free lodging for those who travel to receive cancer care. Check your local phone book, or visit their web site at *http://www.cancer.org/.*

The Candlelighters Childhood Cancer Foundation can help you make travel arrangements. In the U.S., call (301) 657-8401 or (800) 366-CCCF. In Canada, call (800) 363-1062. Also on the Web at *http://www.candlelighters.org/.*

Corporate Angel Network helps cancer patients travel to distant health centers for care. Call (914) 328-1313, or visit their web site at *http://www.corpangelnetwork.org/.*

The Leukemia Society of America will reimburse up to $750 per year in travel expenses. Call (800) 955-4LSA, or visit their web site at *http://www.leukemia.org/.*

Mercy Medical Airlift helps cancer patients travel to distant health centers for care. Call (800) 296-1191, or visit *http://www.mercymedical.org/.*

National Association of Hospital Hospitality Houses (NAHHH) can recommend nearby hotels with reduced rates for cancer patients. Call (301) 961-3094, (317) 883-2226, or (800) 542-9730; or visit *http://visit-usa.com/hhh/members.htm.*

The National Cancer Institute in Bethesda, Maryland, will in some cases help pay for the travel and lodging expenses of those being treated at the NCI. Call (800) 4-CANCER.

Ronald McDonald House Coordinator, c/o McDonalds Corporation, provides free lodging for children who are being treated for cancer. Call (630) 623-7048, or visit *http://www.mcdonalds.com/a_community/.*

The Shriners' Hospitals provide free treatment for children who need orthopedic or burn remediation. In the United States, call (800) 237-5055. In Canada, call (800) 361-7256. Also on the Web at *http://www.shrinershq.org/index.html.*

End-of-life resources

Resources for increasing comfort and serenity in the last stage of life are included in this category.

Home and hospice care

Community Health Accreditation Program, Inc.
350 Hudson Street
New York, NY 10014
(800) 669-9656

Provides a list of accredited home care organizations.

National Association for Home Care
519 C Street NE
Washington, DC 20002
(202) 547-7424

Represents all home health care agencies in the U.S. They offer publications on selecting home care.

National Hospice Organization
1901 North Moore Street, Suite 901
Arlington, VA 22209
(800) 658-8898

Offers information on the goals of hospice and how to choose a hospice.

Oley Foundation
214 Hun Memorial
Albany Medical Center A-23
Albany, NY 12208
(800) 776-OLEY

Offers help with parenteral or enteral nutrition—that is, feeding by IV or stomach tube.

Olsten Health Services National Resource Center
175 Broadhollow Road
Melville, NY 11747
(800) 66-NURSE

Offers help with all home health care services.

Visiting Nurse Associations of America
3801 East Florida Avenue, Suite 900
Denver, CO 80210
(800) 426-2547

Provides skilled nurses, aides, and therapists for homecare.

Reading material about dying

Basta, Lofty. *A Graceful Exit: Life and Death on Your Own Terms.* New York: Plenum Press, 1996.

Bernard, Jan, and Miriam Schneider. *The True Work of Dying.* New York: Avon Books, 1996.

Callanan, Maggie, and Patricia Kelley. *Final Gifts: Understanding the Special Awareness, Needs, and Communications of the Dying.* New York: Bantam Books, 1997.

Furman, Joan, and David McNabb. *The Dying Time: Practical Wisdom for the Dying.* New York: Bell Tower, 1997.

Groopman, Jerome. *The Measure of Our Days.* New York: Viking Press, 1997.

Humphry, Derek. *Final Exit: The Practicalities of Self-Deliverance and Assisted Suicide for the Dying.* The Hemlock Society, 1997.

Kramp, Erin Tierney, Douglas H. Kramp, Douglas H. and Emily P. McKhann. *Living with the End in Mind: A Practical Checklist for Living Life to the Fullest by Embracing Your Mortality.* Three Rivers Press, 1998.

Kubler-Ross, Elisabeth. *Death: The Final Stage of Growth.* New York: Simon and Schuster, 1975.

Kubler-Ross, Elisabeth. *Living with Death and Dying.* New York: Touchstone (Simon and Schuster), 1981.

Kubler-Ross, Elisabeth. *On Death and Dying.* Macmillan, 1969.

Kubler-Ross, Elisabeth. *To Live Until We Say Good-bye.* New York: Fireside (Simon and Schuster), 1978.

Lattanzi-Licht, Marcia, John Mahoney, and Galen Miller. *The Hospice Choice: In Pursuit of a Peaceful Death.* New York: Fireside (Simon and Schuster), 1998.

McPhelimy, Lynn. *In the Checklist of Life: A Working Book to Help You Live and Leave Life.* AAIP Publishing Company, 1997.

Nuland, Sherwin. *How We Die: Reflections on Life's Final Chapter.* New York: Alfred A. Knopf, 1993.

Ray, M. Catherine. *I'm with You Now: A Guide Through Incurable Illness for Patients, Families, and Friends.* New York: Bantam Books, 1997.

Weenolsen, Patricia. *The Art of Dying.* New York: St. Martin's Press, 1996.

Blood and Marrow Test Values

The following tables will provide you with approximate quantitative information about certain blood test results. Test results can be influenced by many things, such as how the blood was drawn and stored, whether the patient exercised recently or was dehydrated, how tight the tourniquet was, medications taken by the patient, and so on. Moreover, your lab will display its own norms alongside your test results. These norms may differ from other sources, as each lab recalculates their norms as their data accumulate.

COMPLETE BLOOD COUNTS IN NORMAL ADULTS

Test Name	Low	High
White cell count (WBC) x 10^9/liter blood	3.9	11.3
White Cell Differentials (percents)		
Polys	42%	78%
Bands	0%	4%
Lymphocytes	15%	45%
Monocytes	0%	12%
Eosinophils	0%	7%
Basophils	0%	2%
Atypical lymphocytdes	0%	4%
Platelet count (PLT) x10^9/liter blood	140	450
Mean platelet volume (MPV)	6.3	10.3
Mean corpuscular volume, fl/red cell (MCV)	80.0	100
Mean corpuscular hemoglobin, pg/red cell (MCH)	26.4	34.0
Mean corpuscular hemoglobin conc., g/dl red cells (MCHC)	31.0	36.0
Red cell distribution width (RDW), CV (%)	11.5%	14.5%

COMPLETE BLOOD COUNTS IN NORMAL ADULTS: RED CELL COUNTS BY GENDER

	Men		Women	
Test Name	**Low**	**High**	**Low**	**High**
Red cell count (RBC) x 10^{12}/liter blood	4.52	5.90	4.1	5.10
Hemoglobin (HB) g/dl blood	14.0	18.0	12.3	15.3
Hematocrit (HCT)	0.40	0.52	0.36	0.45

OTHER BLOOD VALUES IN NORMAL ADULTS

Test Name	**Low**	**High**
Beta-2 Microglobulin, g/ml (B2M)	0	2.5
Direct bilirubin, mg/dl (Bili)	0	0.4
Total bilirubin, mg/dl (Bili)	0	1.0
Blood urea nitrogen, mg/dl (BUN)	8	25
Cholesterol	130	200
Creatinine, mg/dl (CRT)	0.6	1.5
Calcium mg/dl (Ca)	8.5	10.5
Chlorine mEq.l (Cl)	95	100
Potassium, mEq/l (K)	3.5	5.0
Phosphate mg/dl (P)	2.5	4.5
Sodium, mEq/l (Na)	135	145
Magnesium, mEq/l (Mg)	1.5	2.5
Erythrocyte Sedimentation Rate mm/hr (ESR)	0	20
Glucose, mg/dl	65	100
Immunoglobulin A (IgA) mg/dl	90	325
Immunoglobulin D (IgD) mg/dl	0.3	30
Immunoglobulin E (IgE) mg/dl	0.002	0.2
Immunoglobulin G (IgG) mg/dl	720	1500
Immunoglobulin M (IgM) mg/dl	45	150
Lactate Dehydrogenase u/l (LDH)	100	190
Albumin gm/dl (Alb)	3.5	5.0
Alkaline Phosphatase (AlkP) u/l	50	135
(ALT, formerly SGPT) u/l	5	40
(AST, formerly SGOT) u/l	10	50
Thyroid TSH	0.5	5.0
Thyroid free T4	1	4
Uric acid, mg/dl	2.5	8.0

Body Surface Area in Square Meters

The chart on the following page shows body surface area for typical heights and weights. Calculations were made using the DuBois & DuBois formula:

$$kg^{.425} \times cm^{.725} \times 0.007184$$

Weight is the horizontal axis, first in pounds, then in kilograms. Height is the vertical axis, first in inches, then in centimeters. Results are body surface areas in square meters.

If your height or weight falls between or outside the ranges of this chart, you can use one of the following web sites to calculate body surface area:

Cornell University: *http://www-users.med.cornell.edu/~spon/picu/bsacalc.htm*

Medical College of Wisconsin: *http://www.intmed.mcw.edu/clincalc/body.html*

Martindalee's HS Guide: *http://www-sci.lib.uci.edu/HSG/Pharmacy.html*

Or, try a web search on the phrase "body surface area." Note that some of these sites use slightly different formulae, so the results will differ slightly.

Lbs/Kg → / In/Cm ↓	100/45	110/49.5	120/54	130/58.5	140/63	150/67.5	160/72	170/76.5	180/81	190/85.5	200/90	210/94.5	220/99	230/103.5	240/108	250/112.5	260/117	270/121.5
60/152.4	1.38	1.44	1.50	1.55	1.60	1.65	1.69	1.74	1.78	1.82	1.86	1.90	1.94	1.97	2.01	2.04	2.08	2.11
61/154.9	1.40	1.46	1.52	1.57	1.62	1.67	1.71	1.76	1.80	1.84	1.88	1.92	1.96	2.00.	2.03	2.07	2.11	2.14
62/157.5	1.42	1.48	1.53	1.59	1.64	1.69	1.73	1.78	1.82	1.86	1.91	1.94	1.98	2.02	2.06	2.09	2.13	2.16
63/160.0	1.43	1.49	1.55	1.61	1.66	1.71	1.75	1.80	1.84	1.88	1.93	1.97	2.01	2.04	2.08	2.12	2.16	2.19
64/162.6	1.45	1.51	1.57	1.62	1.68	1.73	1.77	1.82	1.86	1.91	1.95	1.99	2.03	2.07	2.11	2.14	2.18	2.21
65/165.1	1.47	1.53	1.59	1.64	1.70	1.74	1.79	1.84	1.88	1.93	1.97	2.01	2.05	2.09	2.13	2.17	2.20	2.24
66/167.6	1.48	1.55	1.60	1.66	1.71	1.76	1.81	1.86	1.90	1.95	1.99	2.03	2.08	2.11	2.15	2.19	2.23	2.26
67/170.2	1.50	1.56	1.62	1.68	1.73	1.78	1.83	1.88	1.93	1.97	2.02	2.06	2.10	2.14	2.18	2.21	2.25	2.29
68/172.7	1.52	1.58	1.64	1.70	1.75	1.80	1.85	1.90	1.95	1.99	2.04	2.08	2.12	2.16	2.20	2.24	2.28	2.31
69/175.3	1.53	1.60	1.66	1.72	1.77	1.82	1.87	1.92	1.97	2.01	2.06	2.10	2.14	2.18	2.22	2.26	2.30	2.34
70/177.8	1.55	1.61	1.67	1.73	1.79	1.84	1.89	1.94	1.99	2.03	2.08	2.12	2.17	2.21	2.25	2.29	2.33	2.36
71/180.3	1.56	1.63	1.69	1.75	1.81	1.86	1.91	1.96	2.01	2.05	2.10	2.15	2.19	2.23	2.27	2.31	2.35	2.39
72/182.3	1.58	1.64	1.71	1.76	1.82	1.87	1.93	1.98	2.02	2.07	2.12	2.16	2.21	2.25	2.29	2.33	2.37	2.41
73/185.4	1.60	1.66	1.73	1.79	1.84	1.90	1.95	2.00	2.05	2.10	2.14	2.19	2.23	2.27	2.32	2.36	2.40	2.44
74/188.0	1.61	1.68	1.74	1.80	1.86	1.92	1.97	2.02	2.07	2.12	2.17	2.21	2.26	2.30	2.34	2.38	2.42	2.46
75/190.5	1.63	1.70	1.76	1.82	1.88	1.94	1.99	2.04	2.09	2.14	2.19	2.23	2.28	2.32	2.36	2.40	2.45	2.48
76/193.0	1.64	1.71	1.78	1.84	1.90	1.95	2.01	2.06	2.11	2.16	2.21	2.25	2.30	2.34	2.38	2.43	2.47	2.51
77/195.6	1.66	1.73	1.79	1.86	1.92	1.97	2.03	2.08	2.13	2.18	2.23	2.28	2.32	2.36	2.41	2.45	2.49	2.53
78/198.0	1.67	1.74	1.81	1.87	1.93	1.99	2.05	2.10	2.15	2.20	2.25	2.30	2.34	2.39	2.43	2.47	2.52	2.56

Classification Systems

This chart is based on research published by Harris and colleagues as *A Revised European-American Classification of Lymphoid Neoplasms: A Proposal from the International Lymphoma Study Group*, appearing in the journal *Blood*, Volume 84, No. 5, September 1, 1994. It includes lymphoma classification information upon which a majority of nineteen hematopathologists reached agreement during the April 1993 meeting of the International Lymphoma Study Group. Controversial, little known, or unpublished tumor characteristics were omitted by this group. Entries marked provisional represent disease categories fairly well described in the scientific literature, but lacking enough scientific scrutiny to be clearly defined as distinct categories.

You can use this table to determine whether your tumor might express genes or antigens targeted by certain treatments. Your approach to using this table should include first obtaining the *exact name* of your diagnosis from your biopsy report, and asking your doctor which classification system was used to arrive at your diagnosis. By finding your diagnosis in one of the columns headed Working Formulation, Rappaport, Kiel, or Lukes-Collins, you can locate its proposed equivalent in the REAL system, and can find information on the antigens and genetic characteristics that may be expressed by your tumor. Characteristics and findings that the ILSG currently consider meaningful for diagnosis appear in bold type.

Treatment will never be based solely on information found in this table. The tumor sample must be tested to be certain it expresses a given gene or antigen, and other aspects of the disease must be weighed.

Following is a lexicon of abbreviations that appear in the chart starting on the next page:

Abbreviation	Definition
+	Over 90% of observed cases were positive
+/−	Over 50% of observed cases were positive
−/+	Less than 50% of observed cases were positive
−	Less than 10% of observed cases were positive
TCR	T-cell receptor gene
IgH	Immunoglobulin heavy chain gene
IgL	Immunoglobulin light chain gene
SIg	Contains surface immunoglobulin
CIg	Contains cytoplasmic immunoglobulin
CD	Cluster of differentiation
EMA	Epithelial membrane antigen
bcl-n	Various genes known to be rearranged in some lymphomas
t(nn;nn)	Transposition of a piece of one chromosome onto another (numbers indicate chromosomes)
c-myc	Gene known to be associated with some cancers
EBV	Epstein-Barr virus
INVnn	Inversion of a chromosome onto itself caused by breaking, turning, and rejoining
INVn qnn;qnn	Inversion of a chromosome onto itself from locus nn to locus nn
+0q	Extra copy of the long arm of a chromosome. Lowercase p indicates the short arm; q indicates the long arm
trisomy	Three copies of a chromosome or part of a chromosome. See also +0q
HTLV-1	Human T-cell lymphotropic virus
FDC	Follicular dendritic cells
MLA	Mucosal lymphocyte antigen
TRAP	Tartrate-resistant acid phosphatase

Consensus Classification	CD Antigens	Working Formulation	Rappaport	Kiel	Lukes-Collins	Other Antigens	Genetic Features
				B-Cell Entities			
Precursor B-Lymphoblastic Leukemia/Lym-phoma (B-LBL)	**CD10+/−** **CD19+** **CD79a+** CD20−/+ CD22+ CD34+/−CD13 and CD33 possible	Lymphoblastic	Lymphoblastic (formerly dif-fuse poorly dif-ferentiated lym-phocytic (PDL))	Lymphoblastic, B-cell type	Undefined cell	**TdT+** HLA-DR+ Sig− cMu −/+,	Ig HC usual; Ig LC possible; TCR receptor gene rearrange-ment in minority of cases
B-Cell Chronic Lymphocytic Leukemia (B-CLL) Prolymphocytic Leukemia (B-PLL) Small Lympho-cytic Lymphoma (B-SLL)	**CD5+** **CD19+** **CD20+** **CD23+** **CD79a+** CD43+ CD10− faint CD11c−/+ CD22+ in some subtypes only	Small lympho-cytic, consis-tent with CLL	Well-differenti-ated lympho-cytic, diffuse	B-CLL, B-PLL, immunocy-toma, lymphop-lasma-cytoid type	Small lympho-cyte B, B-CLL	**Faint SIgM** SIgD+/− CIg−/+	Ig HC & LC gene rearranged; trisomy 12 in 33% of cases; abnormality of 13q in 25%; transposition of chromosome 11 to 14; bcl−1 gene rearranged.
LymphoPlasma-cytoid Lym-phoma/Immu-nocytoma	**CD5− CD10−** CD19+ CD20+ CD22+CD79a+ CD43+/− CD11c possible (faint); CD25 possible (faint)	Small lympho-cytic, plasmacy-toid, diffuse mixed small and large cell	Well-differenti-ated lympho-cytic, plasmacy-toid, diffuse mixed lympho-cytic and histio-cytic	Immunocy-toma, lymphop-lasmacytic type	Plasmacytic-lymphocytic	Surface and **cytoplasmic Ig+** (usually IgM); usually IgD−	Ig HC & LC (heavy chain and light chain) gene rearrange-ment

Consensus Classification	CD Antigens	Working Formulation	Rappaport	Kiel	Lukes-Collins	Other Antigens	Genetic Features
				B-Cell Entities			
Mantle Cell Lymphoma	**CD5+ CD19+ CD20+ CD22+ CD79a+ CD23-** CD10-/+ CD11c- CD43+	Small cleaved cell, diffuse or nodular; rarely diffuse mixed or large cleaved cell	Intermediately or poorly differentiated lymphocytic, diffuse or nodular (ILL/IDL/PDL)	Centrocytic (mantle cell) lymphoma	Small cleaved follicular center cell (FCC)	**SIgM+ usually IgD+** lambda > kappa; disorganized FDC	Transposition of chromosome 11 to 14 (t(11;14)) w/Ig HC and bcl-1 on long arm of chr. 11
Follicle Center Lymphoma, Follicular; (B cell) Grades: I (Predominantly Small Cell); II (Mixed); III (Predominantly Large Cell); Provisional Subtype: Diffuse (Predominantly Small Cell)	**CD5- CD19+ CD20+ CD22+ CD10+/- CD43-**CD11c- CD23-/+	Follicular, small cleaved, mixed, or large cell diffuse small cleaved cell	Nodular PDL, mixed lymphocytic-histiocytic, or histiocytic poorly differentiated diffuse lymphocytic	Centroblastic/centrocytic follicular centroblastic/centrocytic, diffuse	Small cleaved, large cleaved, or large non-cleaved FCC, follicular diffuse small cleaved FCC	SIg+ (M+/-D > G > A) bcl-2+ in follicular	**Transposition of chromosome 14 to 18** with bcl-2 rearranged in 70 to 95% of cases
Marginal Zone B-Cell Lymphoma: 1.Extranodal: Low-grade B-cell lymphoma of MALT type (+/- monocytoid B-cells); 2. Provisional: Nodal: (+/- monocytoid B-cells)	**CD5- CD10-** CD19+ CD20+ CD22+ CD79a+ CD11c+/- CD23- CD43-/+	(Not specifically listed) SLL, (some consistent with CLL, some plasmacytoid) small cleaved, or mixed small + large cell (follicular or diffuse)	(Not specifically listed) well-differentiated lymphocytic (WDL) or WDL-plasmacytoid, IDL, ILL, PDL, mixed lymphocytic-histiocytic (nodular or diffuse)	Monocytoid B-cell immunocytoma (some previously centroblastic-centrocytic or centrocytic)	Small lymphocyte B, lymphocytic-plasmacytic, small lymphoctye B, monocytoid	SIg+ (M >G or A) IgD absent; **Cytoplasmic Ig+ in 40 % of cases**	Trisomy 3 and/or transposition of chromosome 11 to 18 {t(11;18)} reported in extranodal type

Consensus Classification	CD Antigens	Working Formulation	Rappaport	Kiel	Lukes-Collins	Other Antigens	Genetic Features
			B-Cell Entities				
Provisional entity: Splenic Marginal Zone Lymphoma, with or w/o Villous Lymphocytes	**CD5– CD10–** CD19+ CD20+ CD22+ CD79a+ CD11c+/– CD23– CD43–/+	(Not specifically listed) SLL	(Not specifically listed) WDL or WDL-plasmacytoid	(Not specifically listed)	Small lymphocyte B, lympho-cytic-plasma-cytic, small lymphocyte B monocytoid	SIg+ (M>G or A; lack IgD) **Cytoplasmic Ig+ in 40% of cases**	Not well studied; trisomy 3 not detected
Hairy Cell Leukemia	**CD5– CD10– CD11c+strong CD23– CD25+ strong CD103+ (MLA)** CD19+ CD20+ CD22+ CD79a+	—	—	—	—	SIg+ (M+/– D, G, or A) **FMC7+** TRAP+ in majority of cases	Ig HC & LC genes rearranged
Plasmacytoma/Plasma Cell Myeloma	**CD19, CD20, CD22 absent** CD30 possible; CD38+ CD43+/– CD45–/+ CD56+/– CD79a+/–	—	—	—	—	**SIg–** **CIg+ (G, A, rare D/E; or LC only)** HLA-DR–/+ EMA–/+	Ig HC & LC (heavy chain and light chain) rearranged or deleted
Diffuse Large B-Cell Lymphoma	**CD19+ CD20+ CD22+ CD79a+ CD45+/–** CD5–/+ CD10–/+	Diffuse large cell cleaved, noncleaved or immunoblastic; occasionally diffuse mixed small + lg cell	Diffuse histiocytic, occasionally diffuse mixed lymphocytic-histiocytic	Centroblastic, B-immunoblastic, large cell anaplastic (B-cell)	Large cleaved or large non-cleaved FCC, B-immunoblastic	SIg+/– CIg–/+	Bcl-2 gene rearrangement in 30% of cases c-myc rearrang. in some cases

Consensus Classification	CD Antigens	Working Formulation	Rappaport	Kiel	Lukes-Collins	Other Antigens	Genetic Features
				B-cell entities			
Large B-Cell Lymphoma Subtype: Primary Mediastinal (Thymic) Large B-Cell Lymphoma	**CD19+** **CD20+** **CD22+** **CD79a+** CD45+/− CD15− CD30−/+					Often Ig neg.	Ig HC & LC (heavy and light chain) rearrangement
Burkitt's Lymphoma	**CD5− CD10+** **CD19+** **CD20+** **CD22+** **CD79a+** CD23−	Small non-cleaved cell, Burkitt's type	Undifferentiated lymphoma, Burkitt's type	Burkitt's lymphoma	Small non-cleaved FCC	**SIgM+**	Transpositions: t(8;14), t(2;8), or t(8;22) of c-myc gene; EBV+ in most African cases; EBV+ in 25% to 40% of AIDS
Provisional entity: High-Grade B-Cell Lymphoma, Burkitt-like	CD5− CD10− (usually) CD19+ CD20+ CD22+ CD79a+	Small non-cleaved cell, non-Burkitt	Undifferentiated, non-Burkitt	—	Small non-cleaved FCC	SIg+/− CIg possible	bcl-2 gene rearrang. in 30% of cases
		T-Cell Entities and Putative Natural Killer Cell (NK) Neoplasms					
Precursor T-cell Lymphoblastic Lymphoma/Leukemia (T-LBL)	**CD3+ CD7+** **B cell antigens absent** either CD4+/CD8+ or CD4−/CD8− CD1a+/− CD2 (varies) CD5 (varies) CD16 occas. CD57 occas.	Lymphoblastic, convoluted or nonconvoluted	Poorly differentiated lymphocytic, diffuse (modified to lymphoblastic)	T lymphoblastic	Convoluted T lymphocytic	**TdT+** **Ig−** alpha-beta, or gamma-delta, or no TCRs	TCR gene rearrangement varies Ig HC rearrangement might be found variable cytogenic abnormalities reported

T-Cell Entities and Putative Natural Killer Cell (NK) Neoplasms

Consensus Classification	CD Antigens	Working Formulation	Rappaport	Kiel	Lukes-Collins	Other Antigens	Genetic Features
T-Cell Chronic Lymphocytic Leukemia (T-CLL) or T-Cell Prolymphocytic Leukemia (T-PLL)	**CD2+ CD3+ CD5+ CD7+** CD4+/CD8− (65% of cases) CD4+/CD8+ (21% of cases) CD4−/CD8+ rare; CD25−	Small lymphocytic, consistent with CLL; diffuse small cleaved cell-FAB: T-PLL	WDL, PDL	T-cell CLL/PLL	Small lymphocyte T, prolymphocytic		TCR gene rearrangement; inversion of chromosome 14 on long arm, loci 11 to 32, in 75% of cases; trisomy 8q (three copies of the long arm of chromosome 8)
Large Granular Lymphocyte Leukemia (T-cell LGL) FAB system: T-CLL, T-LGL	**CD2+ CD3+ CD16+ CD56− CD57+**/−CD4− /CD8+CD5− CD7− CD25−	Small lymphocytic, consistent with CLL	SLL, CLL	T-CLL	Small lymphocyte, T	TCR alpha/ beta+	TCR gene rearrangement EBV positive in aggressive Asian cases
NK-Cell Large Granular Lymphocyte (LGL) Leukemia (NK-LGL) FAB system: T-CLL, T-LGL	**CD2+ CD3− CD16+ CD56+**/− **CD57+**/−CD4− /CD8+/−	Small lymphocytic, consistent w/CLL	SLL, CLL	T-CLL	Small lymphocyte, T	TCR alpha/ beta−	EBV positive in aggressive Asian cases
Mycosis Fungoides/ Sezary Syndrome (MF/SS)	**CD2+ CD3+ CD5+ CD7−/+ CD4+/CD8−** CD25− usually CD8+ rarely	Mycosis fungoides	Mycosis fungoides/ Sezary syndrome	Small cell, cerebriform	Cerebriform T	S-100+ CD1a+ interdigitating & Langerhans' cells present	TCR gene rearrangement

Consensus Classification	CD Antigens	Working Formulation	Rappaport	Kiel	Lukes-Collins	Other Antigens	Genetic Features
T-Cell Entities and Putative Natural Killer Cell (NK) Neoplasms							
Peripheral T-Cell Lymphomas, Unspecified Provisional: (Medium-Sized Cell, Mixed Medium and Large-Cell, Large-Cell)	**CD2+/-** **CD3+/-** **CD5+/-** **CD7-/+** **no B-cell CD antigens** CD4+ > CD8+ CD4-/ CD8- possible; may express CD45RA but lack CD45RO CD20+ rarely	Diffuse small cleaved cell, diffuse mixed small and large cell, large cell immunoblastic (polymorphous or clear cell)	Diffuse PDL, diffuse mixed lymphocytic-histiocytic, histiocytic	T-zone lymphoma, lymphoepithelioid cell lymphoma, pleomorphic, small, medium and large cell, T-immunoblastic	T-immunoblastic lymphoma		TCR gene rearrangement is usual
Peripheral T-Cell Lymphoma variant: Angioimmunoblastic T-Cell Lymphoma	CD2+ CD3+ CD5+ CD7+ CD4+	Not listed (diffuse mixed small and large cell, diffuse large cell, large cell immunoblastic)	Not listed (diffuse mixed lymphocytic-histiocytic)	T-cell, angioimmunoblastic (AILD)	IBL-like T-cell lymphoma	Expanded follicular dendritic cells (FDC) surrounding proliferating venules	TCR gene rearrang. 75% of cases; Ig HC rearrang. 10% of cases; EBV genome often found; trisomy 3 and/or 5 poss.
Peripheral T-cell Lymphoma variant: Angiocentric Lymphoma	**CD2+** **CD3-** **CD56+** CD5+/- CD7+/- may be CD4+ or CD8+ pulmonary cases may express B cell CD antigens	Not listed (diffuse small cleaved, mixed small and large, diffuse large cell, large cell immunoblastic)	Not listed (diffuse mixed lymphocytic-histiocytic, diffuse PDL)	Not listed (T, pleomorphic small, medium and large)	Not listed (T-immunoblastic sarcoma)	No additional antigens known	EBV+ usually; pulmonary cases may have gene rearrangement & EBV in B cells

Other previous categories : angiocentric, immunoproliferative lesion (grades 2 + 3); polymorphic reticulosis; lethal midline granuloma; midline malignant reticulosis; nasal T-cell lymphoma; lymphomatoid granulomatosis (some cases)

T-Cell Entities and Putative Natural Killer Cell (NK) Neoplasms

Consensus Classification	CD Antigens	Working Formulation	Rappaport	Kiel	Lukes-Collins	Other Antigens	Genetic Features
Intestinal T-Cell Lymphoma (with or without enteropathy)	**CD3+** **CD7+** **CD103+ (MLA)** CD8+/− CD4−	Not listed (diffuse small cleaved, mixed small and large, diffuse large cell, large cell immunoblastic)	Not listed (diffuse mixed lymphocytic-histiocytic, histiocytic, diffuse PDL)	Not listed (T, pleomorphic small, medium and large)	Not listed (T-immunoblastic sarcoma)	No additional antigens known	TCR beta genes rearranged
		Other previous categories: malignant histiocytosis of intestine, ulcerative jejunitis					
Adult T-Cell Lymphoma/Leukemia (ATL/L)	**CD2+** **CD3+** **CD5+** CD4+ CD25+ CD8+ rarely	Not listed (diffuse small cleaved, mixed small and large, diffuse large cell, large cell immunoblastic)	Diffuse PDL, mixed lympho-cytic-histio-cytic, or histio-cytic	Pleomorphic small, medium, and large cell type (HTLV-1+)	Not listed (T-immunoblastic sarcoma)	**Caused by HTLV-1**	TCR genes rearranged; **integrated HTLV-1 genome in all cases**
Anaplastic Large Cell (ALCL) (CD30+) Lymphoma (T- and Null-Cell Types)	**CD30+** CD3−/+ CD15−/+ CD25+/− varies: CD45+/− CD43−/+ CD45RO−/+ CD68−	Not listed (diffuse large cell immuno-blastic)	Not listed (histiocytic dif-fuse)	Large cell ana-plastic (T and null types)	T-immunoblas-tic sarcoma	**EMA+/−** 50% of cases express H-Y antigens cutaneous cases lack EMA and express CLA	**Transposition of chromo-some 2 to 5;** TCR gene rearrangement in 50 to 60% of cases
		Other previous categories: malignant histiocytosis, sinusoidal LCL, regressing atypical histiocytosis					

Consensus Classification	CD Antigens	Working Formulation	Rappaport	Kiel	Lukes-Collins	Other Antigens	Genetic Features
T-Cell Entities and Putative Natural Killer Cell (NK) Neoplasms							
Provisional entity: Anaplastic Large Cell (ALCL), Hodgkin's-Like/Hodgkin's-related	**CD30+** CD3-/+ CD15-/+ CD25+/- varies: CD45+/- CD43-/+ CD45RO-/+ CD68-	Not listed (diffuse large cell immunoblastic)	Not listed (histiocytic diffuse)	Large cell anaplastic (T and null types)	T-immunoblastic sarcoma	**EMA+/-** 50% express H-Y antigens cutaneous lack EMA and express CLA usually EBV negative	Unknown
Hodgkin's-Lymphocyte Predominance (Paragranuloma)(LPHD)	**CD15– CD19+ CD20+ CD22+ CD79a+ CD45+ CD57+** CD30-/+ CDw75+	—	—	—	Lymphocytic and/or histiocytic, nodular or diffuse	T-cells surround L&H cells; EMA+/-; **Ig–** (usually); prominent FDC mesh in nodules	EBV negative in majority of large cells Ig and TCR genes not rearranged
Hodgkin's-Nodular Sclerosis	**CD15+/- CD30+ CD45–**	—	—	—	—	EMA– usually B- and T-cell antigens are negative	EBV+ in 40% of cases; occas. bcl-2 gene rearr. in benign cells
Hodgkin's-Mixed Cellularity	**CD15+/- CD30+ CD45–**	—	—	—	—	EMA– usually B- and T-cell antigens are negative	EBV+ in 60–70% of cases
Hodgkin's-Lymphocyte Depletion	**CD15+/- CD30+ CD45– B- and T-cell antigens neg.**	—	—	—	—	**EMA–**	No rearrangement of Ig and TCR genes
Provisional entity: Hodgkin's Lymphocyte-Rich Classical	**CD15+/- CD30+ CD45–**	—	—	—	Subset of diffuse lymphocyte predominent	EMA– usually B- and T-cell antigens are negative	Resembles Nodular Sclerosis and Mixed Cellularity

Unclassifiable lymphomas

There are times when a lymphoma is unclassifiable for various reasons. The authors of this paper list the following possibilities:

- Unclassifiable B-cell:
  - Low-grade predominantly small cell
  - High-grade mixed small and large cell, or predominantly large cell
- Unclassifiable T-cell:
  - Low-grade predominantly small cell
  - High-grade mixed small and large cell, or predominantly large cell
- Unclassifiable Hodgkin's
- Unclassifiable malignant lymphoma, low grade or high grade

Common Chemotherapies

Many of the chemotherapy regimens shown below are recombinations of CHOP drugs with additional agents, different timing, or different doses. Some, such as LSA2L2 or NHL-BFM, are quite different from CHOP, instead resembling regimens for childhood acute lymphoblastic leukemia, spread over long time periods. Others are unique agents used against specific NHLs, such as psoralen for cutaneous T-cell lymphoma.

Two tables are provided below.

Multi-drug regimen acronyms and their component drugs are shown in the first table. Unfortunately, acronyms have been created over time following few, if any, rules. In a few cases, such as BFM or POG, the acronym stands for a study group, but most often an acronym is assembled from either:

- The first letters of the *generic names* of the drugs used

- The first letters of the *abbreviations* for the drug names, such as V used for etoposide (VP-16)

- Less often, the first letters of the registered *trade names*, such as Adriamycin for doxorubicin, or Oncovin for vincristine

Single drug names, abbreviations, trade names, and modes of action are supplied in the second table

Dose amounts and schedules are not given below, because these may be altered by your doctor to suit your circumstances. In the absence of these amounts and schedules, many of these regimens appear to be almost identical, but dose and schedule do indeed make a considerable difference in tumor response.

Common multidrug regimens

Acronym	Drugs Included
ACOP+	Adriamycin (doxorubicin; DOX), cyclophosphamide (CTX), Oncovin (vincristine; VCR), prednisone (Pred), methotrexate (MTX), hydrocortisone (HC)
ACOP-B	Adriamycin (doxorubicin; DOX), cyclophosphamide (CTX), Oncovin (vincristine; VCR), prednisone (Pred), bleomycin (BLEO)
ACVB	Adriamycin (doxorubicin; DOX), cyclophosphamide (CTX), vindesine (VDS), bleomycin (BLEO)
APO	Adriamycin (doxorubicin; DOX), prednisone (Pred), Oncovin (vincristine; VCR), methotrexate (MTX), l-asparaginase (A-ase), 6-mercaptopurine (6-MP)
BACOP	bleomycin (BLEO), Adriamycin (doxorubicin; DOX), cyclophosphamide (CTX), Oncovin (vincristine; VCR), prednisone (Pred)
BACT	carmustine (BCNU), cytarabine (ARA-C), cyclophosphamide (CTX), 6-thioguanine (6-TG)
BEAC	carmustine (BCNU), etoposide (VP-16), cytarabine (ARA-C), cyclophosphamide (CTX)
BEAM	carmustine (BCNU), etoposide (VP-16), cytarabine (ARA-C), melphalan
BFM (Berlin-Frankfurt-Munster study)	prednisone (Pred), vincristine (VCR), daunorubicin (DNR), asparaginase, cyclophosphamide (CTX), cytarabine (ARA-C), methotrexate (MTX), mercaptopurine (6-MP) (See also NHL-BFM 86/90)
BMV-VIP	bleomycin (BLEO), methylprednisone (Pred), vindesine, ifosfamide (IFF), etoposide (VP-16)
CAPOMEt	CHOP with methotrexate and etoposide added
CEPP-Bleo	cyclophosphamide (CTX), etoposide (VP-16), procarbazine (PCB), prednisone (Pred), bleomycin (BLEO)
CHOP	cyclophosphamide (CTX), hydroxorubicin (doxorubicin; DOX), Oncovin (vincristine; VCR), prednisone (Pred)
CHOP-BLEO	CHOP with bleomycin (BLEO) added
CHOP plus MTX	CHOP alternating with infusional methotrexate (MTX)
CHVP	cyclophosphamide (CTX), hydroxorubicin (doxorubicin; DOX), teniposide (VM-26), prednisone (Pred)
COMLA	cyclophosphamide (CTX), Oncovin (vincristine; VCR), methotrexate (MTX), leucovorin (Leu), cytarabine (ARA-C)
COMP	cyclophosphamide (CTX), Oncovin (vincristine; VCR), methotrexate (MTX), prednisone (Pred)
COP	CHOP without hydroxorubicin (DOX)
COPAD	Cyclophosphamide (CTX), Oncovin (vincristine; VCR), prednisone (Pred), ADriamycin (doxorubicin; DOX)
COPAD-M	COPAD with methotrexate (MTX) added
CVP-1	COP with different doses, different timing
DHAP	dexamethasone (DEX), high-dose cytarabine (ARA-C), and cisplatin (CDDP)
DICE	dexamethasone (DEX), ifosfamide (IFF), cisplatin (CDDP), etoposide (VP-16)
EPOCH	etoposide (VP-16), prednisone (Pred), Oncovin (vincristine; VCR), cyclophosphamide (CTX), hydroxorubicin (doxorubicin; DOX)

Acronym	Drugs Included
ESAP	etoposide (VP-16), methylprednisolone (SOL), cytarabine (ARA-C), cisplatin (CDDP)
ESHAP	ESAP with prednisone (Pred) added
ICE	ifosfamide (IFF), carboplatinum, etoposide (VP-16)
IDA/Ara-C	idarubicin (IDA), cytarabine (ARA-C)
IM-VP16	ifosfamide (IFF), methotrexate (MTX), etoposide (VP-16)
LSA2L2	cyclophosphamide (CTX), intrathecal methotrexate (MTX IT), vincristine (VCR), daunomycin (DNR), prednisone (Pred), cytarabine (ARA-C), asparaginase (A-ase), thioguanine (6-TG), carmustine (BCNU), and hydroxyurea (HU)
LSA2L2 + MTX	The LSA2L2 regimen supplemented by 10 courses of high-dose methotrexate (MTX)
MACOP-B	methotrexate (MTX), Adriamycin (doxorubicin; DOX), cyclophosphamide (CTX), Oncovin (vincristine; VCR), prednisone (Pred), bleomycin (BLEO), leucovorin (Leu)
m-BACOD	methotrexate (MTX), bleomycin (BLEO), Adriamycin (doxorubicin; DOX), cyclophosphamide (CTX), Oncovin (vincristine; VCR), dexamethasone (DEX), leucovorin (Leu)
M-BACOD	Same as m-BACOD, but with higher doses
Milan protocol	prednisone (Pred), vincristine (VCR), cyclophosphamide (CTX), doxorubicin (DOX), high-dose methotrexate (MTX), cytarabine (ARA-C), bleomycin (BLEO), 6-thioguanine (6-TG), methotrexate (MTX), 6-mercaptopurine (6-MP)
MIME	mitoguazon, ifosfamide (IFF), methotrexate (MTX), etoposide (VP-16)
MINE	MESNA, ifosfamide (IFF), mitoxantrone (DHAD), etoposide (VP-16)
MIV	mitoxantrone (DHAD), ifosfamide (IFF), etoposide (VP-16)
NHL-BFM 86/90 (Berlin-Frankfurt-Munster study)	vincristine (VCR), doxorubicin (DOX), prednisone (Pred), cyclophosphamide (CTX), dexamethasone (DEX), etoposide (VP-16), cytarabine (ARA-C), methotrexate (MTX), vindesine, ifosfamide (IFF)
POG 8106 (Pediatric Oncology Group)	high-dose methotrexate (MTX), high-dose cyclophosphamide (CTX), vincristine (VCR), prednisone (Pred)
PROMACE-cytaBOM	prednisone (Pred), Adriamycin (doxorubicin; DOX), cyclophosphamide (CTX), etoposide (VP-16), cytarabine (ARA-C), bleomycin (BLEO), Oncovin (vincristine; VCR), methotrexate (MTX), leucovorin (Leu)
PROMACE/MOPP	prednisone (Pred), methotrexate (MTX), Adriamycin (doxorubicin; DOX), cyclophosphamide (CTX), etoposide (VP-16), mustargen, Oncovin (vincristine; VCR), procarbazine (PCB)
VACOP-B	etoposide (VP-16), Adriamycin (doxorubicin; DOX), cyclophosphamide (CTX), Oncovin (vincristine; VCR), prednisone (Pred), bleomycin (BLEO)
VIM	etoposide (VP-16), ifosfamide (IFF), mitoxantrone (DHAD), prednisone (Pred)
VIM-Bleo	etoposide (VP-16), ifosfamide (IFF), methotrexate (MTX), bleomycin (BLEO)

Common drug names and abbreviations

Listed below in alphabetic order are drug names, abbreviations, their trade names, and modes of action.

Generic Name, Abbreviation	Trade Names	Mode of Action and Comments
Allopurinol	Lopurin Zyloprim	Rescue drug used to protect kidneys from certain chemotherapeutic drugs
9-aminocamp-toth-ecin (9-AC)	(still in clinical trials)	See Camptothecin
Asparaginase (l-asparaginase (A-ase)	Elspar Oncas-par	Antimetabolite
Bleomycin (BLEO)	Blenoxane	Idiosyncratic agent; joins with one form of iron, breaking DNA strands
Busulfan (BU)	Myleran	Alkylating agent
Camptothecin (CPT11)	(still in clinical trials)	Topoisomerase inhibitor; a plant-derived alkaloid
Carmustine; nitro-surea (BCNU)	BiCNU or Gliadel	Alkylating agent
Chlorambucil (Chl)	Leukeran	Alkylating agent
2-chlorodeoxy-ade-nosine (2-CDA)	Cladribine	Antimetabolite
Cisplatin (CDDP)	Platinol	Idiosyncratic alkylating agent
Cyclophospha-mide (CTX)	Cytoxan or Neosar	Alkylating agent
Cytarabine or cytosine arabino-side (ARA-C)	Cytosar-U, Depo-Cyt, Tarabine	Antimetabolite
Cytoxan®		See cyclophosphamide
Dacarbazine (DTIC)	DTIC-Dome	Alkylating agent
Daunorubicin or daunomycin (DNR)	Cerubidine or DaunoXome	Topoisomerase inhibitor
Dexamethasone (DEX)	Decadron, Decaspray, Aeroseb-Dex, Hexadrol	Immunosuppressive agent
Doxorubicin (DOX)	Adriamycin, Doxil, Rubex	Topoisomerase inhibitor
Erythropoietin, Epoietin alfa (EPO)	Epogen, Procrit	Biological therapy; stimulates formation of red blood cells
Etoposide (VP-16)	Toposar, VePesid	Topoisomerase inhibitor
Filgrastim (G-CSF)	Neupogen	See Granulocyte colony stimulating factor
Fludarabine (FLUD)	Fludara	Antimetabolite

Generic Name, Abbreviation	Trade Names	Mode of Action and Comments
5-fluorouracil (5-FU)	Adrucil, Efudex, Fluoroplex	Idiosyncratic agent
Granulocyte colony stimulating factor (G-CSF)	Neupogen	Biological therapy; stimulates growth of white blood cells
Granulocyte-macrophage colony stimulating factor (GM-CSF)	Leukine	Biological therapy; stimulates growth of white blood cells and macrophages
Hydrocortisone (HC)	A-hydroCort, Cortef, Hydro-cortone Hytone, Locoid, Pan-del, Solu-Cortef, Westcort	Immune suppressant
Hydroxorubicin	Adriamycin	See doxorubicin
Hydroxyurea (HU)	Droxia, Hydrea	Antimetabolite
Idarubicin (IDA)	Idamycin	Topoisomerase inhibitor
Ifosfamide (IFF)	Ifex	Alkylating agent
Interferon (IFN)s	Roferon A, Intron A, Alf-eron N	Biological therapies
Interleukin-2 (IL-2)		Biological therapy
Irinotecan	Camptosar	Topoisomerase inhibitor (soluble metabolite of camptothecin)
Leucovorin (Leu)	Wellcovorin	Rescue drug
Lomustine (CCNU)	CeeNU	Alkylating agent
Mechloreth-amine, Nitrogen Mustard, (HN2)	Mustargen	Alkylating agent
Melphalan	Alkeran	Alkylating agent
Mercaptopurine (6-MP)	Purinethol	Antimetabolite
Methotrexate or amethopterin (MTX)	Methotrexate	Antimetabolite
Methylpredniso-lone (SOL)	Medrol, A-methaPred, Depo-Medrol, Solu-Medrol, SOL	Immune suppressant
Mitoguazone, methyl-GAG, meth-ylglyoxal (bis)-gua-nylhydrozan	(still in clini-cal trials)	Inhibitor of polyamine biosynthesis
Mitoxantrone (DHAD)	Novantrone	Topoisomerase inhibitor

Generic Name, Abbreviation	Trade Names	Mode of Action and Comments
Monoclonal antibody (mab, moab)	Rituxan, Bexxar	Biologic therapy; manmade copy of protein secreted by white blood cell to attack invading organisms
Nitrosurca		See Carmustine
Pentostatin or deoxycofor-mycin	Nipent	Antimetabolite
Phosphocholine or hexadecylphosphocholine	Phosphocol P32	Antimetabolite
Prednisone (Pred)	Deltasone®, Orasone®, prednisone	Immune suppressant
Prednisolone	Econopred, Hydeltrasol, Inflamase, Pediapred, Pred Forte, Pred Mild, Prelone	Immune suppressant
Procarbazine (PCB)	Matulane	Alkylating agent
Psoralen	methoxsalen	UV therapy; embeds in DNA, making it more sensitive to UVA light
Rituxan	See monoclonal antibody	Biological therapy
Sargramostim (GM-CSF)	Leukine	See granulocyte-macrophage colony stimulating factor
Teniposide (VM-26)	Vumon	Topoisomerase inhibitor
Thioguanine (6-TG)		Antimetabolite
Thrombopoietin (TPO)	(still in clinical trials)	Biological therapy; manmade copy of a natural body substance that stimulates the production of platelets
Topotecan	Hycamtin	Topoisomerase inhibitor (soluble metabolite of camptothecin)
Tumor necrosis factor (TNF)	(still in clinical trials)	Biological therapy; manmade copy of a natural body substance that exhibits antiviral and anti-tumor activity
Vinblastine (VLB)	Velban, Vinblastine	Vinca alkaloid; tubulin binding agent
Vincristine (VCR)	Oncovin	Vinca alkaloid; tubulin binding agent
Vindesine (VDS)		Vinca alkaloid; tubulin binding agent
Vinorelbine	Navelbine	Vinca alkaloid; tubulin binding agent

Resources

Clinical Pharmacology Online: *http://www:cponline.gsm.com/*

RxMed: *http://www.rxmed.com/*

PharmInfoNet: *http://pharminfo.com/*

Glaxo Wellcome's DoseCalc: *http://www.meds.com/DChome.html*

Notes

Chapter 4: *Prognoses*

1. H. M. Prince et al., "The role of intensive therapy and autologous blood and marrow transplantation for chemotherapy-sensitive relapsed and primary refractory non-Hodgkin's lymphoma: identification of major prognostic groups," *British Journal of Haematology* 92, no. 4 (March 1996): 880–889.

2. M. Shiota and S. Mori, "The clinicopathological features of anaplastic large cell lymphomas expressing p80 NPM/ALK," *Leukemia and Lymphoma* 23, nos. 1–2 (September 1996): 25–32.

3. M. Osada et al., "Mutation of p53 does not determine prognosis in non-Hodgkin's lymphoma," *Gan To Kagaku Ryoho,* 24, no. 4 (February 1997): 471–475.

4. F. d'Amore et al., "Epstein-Barr virus genome in non-Hodgkin's lymphomas occurring in immunocompetent patients: highest prevalence in nonlymphoblastic T-cell lymphoma and correlation with a poor prognosis. Danish Lymphoma Study Group, LYFO" *Blood* 87, no. 3 (1 February 1996): 1045–1055.

5. S. Tsunoda et al., "Clinical and prognostic significance of femoral marrow magnetic resonance imaging in patients with malignant lymphoma," *Blood* 89, no. 1 (1 January 1997): 286–290.

6. W. H. Wilson et al., "Relationship of p53, bcl-2, and tumor proliferation to clinical drug resistance in non-Hodgkin's lymphomas," *Blood* 89, no. 2 (15 January 1997): 601–609.

7. M. E. Hill et al., "Prognostic significance of BCL-2 expression and bcl-2 major breakpoint region rearrangement in diffuse large-cell non-Hodgkin's lymphoma: a British National Lymphoma Investigation Study," *Blood* 88, no. 3 (1 August 1996): 1046–1051.

8. M. H. Kramer et al., "Clinical significance of bcl2 and p53 protein expression in diffuse large B-cell lymphoma: a population-based study," *Journal of Clinical Oncology* 14, no. 7 (14 July 1996): 2131 to 2138.

9. M. Davidge-Pitts, R. Dansey, and W. R. Bezwoda, "Prolonged survival in follicular non-Hodgkins lymphoma is predicted by achievement of complete remission with initial treatment: results of a long-term study with multivariate analysis of prognostic factors," *Leukemia and Lymphoma* 24, nos. 1–2 (December 1996): 131–140.

Chapter 11: *Stress and the Immune System*

1. W. Neuhaus et al., "A prospective study concerning psychological characteristics of patients with breast cancer," *Archives of Gynecology and Obstetrics* 255, no. 4 (1994): 201–209; and R. Schwarz and S. Geyer, "Social and psychological differences between cancer and noncancer patients: cause or consequence of the disease?" *Psychotherapy and Psychosomatics* 41, no. 4 (1984): 195–199.

Chapter 13: *Getting Support*

1. Ellen E. Schultz, "If You Use Firm's Counselors, Remember Your Secrets Could Be Used Against You," *Wall Street Journal*, 26 May 1994.

Chapter 17: *Sexuality, Fertility, and Pregnancy*

1. Z. Blumenfeld and N. Haim, "Prevention of gonadal damage during cytotoxic therapy," *Ann Med* 29, no. 3 (June 1997): 199–206.

2. F. Aubier et al., "Male gonadal function after chemotherapy for solid tumors in childhood," *Journal of Clinical Oncology* 7, no. 3 (March 1989): 304–309.

Chapter 22: *If All Treatments Have Failed*

1. Sherwin B. Nuland, M.D. *How We Die: Reflections on Life's Final Chapter.* New York: Alfred A. Knopf, 1994.

Glossary

This glossary lists only terms specific to NHL. For a comprehensive glossary of cancer medical terminology, see Roberta Altman's *The Cancer Dictionary.* For more general medical terms, any one of several inexpensive medical dictionaries available in bookstores and libraries should suffice.

Guides to pronunciation are included.

But first: unusual phrases

Before we list terms you may find when reading about NHL, we must point out that there are a few specific words and phrases that may be jarring because they mean something other in medicine than they do in everyday usage:

Anecdotal
> When used in a medical context, it does not mean a funny story. It means a single case report not yet substantiated by studies using large numbers of people.

Impressive or not impressive
> When used in a medical context, it does not mean anything derogatory. It means that, when the patient was examined, a particular feature did not strike the examiner as overwhelmingly unusual. For instance, after palpating your abdomen, the doctor may note in your medical record that your spleen was "not impressive." This means it did not feel enlarged, and that you did not report pain when she pressed on it.

Morbid or morbidity
> In a medical context, they do not mean that you have a neurotic outlook. They simply mean illness, and are somewhat the opposite of mortality. You might read, for example, that a treatment resulted in 20 percent low-level morbidity, but only 2 percent mortality. Likewise, comorbidity means the illnesses a person has in addition to cancer, such as high blood pressure or diabetes.

The patient denies

This phrase does not mean that the doctor thinks you're lying. It's just used as the opposite of "the patient reports." For instance, your medical record might read, "The patient reports frequent morning cough, but denies the presence of phlegm."

Tolerable

A word often used by medical staff to describe the side effects of treatment. Your idea of what is tolerable may be much lower than their definition, because medicine defines a tolerable side effect as one that can be ameliorated with supportive care and that does not result in permanent organ damage. For you, these side effects may be intolerable.

NHL terminology

Absolute neutrophil count (NEW-tro-fil), also called ANC

The total number of neutrophils in the blood, a measure of one's ability to fight infection. Also called absolute granulocyte count or AGC.

Allogeneic transplant (al-lo-jeh-NAY-ic)

Marrow or stem cell transplant using donor stem cells of the same species that are immunologically different from the patient's.

Anemia (an-KNEE-me-uh)

A lack of adequate numbers of oxygen-carrying red blood cells.

Apheresis (AFF-er-EE-sis)

The channeling of blood out of the body and through specialized single-use tubing and equipment in order to extract various blood cell types, such as platelets or stem cells, from the bloodstream. After these cells are extracted, the blood is returned to the body. Also called hemapheresis, or leukapheresis for the extraction of white blood cells.

Apoptosis (app-uh-TOE-sis; variant: a-pup-TOE-sis)

Orderly cell death characterized by slow dissolving and reuse of cell parts by neighboring tissue. Some chemotherapy drugs induce apoptosis; others cause cell lysis or bursting.

Autologous transplant (aw-TAHL-uh-gus)

A marrow or stem cell transplant using the patient's own blood products.

B cells

White blood cells that have not traveled to the thymus (see T cells). B cells are responsible for many immune functions, such as producing proteins called antibodies that tag invaders for destruction.

Bone marrow

The soft, spongy matrix of all bones that produce blood cells. As we age, some marrow is replaced by fat cells or fibres.

Bulky disease

A cancer-specific phrase found often in the literature on lymphomas. Bulky disease is any cancerous lymph node or extranodal tissue that measures greater than ten centimeters in any dimension.

Centigrey or cGy

A measurement of radiation dose absorbed by the body.

Complete blood count or CBC

A count of the red, white, and platelet cells in peripheral blood.

Complete remission

The disappearance of all disease for longer than one month.

Consolidation therapy

Chemotherapy or radiotherapy intended to destroy all remaining cancer cells. Consolidation therapy frequently follows induction therapy.

Cytomegalovirus or CMV (sigh-toe-MEG-uh-low-virus)

One of a group of herpesviruses that can cause serious or fatal infection among the immune-suppressed.

-cytosis (sigh-TOE-sis)

A suffix denoting an abnormally high number of blood cells: Lymphocytosis, erythrocytosis, or thrombocytosis. See also -penia.

Cytotoxic (sigh-toe-TOX-ic)

A term for anything that kills cells. Many chemotherapy and radiotherapy regimens are cytotoxic to both healthy and cancerous cells.

Differentiation (diff-er-en-she-A-shun)

The term used to describe cells maturing and developing for a particular task. For lymphomas, differentiation generally refers to white blood cells. In general, the less differentiated a cancer cell, the younger and more aggressive it is.

Erythrocyte (eh-REETH-ro-site)

A red blood cell. Red blood cells are responsible for carrying oxygen to body tissues.

Erythrocytosis (eh-REETH-ro-sigh-TOE-sis)

The condition of having abnormally high numbers of red blood cells.

Erythropenia (eh-REETH-ro-PEA-nee-uh)

The condition of having abnormally low numbers of red blood cells.

Event-free survival
> The total amount of time that a patient survives, without relapse, following treatment. See *Overall survival*.

Graft-versus-host disease or GVHD
> The phenomenon of donor marrow attacking the patient's body. GVHD can be mild, moderate, severe, or fatal.

Granulocytes (GRAN-you-lo-sites)
> Types of white blood cells that attack bacteria by engulfing them. Eosinophils, neutrophils, basophils, and mast cells are types of granulocytes.

Hematocrit or Hct (he-MAH-to-crit)
> Describes the percentage by volume of red blood cells in whole blood drawn for a CBC.

Hemaglobin (HE-muh-glow-bin)
> The iron-containing protein found in the center of a red blood cell that can bind to and transport oxygen.

Human leukocyte antigens or HLAs
> The proteins on the surfaces of white blood cells that characterize white blood cells from different individuals.

Induction therapy
> Chemotherapy or radiotherapy intended to induce a remission.

Leukemia
> The uncontrolled growth of white bloods cells in bone marrow, often overflowing to the circulating blood. As cancers of white blood cells, some leukemias and lymphomas are related; some are distinguished from each other only by their relative presence in marrow versus lymph nodes.

Leukocyte (LU-ko-site)
> A general term for all white blood cells.

Leukopenia (LU-ko-PEA-nee-uh)
> The condition of having abnormally low numbers of white blood cells. See also *-penia*.

Lymphocytes (LIM-foe-sites)
> A subtype of white blood cells that have migrated to the lymph nodes or other lymphoid organs to await the signal to fight infection.

Lymphocytopenia (lim-foe-sit-o-PEA-ne-uh)
> The condition of having abnormally low numbers of certain white blood cells called lymphocytes. See also *-penia*.

Lymphocytosis (lim-foe-sigh-TOE-sis)
The condition of having abnormally high numbers of certain white blood cells called lymphocytes. See also *-cytosis.*

Mean
The same as an average.

Median
The midpoint. If eighty-one patients were treated with drug XYZ, and the time for white blood cell counts to recover following this treatment ranged from two to sixty days, after you rank the patients by the number of days required for their white blood cells to recover, the median is the number of days that it took patient number forty-one's white blood cells to recover.

Neutropenia (nu-trow-PEA-nee-uh)
The condition of having abnormally low numbers of one type of white blood cell called neutrophils.

Overall survival
The total amount of time that a patient survives following treatment, including relapses that were successfully retreated. See *Event-free survival.*

Partial response or partial remission
Describes a tumor's response to treatment that is 50 percent smaller or more, but still remains. It's not unusual to see a partial response on imaging halfway through treatment, and a total response by the end of treatment. See *Complete response.*

-penia
A suffix denoting abnormally low numbers of blood cells: leukopenia, erythropenia, or thrombocytopenia. See also *-cytosis.*

Peripheral blood (pe-RIFF-er-al)
Blood circulating in the body as opposed to bone marrow. Peripheral blood usually is withdrawn from an arm vein or central catheter.

Petechiae (pe-TEA-key-ah)
Small red or brown spots on the skin which are actually tiny hemorrhages. They may indicate abnormally low numbers of platelets or thrombocytes.

Platelet
A blood cell called a thrombocyte, important in the blood clotting process.

Prognosis (prog-KNOW-sis)
The expected or probable outcome.

Remission

The tumor-free time period, and is dated from the first, not the last, therapy session. Patients with tumors that recur within one month of treatment ending are considered to have had no remission. Disappearance of all disease is complete remission; reduction of tumor size by more than 50 percent is considered partial remission.

Stable disease

One or more tumors still visible on imaging that are not growing. Stable disease for months or years is common among low-grade NHLs.

Stem cells

Young blood cells from which all blood cells develop.

T cells

Lymphocytes that have traveled to and resided in the thymus or are descended from those that have done so. T-cell function is immensely complex and is best described in immunology textbooks.

Thrombocyte (THROM-bow-site)

A blood cell commonly called a platelet.

Thrombocytosis (throm-bow-sigh-TOE-sis)

The condition of having abnormally high numbers of platelets.

Thrombocytopenia (throm-bi-sigh-toe-PEA-nee-uh)

The condition of having abnormally low numbers of platelets.

Total response or total remission

Describes a tumor's response to treatment. The tumor has either completely disappeared, or is so small and stable it may just be scar tissue. See also *Partial response, Complete response,* and *Remission.*

Tumor lysis syndrome

Arises from the death of certain large tumors and may arise shortly after chemotherapy is started. It is characterized by symptoms of kidney failure owing to excessive amounts of calcium, phosphate, and potassium being released by dying tumors. See "Metabolic Imbalances" in Chapter 9, *Side Effects of Treatment.*

Vancomycin-resistant enterobacteria or VRE

Intestinal bacteria that are no longer killed by one of the strongest antibiotics, Vancomycin.

Veno-occlusive disease

The closure of veins in the liver following high-dose therapy that may or may not accompany transplantation. See Chapter 9.

Bibliography

Space limitations preclude the listing of the many medical journal articles referred to during the preparation of this book. These articles, along with the bibliography that follows, are listed in chapter order on the web site at *http:// www.patientcenters.com/lymphoma/*.

The Alpha Book on Cancer and Living. Alameda, California: The Alpha Institute, 1993.

Altman and Sarg. *The Cancer Dictionary.* Facts on File, 1992.

American Medical Association Directory of Physicians in the U.S. Published by the American Medical Association, 1996.

Andrews, Maraca, and Michael Shaw. *Everything You Need to Know About Medical Tests.* Springhouse, 1996. An excellent comprehensive reference written for the patient in a readable and respectful style.

Barry, L., editor. *The Patient's Guide to Medical Tests.* Houghton Mifflin Co., 1997.

Basta, Lofty. *A Graceful Exit: Life and Death on Your Own Terms.* New York: Plenum Press, 1996.

Bernard, Jan, and Miriam Schneider. *The True Work of Dying.* New York: Avon Books, 1996.

"Best Hospitals." *U.S. News and World Report, Annual edition.* Washington, DC 20037 to 1196; (202) 955 to 2000.

Boberg, Eric, David Gustafson, and Robert Hawkins, et al. "CHESS: The Comprehensive Health Enhancement Support System," in *Information Networks for Community Health.* Edited by Patricia Brennan. New York: Springer-Verlag, 1997.

Brallier, Jess M. *Medical Wit and Wisdom.* Ontario: General Publishing, 1993.

Brenner and Hall. *Making the Radiation Therapy Decision.* RGA Publishing Group, 1996

Brodin, Michael B. *The Encyclopedia of Medical Tests*. Pocket Books, 1997. A 1982 book with the same title written by Pinckney and Pinckney should be passed over in favor of this newer book.

Callanan, Maggie, and Patricia Kelley. *Final Gifts: Understanding the Special Awareness, Needs, and Communications of the Dying*. New York: Bantam Books, 1997.

Cancer Rates and Risks, 1996. The National Cancer Institute. (800) 4-CAN-CER.

Carlson, Richard. *Don't Sweat the Small Stuff...And It's All Small Stuff*. New York: Hyperion, 1997.

Cash, Connaght. *The Medicare Answer Book: What You and Your Family Need to Know Now!* Provincetown, Massachusetts: Race Point Press, 1997.

Cassell, Eric, M.D. *The Healer's Art: A New Approach to the Doctor-Patient Relationship*. Philadelphia: J. B. Lippincott Co., 1979.

Cavalli-Sforza, L., P. Menozzi, and A. Piazza. *History and Geography of Human Genes*. Princeton: University Press, 1996.

Cooper, Cary, and Maggie Watson. *Cancer and Stress: Psychological, Biological and Coping Studies*. New York: John Wiley & Sons, 1996.

Cousins, Norman. *Anatomy of an Illness as Perceived by the Patient*. New York: W. W. Norton, 1979.

Crane, Judy B. *How to Survive Your Hospital Stay*. Westlake Village, California: The Center Press, 1997.

Cukier, Daniel, and Virginia McCullough. *Coping with Radiation Therapy: A Ray of Hope*. Los Angeles: Lowell House, 1997.

Detlefs, Dale, Robert Myers, and J. R. Robert. *1997 Mercer Guide to Social Security & Medicare*. William M. Mercer, Inc.

Dollinger, M., E. Rosenbaum, and G. Cable, editors. *Everyone's Guide to Cancer Therapy*. Toronto: Somerville House Books Limited, 1991.

Dollinger, M., E. Rosenbaum, and G. Cable, editors. *Everyone's Guide to Cancer Therapy*. Andrews & McMeel, 1994.

Drum, D. *Making the Chemotherapy Decision*. Los Angeles: Lowell House, 1997.

Enteen, Robert. *Health Insurance: How to Get It, Keep It, or Improve What You've Got*. New York: Paragon House, 1992.

Foster, George, and Barbara Anderson. *Medical Anthropology*. New York: John Wiley & Sons, 1978.

Friedman, A., T. Klein, and H. Friedman. *Psychoneuroimmunology, Stress, and Infection*. New York: CRC Press, 1996.

Furman, Joan, and David McNabb. *The Dying Time: Practical Wisdom for the Dying*. New York: Bell Tower, 1997.

Glaser, Ronald, and Janice Kiecolt-Glaser. *Handbook of Human Stress and Immunity*. New York: Academic Press, 1994.

Goleman, Daniel. *Emotional Intelligence*. Bantam, 1995.

Groopman, Jerome. *The Measure of Our Days*. New York: Viking Press, 1997.

Hakin, Cliff. *When You Lose Your Job*. San Francisco: Berrett-Loehler Publishers, 1993.

Handler, Evan. *Time on Fire: My Comedy of Terrors*. New York: Little, Brown & Co., 1996.

Harpham, Wendy Schlessel. *After Cancer: A Guide to Your New Life*. New York: W. W. Norton, 1994.

Harpham, Wendy Schlessel. *Diagnosis: Cancer*. New York: W. W. Norton, 1998.

Harpham, Wendy Schlessel. *When a Parent Has Cancer: A Guide to Caring for Your Children*. HarperCollins, 1997.

Heymann, Jody, M.D. *Equal Partners: A Physician's Call for a New Spirit of Medicine*. New York: Little, Brown & Co., 1995.

Hoffman, Barbara, editor. *A Cancer Survivor's Almanac*. The National Coalition for Cancer Survivorship. Minneapolis: Chronimed, 1996.

Humphry, Derek. *Final Exit: The Practicalities of Self-Deliverance and Assisted Suicide for the Dying*. The Hemlock Society, 1997.

Inlander, Charles, B., editor. People's Medical Society Health Desk Reference: *Information Your Doctor Can't or Won't Tell You*. New York: Hyperion, 1996.

Inlander, Charles B., and Michael Donio. *Medicare Made Easy*. Allentown, Pennsylvania: People's Medical Society, 1998.

Johnson, J., and L. Klein. *I Can Cope: Staying Healthy with Cancer*. Minneapolis: Chronimed, 1994.

Katz, Jay. *The Silent World of Doctor and Patient*. New York: The Free Press, 1984.

Keene, Nancy. *Childhood Leukemia: A Guide for Families, Friends, and Caregivers*. Sebastopol, California: O'Reilly & Associates, 1997.

Keene, Nancy. *Working with Your Doctor: Getting the Healthcare You Deserve*. Sebastopol, California: O'Reilly & Associates, 1998.

Kubler-Ross, Elisabeth. *Death: The Final Stage of Growth*. New York: Simon and Schuster, 1975.

Kubler-Ross, Elisabeth. *Living with Death and Dying*. New York: Touchstone (Simon and Schuster), 1981.

Kubler-Ross, Elisabeth. *On Death and Dying*. Macmillan, 1969.

Kubler-Ross, Elisabeth. *To Live Until We Say Good-bye*. New York: Fireside (Simon and Schuster), 1978.

Kushner, Harold. *When Bad Things Happen to Good People*. G. K. Hall, 1982.

Lattanzi-Licht, Marcia, John Mahoney, and Galen Miller. *The Hospice Choice: In Pursuit of a Peaceful Death*. New York: Fireside (Simon and Schuster), 1998.

Lerner, Michael. *Choices in Healing: Integrating the Best of Conventional and Complementary Approaches to Cancer*. Cambridge: MIT Press, 1996.

Mayer, Musa. *Advanced Breast Cancer: A Guide to Living with Metastatic Disease*. Sebastopol, California: O'Reilly & Associates, 1998.

Magrath, Ian. *The Non-Hodgkin's Lymphomas, Second Edition*. London: Arnold and Oxford University Press, 1997.

McAllister, Horowitz, and Gilden. *Cancer*. BasicBooks, HarperCollins, 1993.

McElroy, Susan. *Animals as Teachers and Healers*. New York: Ballantine, 1997.

McKay, J., and N. Hirano. *The Chemotherapy Survival Guide*. New Harbinger Publications, 1993.

McKay, J., N. Hirano, and M. Lampenfeld. *The Chemotherapy & Radiation Therapy Survival Guide*. New Harbinger Publications, 1998.

Morris, Desmond. *The Human Animal: A Personal View of the Human Species*. New York: Crown Publishers, 1994.

Motulsky, Harvey. *Intuitive Biostatistics*. New York: Oxford University Press, 1995.

Murphy, G., L. Morris, and D. Lange, editors. *Informed Decisions—The Complete Book of Cancer Diagnosis, Treatment and Recovery*. The American Cancer Society. New York: Viking Press, 1997.

The National Cancer Institute's *PDQ State-of-the-Art Treatment Statements for Physicians* on: Anxiety Disorder; Constipation, Impaction, and Bowel Obstruction; Depression; Lymphedema; Post-Traumatic Stress Disorder; Radiation Enteritis; Skin Integrity Changes Secondary to Cutaneous Metastases; Sleep Disorders.

The National Cancer Institute's *PDQ State-of-the-Art Treatment Statements for Physicians* on: Adult Non-Hodgkin's Lymphoma; Childhood Non-Hodgkin's Lymphoma; Breast Cancer and Pregnancy; Non-Hodgkin's Lymphoma During Pregnancy; AIDS-Related Lymphomas; Cutaneous T-Cell Lymphoma; Primary Central Nervous System Lymphoma.

The National Cancer Institute's *PDQ State-of-the-Art Treatment Statements for Physicians* on: Delirium; Fatigue; Fever, Chills, and Sweats; Hypercalcemia; Nausea and Vomiting; Nutrition; Oral Complications Secondary to Cancer Therapy; Pain; Pruritus (itching).

Nickel, Gudrun Maria, Esq. *Debtors' Rights.* Clearwater, Florida: Sphinx Publishing, 1998.

Nuland, Sherwin. *How We Die: Reflections on Life's Final Chapter.* New York: Alfred A. Knopf, 1993.

Olson, Kaye, RN. *Surgery and Recovery: How to Reduce Anxiety and Promote Healthy Healing.* Traverse City, Michigan: Rhodes and Easton, 1998.

Pagana, Kathleen, and Timothy Pagana, editors. *Mosby's Diagnostic and Laboratory Test Reference.* Mosby, 1992.

Porter, Steven L. *Save Your Home!: How to Protect Your Home and Property from Foreclosure.* Colorado Springs: Java Publishing Co., 1990.

Radiation Therapy and You. A fifty-page booklet available from the U.S. National Cancer Institute, (800) 4-CANCER.

Ray, M. Catherine. *I'm with You Now: A Guide Through Incurable Illness for Patients, Families, and Friends.* New York: Bantam Books, 1997.

Rosenbaum, Edward, M.D. *A Taste of My Own Medicine.* New York: Random House, 1998.

Rosenfeld, Isadore, M.D. *Second Opinion: Your Medical Alternatives.* New York: Simon & Schuster, 1981.

Schover, L. *Sexuality and Fertility After Cancer.* New York: John Wiley & Sons, 1997.

Shernoff, William M., Esq. *How to Make Insurance Companies Pay Your Claims and What to Do if They Don't.* Norwalk, Connecticut: Hastings House, 1990.

Shtasel, Philip. *Medical Tests and Diagnostic Procedures—A Patient's Guide to Just What the Doctor Ordered.* Harper and Row, 1990.

Siebert, Al. *The Survivor Personality.* Practical Psychology Press, 1994.

Spiegel, David. *Living Beyond Limits: New Hope and Health for Facing Life-Threatening Illness.* New York: Fawcett Columbine, 1994.

Stauffer, Joseph, and Joseph C. Segen. *The Patient's Guide to Medical Tests: Everything You Need to Know About the Tests Your Doctor Prescribes, Fourth Edition.* Facts on File, 1997.

Stern, Ken. *Comprehensive Guide to Social Security and Medicare.* Hawthorne, New Jersey: The Career Press, 1995.

Stewart, Susan L. *Bone Marrow Transplants: A Book of Basics for Patients.* Highland Park, Illinois: BMT Newsletter, 1992.

Ventura, John. *Fresh Start!: Surviving Money Troubles.* Dearborn Financial Publishing, Inc., 1992.

Weenolsen, Patricia. *The Art of Dying.* New York: St. Martin's Press, 1996.

Westhem, Andrew, and Donald J. Korn. *Protecting What's Yours: How to Safeguard Your Assets and Maintain Your Personal Wealth.* New York: Carol Publishing Group, 1995.

Youngson, Robert. *The Surgery Book.* New York: St. Martin's Press, 1993.

Zakarian, Beverly. *The Activist Cancer Patient.* New York: John Wiley & Sons, 1996.

Zukerman, Eugenia, and Julie Ingelfinger. *Coping with Prednisone (and other cortisone-related medicines).* New York: St. Martin's Press, 1997.

Index

A

abdominal pain, 169
acupuncture, 216–217
acute graft-versus-host disease, 400–401
adoptive immunotherapy, 388
adrenal dysfunction, 314
adult Burkitt's, 60
adult T-cell lymphoma/leukemia (ATLL), 137–138
age as factor in NHL, 31, 34, 43, 62, 125
aggressive NHLs (intermediate- or high-grade), 130–132
AGM-1470 (TNP-470), 440–441
AIDS, 37, 327
Ali, Karen, advice on asking for help, 277
alkaline phosphatase, 83
alkylating agents, 340, 439
all-trans retinoic acid (ATRA), 445
allogeneic transplants, 386–387
allopurinol, 319
alopecia (hair loss), 176–177, 318
alternative therapies, questions about, 71
Ambien, 233
amifostine (Ethyol), 442
aminocamptothecin (9-AC), 450
anaplastic large-cell lymphoma (ALCL), 32, 60–61
Ann Arbor system
  divisions of, 46–47
  use in NHL staging and grading, 44
antiangiogenesis therapy, 439–440
antibody therapy, 440–441
anticytokine therapy, 441
antimetabolite therapy, 441–442
antisense molecules (antisense oligonucleotides), 452–453
anxiety, 304
  causes of, 208–210
  fear distinguished from anxiety, 207
  immune system, impact on, 209–210
  medications for, 231–232
apoptosis induction therapy, 442
appetite or taste changes, 169–170
Association of Cancer Online Resources (ACOR), 272
Ativan, 70, 231–232
autologous graft-versus-lymphoma responses, 453
autologous transplants. See transplantation
azacytidine, 441

B

baldness, 176–177, 318
bcl-2 or bcl-6 gene rearrangements, 83
beta-2 microglobulin (B2M), 83
bilirubin, 83

biofeedback, 217–218
biological therapies, 121–123
    colony stimulating factors, 122–123
    cytokines, 122
    monoclonal antibodies, 121–122
    tumor vaccines, 123
biological/natural anticancer
            substances, 435–437
biopsy samples, need for storage of,
            293
bladder damage, 319
bleomycin, 119, 179, 320
blinded trial, 360
blood and marrow test values, table of,
            505–506
blood clots, pulmonary embolism,
            170
blood counts
    low counts, 319–320
    testing before chemotherapy, 145
body surface area, calculation of, table,
            507–508
bone marrow transplantation. See
            transplantation
bone pain, 170
breathing problems, 171
broxuridine, 449
bryostatin 1 (one), 443, 445
buffy-coat infusion, 388
Burkitt's lymphoma, 32
Buspar (buspirone), 231–232
busulfan, 320
Butler, Mary, assertiveness in
            resolution of conflict
            with medical personnel,
            244–245

C
cancer
    causes of, 35–43, 433–434
    prevention of, 35–43, 433–434,
            438
    resources, 481–504

carboxyamidotriazole, 440–441, 446
carmustine (BCNU), 320
carzelesin, 439
catheters, 88–91
    removal at end of treatment, 306
causes of NHL, 35–43, 433–434
CBC (complete blood counts). See
            blood counts
CD34+ cell separation devices, 451
cellular matrix exploitation, 453
central catheter/central line, 88–91
CGP-48664, 442
chemoprevention, 453
chemoprotectants, 442–443
chemosensitization/potentiation, 443,
            445, 449
chemotherapy
    drugs
        antimetabolites, 118–119,
            441–442
        breast milk, in, 346
        dosages, 151
        idiosyncratic agents
            (miscellaneous drugs),
            119
        immune suppressants, 119
        rescue drugs, 119
        table of, 524–531
        topoisomerase inhibitors, 117
        tubulin binding agents, 117
    during pregnancy, 345–346
    effects on fertility, 326, 340–341
    events at departure after
            administration, 151–152
    events on arrival for
            administration, 146
    immune system, impact on, 215
    methods of administration
        intravenous therapy, 147–149
        oral therapy, 149
        portable (ambulatory
            pumps), 151
        spinal or intrathecal therapy,
            150

chemotherapy
    methods of administration
            (*continued*)
        subcutaneous injections, 150
        topical therapy
                (photochemotherapy),
                149–150
    preparation for, 143–144
    resources, 524–531
    scheduling of, 144–145
    setting for administration, 147
    side effects, 165–188
        drugs for, 167
    See also clinical trials; drugs;
                prednisone
childhood Burkitt's lymphoma, 60
children
    communication with about death
                and dying, 421–423
    control of pain, 70
    growth impairment (short stature,
                precocious puberty), 318
    hugging, kissing, snuggling,
                importance of, 229
    NHL in, 35
    resources for, 487–490
    sexual development of, 346–347
    side effects of treatment in, 120,
                318
    treatment of, 124–125
CHOP (multidrug chemotherapy
                regimen), 130–138, 325
chronic graft-versus-host disease,
                404–405
    See also graft-versus-host disease
cisplatin, 119, 178, 319, 323, 334
classification of NHLs
    determination of, in general, 9–
                10, 30–32
    importance of precision in, 27, 69
    specific tests for, 77–112
    systems for, table of, 509–523
clinical relapse, 350

clinical trials
    admission, 373–374
    description, 359–361
    experimental drugs outside, 377
    finding, 19–22, 369–370, 471
    National Cancer Institute,
                recommendation of, 380
    payment for, 378–379
    phases of, described, 364–369
    physical characteristics of
                participants, 55
    placebo used in, 21, 360, 363
    reasons for patient participation,
                361–363
    research by patients, 371–373,
                471–473
    resources, 370, 379–380, 498
cognitive changes, 171, 315
COL-3 (antiangiogenesis substance),
                440–441, 446
colony stimulating factors, 122–123
comfort, as patient priority, 71
communication
    family and friends, 257–266
    HMO case managers, 241
    medical/oncology personnel,
                234–247
    need for support, 249–251, 255–
                257
    test results, 71
    See also friends and family;
                support and self-help
                groups
complete blood count (CBC), 84
complications of treatment. *See* late
                side effects of treatment;
                side effects of treatment
computer, use in patient research. *See*
                Internet
computerized self-help programs,
                Comprehensive Health
                Enhancement Support
                System (CHESS), 276

conflict between patient and medical personnel, resolution of, 244–247

constipation, 172

continuous antigenic stimulation, 43

coping with illness. *See* communication; friends and family; support and self-help groups

counseling, 218
    Spiegel, Dr. David
        work with breast cancer survivors, 218

Cousins, Norman
    Anatomy of an Illness as Perceived by the Patient, 222
    stress of illness, need for humor in coping with, 222

creatinine (serum creatinine), 84

Cushing's syndrome, 314, 330

cutaneous T-cell lymphoma, 59, 139–140

cyclin-dependent kinase inhibitor therapy, 443

cyclophosphamide (alkylating agent), 147, 179, 319–320, 325–326, 340

cyclosporine, 445

cytarabine, 447

cytogenic relapse, 350

cytokines, 122, 441, 443

D

DAB389-IL2, 441

dance, as stress reducer, 225–226

deafness, 322–323

death and dying
    communications with children, 421–422, 424
    decisions to end treatment, 428–429
    family issues, 421
    honesty about important, 421
    hospice/hospice home care, 428
    letting go, 423–425
    memorial service planning, 429–431
    pain management, 427–428
    physical aspects, questions about, 425–427
    resources for coping with, 490, 504
    spiritual and religious considerations, 423–424
    Tyler, Marilyn, survivor's perspective, 419–420

death receptors, 453–454

definitions of terms, 529–534

dehydration, 173

Demerol, 70

demethylating agents, 444

demographics of NHL patients, ix, 33–35

denial, as stress reducer, 225

dental problems, 322

deoxycytidine, 444

depression
    causes of, 211
    medications for, 232
    relationship to immune system function, 210
    symptoms of, 210–211

desferoxamine, 442

dexrazoxane (Zinecard), 442

diabetes, 315

diagnosis of NHL
    definitive, 8–9
    early guess, 7
    effect on treatment plan, 10
    emotional responses to, 10–15
    importance of tests in, 69
    narrowing of, 8
    symptoms, 2–3
    type of lymphoma, determination of, 69
    See also classification of NHLs; tests, specific

diarrhea, 173, 184

diaziquone (AZQ), 439

differentiation therapy, 444–445
diffuse large-cell lymphoma, 59
disability income, 290–292
    See also insurance
dizziness, 322–323
DNA, 115–116
    See also genetics
doctors. *See* oncologists
donor leukocyte infusion (buffy-coat infusion, adoptive immunotherapy), 388
double-blinded trial, 361
doxorubicin (adriamycin), 318, 447
drug modulation, 443, 445
drug resistance inhibition, 445
drugs
    chemotherapy drugs, 117–119, 524–531
    dosage, verification of, 151, 507
    stress, medications for, 231–233
    treatment of side effects, 346
    See also clinical trials
dry mouth, difficulty swallowing, 174, 322

E

elderly patients
    Medicare/Medicaid, 286
    treatment of, 125
electrolytes, 84
EMLA (topical anesthetic), 70, 82–83
emotions
    end of treatment, responses to, 297–304
    fears
        of abandonment at end of treatment, 299–300
        of relapse, 300
        from symptoms to diagnosis, 10–15
    preparation for end of life, responses to, 420–424
    prognoses, responses to, 66–68

stress, responses to, 206–211
    workplace, re-entrance at end of treatment, responses to, 309–310
employment issues, 292–293
    employee assistance programs (EAP), 275–276
    re-entering workplace at end of treatment, 309–310
    resources, 499–501
    See also insurance
end of treatment
    emotional responses to, 297–304
    medical monitoring, 304–306
    social and professional after-effects, 307–311
    unused drugs or equipment, donation of, 310–311
engraftment, 401–402
Epstein-Barr virus (EBV), 36–37, 42, 62
erythrocyte sedimentation rate (sed rate), 84
etoposide, 325
euthanasia, 428–429
exercise, as stress reducer, 218–219
extravasation, 174
eye problems, 174–175, 316

F

faith. *See* spirituality and faith
family. *See* friends and family
fatigue and sleep disorders, 175–176, 316–317, 320
fertility
    discussion with oncologist, 331, 337
    effects of chemotherapy on, 331, 338–341
    effects of radiotherapy on, 331, 341–343
    effects of surgery on, 331, 343–344

fertility (*continued*)
  Suhadolc, Nan, questions for
      doctor, 332–333
  treatments for, 344
fever, chills, sweats, 176
financial issues, 288–289
  resources about, 499–502
FISH (fluorescence in situ
      hybridization), 84, 350
flavopiridol, 443
flow cytometry, 85, 350
fludarabine, 320
folate agonist therapy, 445
follicle-stimulating hormone (FSH),
      341–342
follicular lymphomas, 59, 62
friends and family
  acceptance of death by family,
      421
  communicating needs to, 257–
      268
  communication with medical
      personnel, 241
  coping with stress role in, 219–
      220
  diagnosis, reactions to, 15
  end of treatment, reactions to,
      307–309
  needs for support, reactions to,
      252–258
  permission to die, as gift from
      family, 424
  relapse, reactions to, 356
fungal infection, 400
fusion protein therapy, 445–446

G

gemcitabine (difluorodeoxycytidine),
      441
gene therapy, 454–455
genetics
  characteristics of tumors, 61–62
  development of tumors, 35–36

explanation of treatments for
      NHL, 115–116
predisposition to NHL, possible
      role in, 40–42
transplantation, role in, 384–388
gonadotropin-releasing hormone
      agonists (GnRH-a), 340
Gould, Stephen Jay
  "The Median Isn't the Message,"
      53
  statistics for cancer, interpreting,
      53
grading NHLs, 44–45
graft-versus-host disease, 317, 397,
      440
  immunosuppressive drugs used to
      control, complications,
      405
  See also acute graft-versus-host
      disease; chronic graft-
      versus-host disease
growth factor agonist therapy, 446

H

hair loss (alopecia) and growth, 176–
      177, 318
heart damage, 177, 318–319
hematologic oncologist, 16–17
hematopathologist, 9
herpesviruses, 326–327
high-dose therapy
  side effects of, after marrow
      transplantation, 399–401
  with bone marrow
      transplantation, 58
  See also transplantation
high-grade NHLs. See staging NHL
histologic grade, 45
histology (cell appearance), 59–60,
      114–115
HIV, 63, 337
HMOs (health maintenance
      organizations). See
      insurance

hobbies, as stress reducer, 221
Hodgkin's lymphoma (HL),
          distinguished from
          NHLs, 31–32
hormone therapy, 446
hormones, 334
    follicle-stimulating, pituitary
          (FSH), 341–342
    gonadotropin-releasing hormone
          agonists (GnRH-a), 340
    luteinizing (LH), 341–342
hospice/hospice home care, 428
hospitalization, 189–204
    resources, 494–495
HTLV-1 (human T-cell lymphotropic
          virus I), 337
hugging, kissing, as stress reducers,
          229
hyper-/hypothyroidism, 329–330
hypercalcemia, 180

I

ICI D1694 (ZD1694), 445
idiotype vaccines, 450
ifosfamide, 318–319
immune system
    developing NHL, role in, 34
    functions of, xi–xiii
    impact of age on, 43
    stress and, 205–233
immune-compromised patients
    treatment of, 126–127
    viral links to NHL, 36–37
immunoglobulin studies (IgM, IgA,
          IgD, IgF, IgH, IgE), 85
immunophenotype, 47–49, 60–61
immunosuppressant therapy, 446–
          447
impotence, 333, 336
in vitro sensitivity-directed
          chemotherapy, 455
incidence of NHL, ix, 29–30
indolent NHLs, 127–130
induction therapy, 394

infection, 177–178
infertility. *See* fertility
insurance, 282–287
    approval of transplantation by
          company, 407–408
    health and disability insurance,
          283–287
    HMO case managers,
          communication with,
          241
    life insurance, 286–287
    long-term care insurance, 287
    Medicare/Medicaid, 286
    payment for clinical trial or
          investigational drug,
          378–379
    resources, 499–501
    unemployment insurance, 286
interacting with medical personnel,
          234–247
interferons, 122, 443
interleukin-12 (IL-12), 443
interleukin-2 (IL-2), 443
Internet
    Association of Cancer Online
          Resources, 272
    NHL support groups on the Web,
          271–272
    oncologists/treatment centers, use
          of in finding, 18, 22–23
intestinal distress, 328
investigational new drugs (IND), 377
    See also clinical trials
irinotecan, 450
isolation, as protection against
          infection, 399

K

keratinocyte growth factor (KGF), 443
kidney damage, 178, 319
Kiel system, use in NHL classification,
          44

L

lactate dehydrogenase (LDH), 85
large-cell lymphomas, 62, 136–137
late side effects of treatment
    adrenal dysfunction, 314
    bladder damage, 319
    cognitive and psychological
        damage, 315
    Cushing's syndrome, 314
    deafness, 322–323
    diabetes, 315
    distinguished from relapse, 349
    distinguished from side effects,
        313–314
    dizziness, 322–323
    eyes, 316
    fatigue, 316–317
    graft-versus-host disease, 317,
        397
    growth impairment (short stature,
        precocious puberty), 318
    hair loss (alopecia), 318
    heart and vascular damage, 318–
        319
    kidney damage, 319
    liver damage, 319
    low blood counts, 319–320
    lung damage, 320–321
    lymphedema, 321
    mouth, teeth, throat problems,
        322
    numbness, tingling, 322–323
    pain, 323–324
    paralysis, 322–323
    radiation fibrosis, 324
    recall sensitivity, 324–325
    recent phenomena, as, 313
    sexuality and fertility issues, 326
    shingles, 326–327
    shortness of breath, 327
    skeletal damage, 327–328
    skin, 328
    stomach or intestinal distress, 328
    surgical complications, 328–329

    swollen arms, legs, hands, feet,
        329
    thyroid dysfunction, 329–330
    transplantation, 315–330, 403–
        406
    treatment-related leukemias (t-
        MDS, t-AML), 325
    treatment-related solid tumors
        (second solid tumors),
        326
    See also side effects of treatment
laughter, as stress reducer, 222–223
legal issues, resources about, 499–501
leucovorin, 445
leukocyte therapy, 447
leutinizing hormone, 341–342
Levin, Lowell S., interactions with
        medical personnel, role
        of friends in, 242
Lhermitte sign, 185
libido. *See* sexuality after treatment
light therapy, 121, 139
liposomal encapsulation, 447
lisofylline, 441
liver enzymes (SGOT, SGPT, ALT,
        AST), 85
liver or gallbladder dysfunction, 178,
        319
loved ones. *See* friends and family
low-grade NHLs (indolent NHLs),
        127–130
    See also staging NHLs
lung damage, 179, 320–321
lymphatic system, description of, 27–
    28
lymphoblastic lymphoma, 32, 133–
    135
lymphocyte-depleted Hodgkin's
        lymphoma (LDHL), 32
lymphokine-activated killer cell
        therapy, 448
lymphoma, definition of, 28–29

M

mabs/moabs. *See* monoclonal antibodies

Magrath, Dr. Ian T., perspective on NHL, ix–xiv

MALT lymphomas, 43, 60, 127, 130, 138, 140, 330

mantle cell lymphoma, 60

mantle zone lymphoma, 60

marrow

  harvest of, 394

  high-dose therapy with, 58

  transplantation

    how it works, 124

    new strategies and tactics, 451

  See also transplantation

marrow purging, 452

marrow test values, table of, 505–506

massage therapy, as stress reducer, 223

matrix metalloprotease inhibitors, 440

medical oncologist, 16–17

medical personnel, interactions with. *See* communication; oncologists

medical treatments

  biological therapies, 121–123

  chemotherapies, 117–119

  marrow or stem cell transplantation, 124

  philosophies of, 115

  phototherapy, 121

  radiotherapy, 120

  surgery, 123

  See also chemotherapy; radiotherapy; transplantation

Medicare/Medicaid, 286

medications. *See* drugs

meditation, as stress reducer, 224–225

Medline, 467–468

melatonin, 233

melphelan, 320

Mesna, 319, 326

metabolic imbalances, 180

methotrexate, 320, 322

mitochondrial DNA, 455–456

mitomycin, 439

molecular oncology, 456

monoclonal antibodies, 121–122, 148–149, 440–441, 449

mouth or rectal pain (mucositis), 180

MRI (magnetic resonance imaging), 100–102

mucosa-associated lymphoid tissue (MALT). *See* MALT lymphomas

mucositis, 180

muscle cramps, 181

music, as stress reducer, 225–226

N

National Cancer Institute, 464–465

National Marrow Donor Program, 408

  See also transplantation

natural anticancer substances, 435–437

nausea and vomiting, 181–182

neurotoxic therapies, 334

neutropenia, 177–178

NHL. *See* non-Hodgkin's lymphoma

non-Hodgkin's lymphoma (NHL)

  causes, 35–37

  causes, unproven, 37–43

  demographics of patients, 33–35

  grading and staging, 44–49

  organizations, 481–482

  resources, 481–504

  unique aspects, overview of, 29–33

noncutaneous T-cell lymphoma, 59

nonspecific immune-modulator therapy, 448, 450

novobiocin, 443, 445

numbness, tingling, 180, 184–185, 322–323

numbness/tingling, 184–185

nutrition, as stress reducer, 226–227

O

O6-Benzylguanine, 443
octreotide, 446
oncologists
    choice of, 8, 23–26
    communication, suggestions for,
        242–244
    finding candidates, 17–26
    resources, 494–495
    styles of interacting with patients,
        238–240
    types/specialties of, 16–17
oncology nurses, 240
Oncovin. *See* vincristine

P

P-Glycoprotein Antagonist PSC 833,
    443
pain, 183, 323–324, 427–428
pancytopenia, 183
paralysis, 184–185
PEG-L asparaginase (pegaspargase,
        polyethylene glycol-L-
        asparaginase), 441
peldesine (BCX-34), 447
penclomedine, 439
pentetic acid calcium, 443
perillyl alcohol, 442
peripheral blood lymphocyte therapy,
    447
peripheral neuropathy, 183, 184–185
peripheral stem cells, 395–396
pets
    as stress reducers, 227–228
    exposure to after transplantation,
        403
phenobarbital, 445
phenylbutyrate, 445
phototherapy, 121
physicians. *See* oncologist
placebo, 21, 360, 363
polymerase chain reaction (PCR), 85
positive thinking, as stress reducer,
    228

positron emission tomography (PET),
    352
prednisone
    depression, cause of, 211
    discontinuing use, 149
    side effects of, 167–168, 187–
        188, 327
pregnancy
    after NHL, 346
    chemotherapy, effects of, 345–
        346
    NHL breast tumors, pregnancy
        related, 345
    radiotherapy, effects of, 346
    treatment by obstetrician/
        gynecologist, 346
    treatment of side effects of
        chemotherapy, during,
        346
primary extranodal sites, 141
procarbazine (alkylating agent), 340
procedures. *See* tests, specific
prognoses
    emotional responses to, 66–68
    limitations on accuracy of, 51–57
    risk factors, relative effects of, 57–
        65
protein kinase C inhibition, 449
proto-oncogenes, oncogenes, and
        tumor suppressor genes,
        456–457
PSC 833, 445
puberty, precocious, as late effect of
        treatment, 318
pulmonary embolism/thrombosis, 170
pyrazoloacridine, 450

Q

questions
    about tests, 71
    rude or hurtful, responses to,
        278–280

R

radiation enteritis, 184

radiation fibrosis, 324

radiation oncologist, 17

radiation pneumonitis, 184

radioimmunotherapy, 121–123, 163, 449

See also antibody therapy

radiosensitization, 449–450

radiotherapy (radiation therapy)

dosages, 164

during pregnancy, 346

effects on fertility, 341–343

events at arrival for administration, 161

events at departure after administration, 164

methods of administration, 162–163

scheduling of, 160–161

setting for, 161–162

side effects, 165–188, 324, 329

in children, 120, 318

simulation of in early visits, 158–159

See also late side effects of treatment; radioimmunotherapy; side effects of treatment

randomized trial, 360

Rappaport system, use in NHL classification, 44

reading, as stress reducer, 228

rebeccamycin, 450

recall sensitivities, 184, 324–325

recombinant viral vaccines, 457

record-keeping

biopsy samples, storage of, 293

importance of, 293

obtaining records for, 293–295

organization of, 295

rectal pain, 180

reinfusion of marrow, 398–399

relapse

causes of, 349

clinical, 350

cytogenic, 350

definition of, 348–349

detection of, 349–350

distinguished from after effects of treatment, 349

emotional responses to, 353–357

low-grade disease, more frequent recurrence of, 350–351

medical issues, 348–352

time of occurrence, 351

treatment options, 352–353

relaxation training, as stress reducer, 228

See also biofeedback; visualization

religion. *See* spirituality and faith

research by patients/non-professionals

chemotherapy dose, calculation of, 475–476

clinical trials, finding, 471–473

drugs, information about, 474–475

empowerment as result of, 459

information needed to begin, 460–461

Internet and web sites, 463–465, 478

medical libraries, 469

medical research papers, obtaining, 465–466

medical textbooks, obtaining, 470–471

Medline, 467–468

methods of finding information, 463–464

National Cancer Institute, obtaining information from, 464–465

perspectives and attitudes during, 461–463

resources, 481–504

search firm, hiring, 469

research by patients/non-professionals
(*continued*)
support groups, finding, 471–473
test results, interpretation of, 477
transplantation, 474
unproven remedies, assessment
of, 477–478
research by professionals
current clinical trials, 439–451
future trials, 452–458
overview of trends in, 434–438
See also clinical trials
Revised European American
Lymphoma system,
(REAL)
distinguished from other
classification systems, 48
use in NHL classification, 44
rhizoxin, 450
Rituxan, 148

S

second and subsequent opinions, 244
second solid tumors (treatment-related
solid tumors), 326
seizures, 180, 184–185
self-help groups. *See* support and self-
help groups
sexual development of children, 346–
347
sexuality after treatment
libido, 334–335
sources of information about, 335
shingles, 326
shortness of breath, 327
side effects of treatment, 165–188
abdominal pain, 169
appetite or taste changes, 169–
170
blood clots, pulmonary embolism,
170
bone pain, 170
breathing problems, 171
cognitive changes, 171, 315

constipation, 172
dehydration, 173
diarrhea, 173
distinguished from late side
effects and
complications, 313–314
drugs for treatment of, 346
dry mouth, difficulty swallowing,
174, 322
extravasation, 174
eye problems, 174–175, 316
fatigue and sleep disorders, 175–
176, 316–317
fever, chills, sweats, 176
hair loss (alopecia) and growth,
176–177, 318
heart damage, 177, 318–319
hypercalcemia, 177
in children, 120
infection, 177–178
kidney damage, 178–179, 319
late effects and complications of
treatment, 312–330
liver or gallbladder dysfunction,
178, 319
lung damage, 179, 320–321
metabolic imbalances, 180
mouth or rectal pain (mucositis),
180
muscle cramps, 181
nausea and vomiting, 181–182
neutropenia (low white counts),
177–178
numbness, tingling, 184–185,
322–323
pain, 183, 323–324
pancytopenia, 183
peripheral neuropathy, 184–185
pulmonary thrombosis, 170
radiation enteritis, 184
radiation pneumonitis, 184
reasons for, 166–167
recall sensitivities, 184, 324–325
resources, 498–499

side effects of treatment (*continued*)
seizures, paralysis, numbness, tingling, 184–185
skin problems, 185–186, 328
sore, red, stiff veins, 186
transplantation, specific to, 399–401
treatment of, during pregnancy, 346
tumor lysis syndrome, 180
urinary bladder, hemorrhagic cystitis, 187
weight gain or loss, 187–188
See also late side effects of treatment
skin problems, 185–186, 328
sleep, as stress reducer, 228–229
small lymphocytic/ lymphoplasmacytoid (immunocytomas), 32, 59
small noncleaved cell lymphomas, 135–136
sore, red, stiff veins, 186
Spiegel, Dr. David
counseling breast cancer survivors, 218
study showing survival value of support groups, 268
spirituality and faith
faith questioned at relapse, 354
life as gift, 68
life tasks, spiritual, completion before death, 423
satisfaction with inner being at death, 423
stress reduction, role in, 229–230
staging NHLs, 44–47, 127–141
standard treatments. *See* medical treatments
statistics for NHL, interpreting, 53
stem cell transplantation, 124
donor's harvest, 396
patient's harvest, 394–396
See also transplantation

steroid drugs, 171
stomach distress, 328
stress
Cousins, Norman, on role of humor in coping with, 222
definition of, 206
emotional responses to, 205–211
immune system, effect on, 211–215
medications for, 231–233
anti-anxiety medications, 231–232
antidepressant medication, 232
sleep medications, 232–233
reduction techniques, 215–231
Suhadolc, Nan
categories of people patients deal with, 249
fertility and sexuality, questions for doctor, 331–332
support and self-help groups
Ali, Karen, advice on asking for help, 277
communication of need for, 255–266
finding support, 268–278
Internet, available on, 271–272
resources, 482
specific needs for support, 249–251
Spiegel, Dr. David, study showing survival value of, 268
stress reduction, role in, 230–231
telephone, available by, 272–273
supportive care, as therapy, 438
suramin (SUR), 441, 446
surgery, 123
effects on fertility, 343–344
surgical complications, 328–329
surgical oncologist, 17
swelling of arms, hands, feet, 329
symptoms, 1–10
syngeneic transplants, 387

T

t-AML (treatment-related leukemia), 325
t-MDS (treatment-related leukemia), 325
tacrolimus (FK506), 447
tallimustine, 439
targretin, 445
Taxol, 324
tecogalan sodium, 440
telomerase inhibitors, 457
temozolomide, 439
terms, glossary, 533–538
test results, communication about, 71
tests, resources about, 498
tests, specific, 77–112
    abdominal surgery (laparotomy), 77–80
    barium enema, 110–112
    blood product transfusion, 80–81
    blood tests, 81–86, 505–506
    bone marrow aspiration/biopsy, 86–87
    bone marrow harvest, 87
    bone scan (scintigraphy), 87–88
    bronchoscopy, 93–94
    catheter insertion (central catheter, central line), 88–91
    colonoscopy, 93–94
    CT scan (computed tomography, "CAT" scan), 91–93
    endoscopy (colonoscopy, bronchoscopy, gastroscopy, sigmoidoscopy), 93–94
    FISH (fluorescence in situ hybridization), 84, 350
    flow cytometry, 85, 350
    gallium scan (scintigraphy, gallium scintigram), 94–96
    GI series, 110–112
    intravenous pyelogram, 96, 110–112
    laparotomy, 77–80
    lumbar puncture, 108–110
    lymphangiogram (bipedal lymphangiography, lymphography), 96–98
    mammogram (mammography, breast x-ray), 98–100
    MRI (magnetic resonance imaging), 100–102
    MUGA scan (multiple gated acquisition scan, gated blood pool scan, radionuclide ventriculography [RNV]), 102–103
    needle biopsy (fine needle aspiration, CT-guided needle biopsy, percutaneous biopsy), 104–105
    node biopsy (excisional biopsy), 106
    PCR (polymerase chain reaction), 85
    sigmoidoscopy, 93–94
    sonogram (ultrasound, sonography), 107–108
    SPECT or SPET (single position positron emission computed tomography), 94–96
    spinal tap (lumbar puncture), 108–110
    thallium scan, 110
    ultrasound (ultrasonography, sonogram), 107–108
    x-rays (radiographic studies), 110–112
thalidomide, 440
thyroid dysfunction, 329–330
tissue engineering, 457–458
TNP-470 (AGM-1470), 440–441, 446

topoisomerase inhibitor therapy, 450
topotecan, 449
transition of NHLs, 351–352
transplantation
    autologous transplants (rescues), 317, 383
    becoming a donor, 408–409
    choice of technique, factors influencing, 388–390
    choice of treatment center, 406–407
    donor transplants
        kinds of, 386–388
    engraftment, 401–402
    finding a donor, 390–392
    harvest of marrow for, 395
    harvest of stem cells for, 395–396
    insurance company approval of, 407–408
    marrow versus peripheral stem cells, 382–383
    new strategies and tactics, 451
    outpatient follow-up, 402–403
    pets after, 403
    rescue versus transplantation, 382
    resources, 406–407, 409, 493–494
    risks and benefits of, 124
    side effects specific to, 399–401
    steps in, 392–399
traveling for care, 410–417
treatment center, choice of, 19–22, 406–407
    resources, 494–495
treatment-related leukemias (t-MDS, t-AML), 325
treatment-related solid tumors (second solid tumors), 326
triplex molecules, 458
tubulin inhibitor therapy, 450
tumor cell derivative vaccines, 450
tumor infiltrating lymphocyte therapy, 458
tumor lysis syndrome, 180
tumor stabilization (stasis), 437–438

tumor vaccines, 123
tumor, characteristics of, as prognostic indicators, 63–65
Tyler, Marilyn, survivor's perspective, 419–420
types and subtypes of NHL
    general description of, 30–31
    table of, 509–523
    See also classification of NHLs

U

UCN-01, 449
umbilical cord blood transplants, 387–388, 451
United States Food and Drug Administration (FDA), role in clinical trials, 359
uric acid, 86
urinary bladder pain, hemorrhagic cystitis, 187

V

Valium, 231
vascular damage, 318
veno-occlusive disease, 400
Versed, 70, 87
vincristine (Oncovin), 148, 185, 318, 323, 328, 334
viral causes of NHL, 36–37
viral hepatitis, 400
visualization, as stress reducer, 228
volunteer work, as stress reducer, 221

W

water, as stress reducer, 229
weight gain or loss, 187–188
whole-body hyperthermia, 452
Working Group system, use in NHL classification, 44

X

Xanax, 231
Xylocaine, 70

Z

Zantac (ranitidine), 81

BECOMING A MARROW DONOR

■ ■ ■

Only 20 to 30 percent of patients needing bone marrow transplants are able to find a donor because there are too few donors in the marrow registries.

A blood sample only—not marrow—is used for testing to find matches. If you volunteer to be a donor and you match, immature marrow cells can be collected from the blood in an arm vein over the course of about two hours. If this procedure is used, you may be asked to have, in the preceding week, two or three injections of a drug that will cause blood cells to develop more quickly.

Some centers still use bone marrow as a source of these immature cells, instead of blood from an arm vein. Harvesting bone marrow from the hipbone is only mildly uncomfortable, but may require a sedative or possibly general anesthesia. You may feel an ache in the hipbone for two to fourteen days after. This pain is easily controlled with drugs such as Tylenol or Advil.

This flyer is being distributed on behalf of _____, who needs a transplant to cure _____

_____

Many who have donated marrow describe it as one of the most fulfilling experiences of their life, second only to becoming a parent. Most say they will do it again, eagerly and without hesitation, if called.

■ ■ ■

YOU CAN JOIN THE NMDP BY CALLING 1-800-MARROW-2.

About the Author

Lorraine Johnston is the wife of an eight-year lymphoma survivor and the daughter of a twenty-year lymphoma survivor. In the years since her husband's diagnosis, she's been involved in a number of support groups that offer emotional and practical support to lymphoma survivors. This is her first book.

In the course of her support group efforts, Lorraine has been interviewed by the *Philadelphia Inquirer* and by National Public Radio's *Marketplace* program regarding the best ways to find reliable medical information using a personal computer and various media such as the Internet. She attempts to dispel the myths that access to sound medical information is cloaked in secrecy and that medical literature is impossible to interpret. Using her lifelong love of biology and her degree in life sciences, she helps cancer survivors evaluate accurately the material they locate, emphasizing resources such as the National Cancer Institute's databases of treatments and clinical trials, and the National Library of Medicine's Medline, a collection of over nine million published medical research studies. Lorraine's years of study have included many courses in psychology, but she found that nothing in her educational background prepared her adequately for facing the terror and heartbreak of cancer. One of her chief interests is helping the newly diagnosed as well as long-term survivors feel less lonely and less afraid as they confront their diagnoses and weigh their options.

Colophon

Patient-Centered Guides are about the experience of illness. They contain personal stories as well as a combination of practical and medical information. The faces on the covers of our Guides reflect the human side of the information we offer.

The cover of *Non-Hodgkin's Lymphomas: Making Sense of Diagnosis, Treatment, and Options* was designed by Edie Freedman using Adobe Photoshop 5.0 and QuarkXPress 3.32 with Onyx BT and Berkeley fonts from Bitstream. The cover photos are from Rubberball Productions and Photodisc, Inc. and are used with their permission. The cover mechanical was prepared by Kathleen Wilson. The interior layout for the book was designed by Nancy Priest, Edie Freedman, and Alicia Cech. The interior fonts are Berkeley and Franklin Gothic. The text was prepared by Mike Sierra using FrameMaker 5.5. The text was copyedited by Lunaea Hougland and proofread by David Futato. Nicole Gipson Arigo, Jane Ellin, Sheryl Avruch, Kim Snow, and Melanie Wang provided quality assurance. The index was written by Katherine J. Wilkinson. Interior composition was done by Claire Cloutier LeBlanc and Sebastian Banker. Whenever possible, our books use RepKover™ or Otabind™ lay-flat binding. If the page count exceeds the limit for lay-flat binding, perfect binding is used.

Patient-Centered Guides™

Questions Answered
Experiences Shared

*We are committed to empowering individuals to evolve
into informed consumers armed with the latest information and heartfelt
support for their journey.*

When your life is turned upside down, your need for information is great. You have
to make critical medical decisions, often with what seems little to go on. Plus you
have to break the news to family, quiet your own fears, cope with symptoms or
treatment side effects, figure out how you're going to pay for things, and sometimes
still get to work or get dinner on the table.

Patient-Centered Guides provide authoritative information for intelligent
information seekers who want to become advocates of their own health. They
cover the whole impact of illness on your life. In each book, there's a mix of:

- **Medical background for treatment decisions**
  We can give you information that can help you to intelligently work with your
  doctor to come to a decision. We start from the viewpoint that modern
  medicine has much to offer and also discuss complementary treatments.
  Where there are treatment controversies, we present differing points of view.

- **Practical information**
  Once you've decided what to do about your illness, you still have to deal with
  treatments and changes to your life. We cover day-to-day practicalities, such as
  those you'd hear from a good nurse or a knowledgeable support group.

- **Emotional support**
  It's normal to have strong reactions to a condition that threatens your life or
  changes how you live. It's normal that the whole family is affected. We cover
  issues like the shock of diagnosis, living with uncertainty, and communicating
  with loved ones.

Each book also contains stories from both patients and doctors—medical
"frequent fliers" who share, in their own words, the lessons and strategies they
have learned when maneuvering through the often complicated maze of
medical information that's available.

We provide information online, including updated listings of the resources that
appear in this book. This is freely available for you to print out and copy to
share with others, as long as you retain the copyright notice on the printouts.

http://www.patientcenters.com

Other Books in the Series

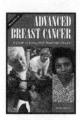

Advanced Breast Cancer
A Guide to Living with Metastatic Disease, 2nd Edition
By Musa Mayer
ISBN 1-56592-522-X, Paperback, 6" x 9", 542 pages, $19.95
"An excellent book ... if knowledge is power, this book will be good medicine."

—David Spiegel, M.D.
Stanford University
Author of *Living Beyond Limits*

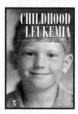

Childhood Leukemia
A Guide for Families, Friends & Caregivers
By Nancy Keene
ISBN 1-56592-191-7, Paperback, 6" x 9", 566 pages, $24.95
"What's so compelling about Childhood Leukemia *is the amount of useful medical information and practical advice it contains. Keene avoids jargon and lays out what's needed to deal with the medical system."*

—The Washington Post

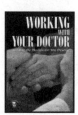

Working with Your Doctor
Getting the Healthcare You Deserve
By Nancy Keene
ISBN 1-56592-273-5, Paperback, 6" x 9", 382 pages, $15.95
"[This book] fills a genuine need for patients and their family members caught up in this new and intimidating age of impersonal, economically-driven health care delivery."

—James Dougherty, M.D.
Emeritus Professor of Surgery,
Albany Medical College

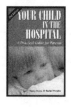

Your Child in the Hospital
A Practical Guide for Parents, 2nd Edition
By Nancy Keene and Rachel Prentice
ISBN 1-56592-573-4, Paperback, 5" x 8", 176 pages, $11.95
"When your child is ill or injured, the hospital setting can be overwhelming. Here is a terrific 'road map' to help keep families 'on track.'"

—James B. Fahner, M.D.
Division Chief, Pediatric Hematology/Oncology
DeVos Children's Hospital, Grand Rapids, Michigan

Patient-Centered Guides
Published by *O'Reilly & Associates, Inc.*
Our products are available at a bookstore near you.
For information: 800-998-9938 • 707-829-0515 • info@oreilly.com
101 Morris Street • Sebastopol • CA • 95472-9902

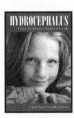

Hydrocephalus
A Guide for Patients, Families & Friends
By Chuck Toporek and Kellie Robinson
ISBN 1-56592-410-X, Paperback, 6" x 9", 384 pages, $19.95

"In this book, the authors have provided a wonderful entry into the world of hydrocephalus to begin to remedy the neglect of this important condition. We are immensely grateful to them for their groundbreaking effort."

—Peter M. Black, M.D., Ph.D.
Franc D. Ingraham Professor of Neurosurgery
Harvard Medical School, Neurosurgeon-in-Chief
Brigham and Women's Hospital, Children's Hospital
Boston, MA

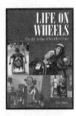

Life on Wheels
For the Active Wheelchair User
By Gary Karp
ISBN 1-56592-253-0, Paperback, 6" x 9", 550 pages, $24.95

"I think a book like this should be given to everyone in the rehab hospital ... it offers the broadest perspective of life on wheels that I've ever seen."

—Michelle Gittler, M.D.
Director, Resident Training Program,
Schwab Rehab Hospital

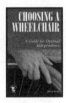

Choosing a Wheelchair
A Guide for Optimal Independence
By Gary Karp
ISBN 1-56592-411-8, Paperback, 5" x 8", 192 pages, $9.95

"I love the idea of putting knowledge often possessed only by professionals into the hands of new consumers. Gary Karp has done it. This book will empower people with disabilities to make informed equipment choices."

—Barry Corbet
Editor, *New Mobility Magazine*

Patient-Centered Guides
Published by O'Reilly & Associates, Inc.
Our products are available at a bookstore near you.
For information: **800-998-9938 • 707-829-0515 • info@oreilly.com**
101 Morris Street • Sebastopol • CA • 95472-9902

Ten Patient Rights

1. Receive considerate and respectful care.

2. Obtain complete information on illness and treatment.

3. Participate in treatment decisions.

4. Give informed consent.

5. Refuse any treatment.

6. Receive reasonable medical care and skill.

7. Wait only a reasonable amount of time.

8. Have your records kept confidential.

9. Get copies of requested records.

10. Have an advocate with you.

Patient-Centered Guides
800-998-9938

We Care About What You Think

Which book did this card come from?

_____

Why did you purchase this book?
☐ I am directly impacted
☐ A family member or friend is directly impacted
☐ I am a health-care practitioner looking for information to recommend to patients and their families
☐ Other _____

How did you first find out about the book?
☐ Recommended by a friend/colleague/family member
☐ Recommended by a doctor/nurse
☐ Saw it in a bookstore
☐ Online
☐ Other _____

☐ *Please send me the Patient-Centered Guides catalog.*

What sources do you use to gather your medical information?
☐ Friends/family   ☐ A library
☐ Your doctor   ☐ Your nurse(s)
☐ Television (which shows?) _____
☐ Newspapers (which newspapers?) _____
☐ Magazines (which magazines?) _____
☐ Newsletters (which newsletters?) _____
☐ The Internet (which newsgroups, mailing lists, or Web sites?) _____
☐ Support groups (which groups?) _____
☐ Other _____

What other medical conditions are of concern to you, your family, and your community?

_____

_____

Name _____ Company/Organization (optional)

Address _____

City _____ State _____ Zip/Postal Code _____ Country

Telephone _____ Internet or other email address (specify network)